2

5

REDUCING BREAST CANCER
RISK IN WOMEN

Developments in Oncology

Volume 75

The titles published in this series are listed at the end of this volume.

REDUCING BREAST CANCER RISK IN WOMEN

Edited by

BASIL A. STOLL
Honorary Consulting Physician to Oncology Department,
St. Thomas' Hospital, London;
Consultant to Joint Breast Clinic,
Royal Free Hospital, London, UK

Introduced by

SUSAN M. LOVE
Director UCLA Breast Center; Associate Professor of Clinical Surgery,
University of California at Los Angeles School of Medicine, California, USA

KLUWER ACADEMIC PUBLISHERS
DORDRECHT / BOSTON / LONDON

Library of Congress Cataloging-in-Publication Data

Reducing breast cancer risk in women / edited by Basil A. Stoll ;
  introduction by Susan M. Love.
       p.   cm. -- (Developments in oncology ; 75)
    Includes index.
    ISBN 0-7923-3064-1 (HB : alk. paper)
    1. Breast--Cancer--Prevention. 2. Breast--Cancer--Risk factors.
 I. Stoll, Basil A. (Basil Arnold) II. Series.
    [DNLM: 1. Breast Neoplasms--prevention & control. 2. Risk
 Factors.   W1 DE998N v. 75 1995 / WP 870 R321 1995]
 RC280.B8R426 1995
 616.99'449052--dc20
 DNLM/DLC
 for Library of Congress   94-29394

ISBN 0-7923-3064-1

Published by Kluwer Academic Publishers,
P.O. Box 17, 3300 AA Dordrecht, The Netherlands.

Kluwer Academic Publishers incorporates
the publishing programmes of
D. Reidel, Martinus Nijhoff, Dr W. Junk and MTP Press.

Sold and distributed in the U.S.A. and Canada
by Kluwer Academic Publishers,
101 Philip Drive, Norwell, MA 02061, U.S.A.

In all other countries, sold and distributed
by Kluwer Academic Publishers Group,
P.O. Box 322, 3300 AH Dordrecht, The Netherlands.

Printed on acid-free paper

Printed in the Netherlands

This book is dedicated to

The courageous smiles of our patients

Contents

Preface

This book is aimed particularly at primary health-care professionals including physicians, medical assistants, nurses and counselors. They are in the front line, answering questions daily from women concerned about their risk of developing breast cancer. Not only is the problem a burning public issue, but very soon we shall see genetic testing for a woman's predisposition to breast cancer. Many close relatives of breast cancer patients will be pressing to know their degree of risk and will need counseling to cope with that information. If they are aware of recent public discussion on the safety of agents on trial for breast cancer prevention, they will be looking for information on all possible options.

To answer such questions, this book has combined a guide to identifying women at increased risk to breast cancer with a balanced review of approaches which aim to reduce that risk. As it is a practical handbook, technicalities have been deliberately kept to a minimum, making the book concise and easy to read.

The first section of the book provides an update on the major clinical, microscopic, family history and genetic criteria used to identify a woman at increased risk, and how these characteristics are combined for risk assessment. The second section sets out the preventive options which are being used or tested, their rationale, possible benefits and disadvantages. The third section evaluates suspected or minor risk factors, and examines lifestyle or personal habits which may affect a woman's risk of developing breast cancer. The final section offers personal views on specific aspects of breast cancer control.

The book is patient-centered and is not intended to be an exhaustive or academic study of past research or current hypotheses. It aims to provide a balanced perspective on the state-of-the-art. For a woman who is at clearly increased risk, the book discusses different protection options with different levels of efficacy and acceptability. For the woman at average risk, the book offers a guide to practical general measures which may reduce her risk, particularly in avoiding substances which are believed to increase breast cancer risk. Slight overlap between sections ensures that each is complete in itself.

Inexact knowledge is responsible for the different criteria used in selecting women for preventive trials. More serious, however, is that clinicians differ also in their attitudes to discussing protective options with a woman who is clearly at increased risk. Many experts tell her that they are unable to suggest a method which is both effective and safe, and advise her to join any trial for which she is eligible.

We need to face up to the situation that it will be many years before the current clinical trials of preventive measures provide meaningful results. Meanwhile, the woman who seeks to decrease her risk of breast cancer needs all the available information and time to digest it. She must be given full responsibility to make an informed decision on her own health care and deserves understanding and counseling, because patients' perspectives are not necessarily the same as those of their clinicians.

London, 1995   *Basil A. Stoll*

List of Contributors

Christopher Bain, MB BS, MPH
Reader
Department of Social and Preventive Medicine
University of Queensland
Australia

Laura Boehnke, Pharm D
Clinical Pharmacy Specialist
MD Anderson Cancer Center
Houston, Texas
USA

H. Leon Bradlow, PhD
Strang-Cornell Medical Center
New York
USA

Rowan T. Chlebowski, MD, PhD
Professor of Medicine
Associate Chief
Division of Medical Oncology
Harbor-UCLA Medical Center
Torrance, California
USA

Graham A. Colditz, MB BS, Dr PH
Channing Laboratory
Department of Medicine
Brigham and Women's Hospital
    and Harvard Medical School
Boston, Massachusetts
USA

Theresa Conway, BSN, RN
Department of Preventive Medicine and Public Health
Creighton University
School of Medicine
Omaha, Nebraska
USA

Alberto Costa, MD
Division of Senology
Istituto Europeo di Oncologia
Milan
Italy

Devra Lee Davis, PhD, MPH
Office of the Assistant Secretary for Health
US Department of Health and Human Services
Washington, DC
USA

Andrea Decensi, MD
Department of Medical Oncology
National Institute for Cancer Research
Genoa
Italy

Nina Entrekin, RN, MN, OCN
Director
Breast Cancer Program Development
American Cancer Society
Florida Division Inc.
Tampa, Florida
USA

Marianne Ewertz, MD, Dr. Med. Sci.
Danish Cancer Society
Division of Cancer Epidemiology
Copenhagen
Denmark

Franca Formelli, PhD
Division of Experimental Oncology B
Istituto Nazionale Tumori
Milan
Italy

A. Lindsay Frazier, MD, MSc
Department of Pediatric Hematology
Dana Farber Cancer Institute
    and Harvard Medical School
Boston, Massachusetts
USA

Constance M. Goldgar, MS
Genetic Epidemiology Group
University of Utah
Salt Lake City, Utah
USA

David E. Goldgar, PhD
Associate Professor
Genetic Epidemiology Group
Department of Medical Informatics
University of Utah
Salt Lake City, Utah
USA

Robert M. Goldwyn, MD
Clinical Professor of Surgery
Harvard Medical School
Chief, Division of Plastic Surgery

Beth Israel Hospital
Boston, Massachusetts
USA

Maureen M. Henderson, MD
Head
Cancer Prevention Research Program
Professor of Epidemiology and Medicine
Fred Hutchinson Cancer Research Center
Seattle, Washington
USA

Robert A. Hiatt, MD, PhD
Assistant Director for Epidemiology
Division of Research
Kaiser Permanente Medical Care Program
Oakland, California
Director of Prevention Sciences
Northern California Cancer Center
Union City, California
USA

Michelle D. Holmes, MD
Department of Epidemiology
Harvard School of Public Health
Instructor Harvard Medical School
    and The Cambridge Hospital
Boston, Massachusetts
USA

Mary Jane Houlihan, MD
Instructor in Surgery
Harvard Medical School
Co-Director Breast Care Center
Beth Israel Hospital
Boston, Massachusetts
USA

George R. Huggins, MD
Chairman
Department of Obstetrics and Gynecology
Francis Scott Key Medical Center
Baltimore, Maryland
USA

David J. Hunter, MB, BS, ScD
Associate Professor
Department of Epidemiology
Harvard School of Public Health
Channing Laboratory
Department of Medicine
Harvard Medical School
    and Brigham and Women's Hospital
Boston, Massachusetts
USA

Elizabeth A. Krecker, MD
Department of Medicine
University of Southern California

School of Medicine
Los Angeles, California
USA

Beth Leedham, PhD
Department of Psychology
University of Southern California
Los Angeles, California
USA

Susan M. Love, MD
Director
UCLA Breast Center
Associate Professor of Clinical Surgery
University of California at Los Angeles
School of Medicine
Los Angeles, California
USA

Henry T. Lynch, MD
Professor and Chairman
and Professor of Medicine
Creighton University
School of Medicine
Department of Preventive Medicine
Omaha, Nebraska
USA

Jane F. Lynch, BSN
Department of Preventive Medicine and Public Health
Creighton University
School of Medicine
Omaha, Nebraska
USA

Kathryn F. McGonigle, MD
Department of Gynecology
City of Hope National Medical Center
Duarte, California
USA

Anne McTiernan, MD, PhD
Cancer Prevention Research Program
Fred Hutchinson Cancer Research Center
Seattle, Washington
USA

Jeanmarie Marshall
Writer/Researcher
Women's Community Cancer Project
Cambridge, Massachusetts
USA

Beth E. Meyerowitz, PhD
Associate Professor and Director of Clinical Training
Department of Psychology
University of Southern California
Los Angeles, California
USA

Anthony B. Miller, MB, FRCP
Director National Breast Screening Study
Professsor and Chairman
Department of Preventive Medicine and Biostatistics
University of Toronto
Canada

Malcolm D. Pike, PhD
Department of Preventive Medicine
University of Southern California
School of Medicine
Los Angeles, California
USA

Kathy L. Radimer, M.Ed, PhD
Senior Research Officer
Department of Social and Preventive Medicine
University of Queensland
Australia

Rena V. Sellin, MD
Associate Internist
Associate Professor of Medicine
Medical Specialties
MD Anderson Cancer Center
Houston, Texas
USA

Darcy V. Spicer, MD
Department of Medicine
University of Southern California
School of Medicine
Los Angeles, California
USA

Basil A. Stoll, FRCR, FFR
Honorary Consulting Physician to
    Oncology Department
St. Thomas' Hospital London
Physician to Joint Breast Clinic
Royal Free Hospital
London
UK

Lisa Summerlot, RN, BA, OCN
Cancer Risk Counselor
South Florida Comprehensive Cancer Centers
Salick Health Care
Florida
USA

Richard L. Theriault, DO, FACP
Associate Internist
Associate Professor of Medicine
MD Anderson Cancer Center
Department of Breast and
    Gynecologic Medical Oncology
Houston, Texas
USA

Hazel Thornton
"Saionara"
31 Regent Street
Rowhedge, Colchester
UK

Rosalba Torrisi, MD
Department of Medical Oncology
National Institute for Cancer Research
Genoa
Italy

Victor G. Vogel, MD, MHS
Associate Professor of Medicine
    and Epidemiology
Chief Section of Clinical Cancer Prevention
University of Texas
MD Anderson Cancer Center
Houston, Texas
USA

Walter C. Willett, MD, DrPH
Professor of Epidemiology and Nutrition
Harvard School of Public Health
    and Professor of Medicine
Channing Laboratory
Harvard Medical School and
Department of Medicine
Brigham and Women's Hospital
Boston, Massachusetts
USA

Introduction

SUSAN M. LOVE

Breast cancer has become an epidemic! The incidence has continued to rise while the mortality rate remains unchanged. Our treatments of surgery, radiation therapy, chemotherapy are crude ways to deal with a disease and have had only a limited impact on this killer. Everyday, women ask me: What can I do to prevent breast cancer? What is the cause? Unfortunately we do not know. As of yet, there are no magic bullets, no sure ways to avoid a disease that most women fear.

Mammography is not prevention. It is only detection. Figuring out risk factors is interesting to those of us in the field, but of little use to most of women who have no risk factors at all. Every day the media are replete with reports regarding possible causes of this disease. These announcements are confusing to most women and have limited applicability. Soon we will be able to test for one of the genes for breast cancer BRCA1. What will this mean? How will we treat these women who are at very high risk? What about the women who test negative and yet still may be at high risk? There are many questions and few answers. This book is an attempt to look at the state of knowledge today in an attempt to set the stage for what is to come.

One way to look at breast cancer and, for that matter, all cancers, is to go back to basics. All cancer is genetic. Not all cancer is hereditary, however. What this means is that all cancer is caused by defects in the genes which control the normal growth and death of cells. There are probably several defects or mutations involved and there may even be more than one combination that will lead to cancer. Suffice it to say that it is these aberrations which are responsible for the overgrowth of cells in tumors, and their invasion into blood vessels and then the rest of the body. Some women (and men) inherit these mutations and others acquire them during their lifetime. Exactly what they are and what causes them is still largely hypothetical but the picture is becoming clearer all of the time. One approach to the mystery of breast cancer is to identify these mutations, genes and oncogenes. Once identified, we can look for ways to reverse the mutations, supply the missing proteins, and block the progression of the disease. These efforts are going on at a fevered pace.

It is possible that by the time this book is being read the BRCA1 gene will have been identified. This is a hereditary (germline) mutation seen in women from families with a strong history of premenopausal breast and ovarian cancer. It is also possible that other women with sporadic breast cancer will have a similar gene. P53 is a tumor suppressor gene which puts a brake on cell growth. Her 2 neu is a growth gene telling cancer cells to keep growing. NM23 may be the gene which blocks metastasis. The steps are falling into place and the picture, although hazy right now, is rapidly coming into focus. Moreover, we don't have to wait for the whole answer to start using this new molecular genetic information. At UCLA we are studying an antibody for the Her 2 neu gene which, when coupled with chemotherapy, has had very promising results. We only have to figure out how to block one important step in this pathway to be able to prevent the disease. It is within our grasp.

The other front for finding the cause and cure is to identify the carcinogens which cause the somatic mutations in susceptible women. This is where hormones, viruses, radiation, diet and pesticides come in. We can stop this disease by preventing the mutations in the first place if we know what causes them, and we can do that without actually knowing what the mutations are. We know for example that smoking causes lung cancer without knowing the exact mutations responsible.

What is causing the breast cancer mutations and when? Breast cancer is a long process and much of the damage may well occur in teenagers and young adults. It may not be what we are eating now but what we ate when we were eighteen which lays the groundwork for our later destruction. These external environmental factors are less well studied. It is time for us to shift the research dollar from treatment and detection to prevention. The variations in breast cancer incidence throughout the world and its increase in the West points to an environmental connection. It is time that we start to investigate it.

Finally there is the attempt at prevention. All of our attempts at prevention at this time are limited by our lack of knowledge about the cause. Nonetheless, we have to proceed with what little we have or allow this epidemic to go on unchecked. Some things are easier than others. Have a good diet, avoid alcohol, eat your broccoli. Others are more complex, such as the new contraceptive which suppresses ovarian function, and Tamoxifen. It is a sad state of affairs when we have to add yet more chemicals to counteract the effects of other chemicals.

This is an exciting time. The fact that this book could be written at all is testimony to the fact that progress is being made. But we are not there yet. Practitioners and patients alike need to join forces demanding an end to this terrible disease. We need more research money and we need a new research direction. We need to find the cause and prevention of a disease which has been around for too many generations. The answers are there for the asking; we need only the courage and the will to look.

PART ONE

RECOGNIZING INCREASED
BREAST CANCER RISK

Chapter 1

Who Develops Breast Cancer?

BASIL A. STOLL

Breast cancer accounts for up to one third of all new cases of women's cancer in North America and Northern Europe. The death rate from the disease has changed very little in the past 50 years, but its incidence has increased by 40 to 70% in the past 30 or 40 years. In some Western populations, the increase has been mostly in premenopausal women while in the USA it has been mainly in older women [1]. These observations suggest that changes in lifestyle, diet or environment may be responsible for the Western increase in breast cancer incidence.

The age-adjusted incidence of breast cancer has also increased in Asia and South America, where previously the incidence was relatively low. In particular, Japan has shown a doubling of a previous low incidence in the past 25 years and there, the increase has been more in postmenopausal women. Decline in fertility rates and Westernization of the diet is suspected of causing the increased incidence in non-Western countries [2]. The question is how they affect breast cancer development.

Initiation and Promotion of Breast Cancer

Cancer of an organ develops as a result of accumulated damage to one or more specific genes in the chromosomes of tissue cells. The damage results from exposure to environmental factors, but increased susceptibility to cancer can also be inherited from one's parents. The accepted model [3] suggests that inherited susceptibility involves transmission of a flawed gene, and further damage to the chromosome results from factors in the cell environment originating either inside on outside the body.

The environmental factors causing such mutations include viruses, a variety of chemicals and physical agents such as ionizing radiation. Genetic damage may involve specific oncogenes which switch on cell division, or tumor suppressor genes which switch it off. By the time a person is an adult, mutations are likely to

3

Basil A. Stoll (ed.), Reducing Breast Cancer Risk in Women, 3–9.
© 1995 *Kluwer Academic Publishers. Printed in the Netherlands.*

have occurred in a majority of body cells but minor ones can be repaired. Mutations in more than one gene in a cell are probably required to initiate cancer development.

Breast cancer is believed to originate from a *series* of genetic changes in a cell. The first change (initiation) transforms a normal cell into a 'dormant' tumor cell. The second group of changes (promotion) activate the dormant cell leading to a precancerous cell. The final genetic change involves the development of invasiveness.

Initiation change is thought to occur either before or after a person's birth. Initiation damage to cells is thought to occur in a high proportion of the population and so far, we have no scientific model on which to base a practical method of reversing genetic mutation. However, once the initiation change has occurred, a step-by-step progression to invasive cancer depends on continued stimulation by chemical or hormonal promoting factors. These factors operate over the 15 to 30 years which are believed to elapse between the initiating damage and the final appearance of cancer. While we are unable to reverse the initiating damage to the DNA of the chromosomes, subsequent promoting changes are reversible. It may therefore be possible to extend the latent interval between first genetic damage and the clinical manifestation of cancer, this being the basis of current attempts at breast cancer prevention.

The atomic bomb explosions in Japan in 1945 provide some precise information on this latent interval. Women aged between 10 and 59 at the time of exposure to the explosions first showed an increased incidence of breast cancer after a mean interval of 14 years. The incidence continued to rise for 30 years after the radiation exposure [4].

The role of ovarian hormones during this latent interval is suggested by the report that those women aged over 50 at the time of the explosions did not show any increased susceptibility to breast cancer. Moreover, girls who were aged under 10 at the time of the explosions, did not begin to show an increased incidence of breast cancer until after a mean interval of 21 years. This suggests that their latent interval was extended because of the need for ovarian hormones to appear and promote the growth of tumors.

Ionizing Radiation and Breast Cancer Risk

Ionizing radiation from outer space and from radioactive materials in the environment undoubtedly have a role in the initiation of human breast cancer. Ionizing radiation is of two varieties – wave-like including electromagnetic radiation such as gamma or X-rays, or particle-like including electrons and alpha particles emitted during radioactive decay. The ability of this type of energy to damage DNA depends on its ability to cause ionization in the tissues.

Ionizing radiation may have acute effects after high levels of exposure, such as that received by the firefighters of Chernobyl. Low level exposure is however of wider concern and its sources include natural background radiation, occupational exposure, or exposure from nuclear power, consumer products or medical procedures [5]. Everyone is continuously exposed to natural background radiation, either from cosmic radiation emanating from outer space, on terrestrial gamma radiation originating in radioactive materials in the environment. Air travel exposes passengers to increased levels of cosmic radiation while exposure to terrestrial radiation depends on geographic location. Radioactive materials are widely distributed but their concentration varies greatly.

Internal exposure to ionizing radiation comes from radioactive materials which are present naturally in the body and of these, carbon–14 and potassium–40 contribute the greatest dose [5]. But by far the greatest source of internal radiation exposure is from inhaled radioactive materials, principally radon and its decay products. The importance of radon as a source of natural background radiation has been recognized only recently. In the USA, it is estimated that 82% of all human radiation exposure is due to background radiation, and two-thirds of it comes from the inhalation of radon and its decay products [5].

The role of radiation in increasing breast cancer risk has long been recognized. Studies of women who received multiple X-ray screening for monitoring lung tuberculosis have shown an increased risk of breast cancer [6]. The tumors tend to occur in the inner half of the breasts in contrast to the general population where they are more common in the outer half. Studies of the women who survived the atomic bomb explosions in Japan showed that breast cancer increased with increasing doses of radiation exposure [7].

Few women would normally be exposed to such high doses of radiation. State-of-the-art mammography results in a dose to breast tissue of between 0.05 and 0.15 rads for a two-view mammogram. If a woman with suspected hereditary susceptibility to breast cancer was exposed to mammography every year from the age of 20 to the age of 70, it has been calculated that her increased risk of developing breast cancer would be 0.0033% [8]. This is negligible in relation to her risk from inherited susceptibility.

Radiation is capable of damaging DNA and causing chromosomal aberrations, and only a few of the changes are reversible. The importance of low doses of radiation on breast cancer risk is probably dependent on the age of the subject. The risk is likely to be greater in teenage and childhood, whereas older women are less at risk [9].

A variety of consumer products may expose the public to ionizing radiation. Thus, it may originate in radioactive materials naturally present in tobacco, domestic water, building materials and fuels. It may also come from luminous watch dials, airport X-ray inspection systems, static eliminators and smoke detectors [5]. Tobacco products normally contain radioactive isotopes of lead and polonium and are the greatest source of radiation exposure among consumer products. However, it is calculated that the radiation dosage from use of tobacco products accounts for only a small proportion of lung cancers.

Table 1. Major markers of increased breast cancer risk in women

---

Relative risk increased more than 4 times
  Evidence of susceptibility gene BRCA1
  Premenopausal breast cancer in mother *and* sister
  Atypical hyperplasia in breast biopsy or aspirate
  In situ cancer – ductal or lobular

Relative risk increased 2 to 4 times
  Premenopausal breast cancer in mother *or* sister
  Hyperplasia without atypia in breast biopsy or aspirate
  History of previous cancer in one breast
  Aging Caucasian women

Prenatal Factors in Breast Cancer Risk

It has recently been suggested that exposure to hormones of the fetus in the womb may influence the risk of subsequent breast cancer and that the high estrogen levels of pregnancy may increase risk [10]. A decreased breast cancer risk among left-handed women has been claimed [11] and left-handedness may be related to exposure of the fetus to relatively lower estrogen levels.

Having an older mother at the time of childbirth has been suggested to increase the risk of breast cancer in the daughter [12]. A similar risk is postulated for having an older father also, independent of the age of the mother [13]. Older parents may possibly have an increased risk of chromosomal abnormalities which may be transmitted to the offspring.

Assessing Individual Risk

Changes in lifestyle, diet or environment have each been blamed for the increasing incidence of breast cancer in many countries. All may play a part. Currently, interest is focused on the role of environmental chemicals but it is uncertain whether they act directly on the breast cell on by affecting the metabolism of estrogen in the body. What is becoming clear, however, is that we cannot afford to wait until the mechanisms of breast cancer development are fully understood before starting trials on the prevention of the disease. Such research should start with women who are at the greatest risk of developing the disease.

Clinical, laboratory and epidemiologic studies over the years have looked for markers to identify such women. These markers are commonly referred to as risk factors, suggesting that they are involved in causing the disease, but this is not always so. Higher socio–economic and educational status are markers of increased breast cancer risk but are only indirect risk factors. It is useful to distinguish two

Table 2. Minor markers of increased breast cancer risk in women. The markers are associated with up to twofold increase in risk in many studies, although not all studies agree

General markers

    Postmenopausal breast cancer in first-degree relative

    Previous cancer of the ovary or uterine endometrium

    Nodular densities in mammogram are predominant

    Obesity (in women over 50)

    Tallness in adult life

    Excess ionizing radiation to chest wall or breasts

    Higher alcohol consumption

    Higher socio-economic status

Hormone-related markers

    Non-childbearing (in women under 40)

    Delayed first childbirth

    Short duration of breast feeding of children

    Onset of menstruation before age 12

    Onset of menopause after age 49

    Prolonged use of oral contraceptives (in women under 45)

    Prolonged estrogen replacement therapy

types of marker–*biological* risk markers which cannot be changed (such as age, race, and family history of breast cancer), and *lifestyle* markers which can be influenced (such as obesity, alcohol intake or age at first childbirth). Most of the lifestyle markers are related to racial, cultural and socio-economic factors. Tables 1 and 2 set out recognized major and minor markers of increased breast cancer risk.

Combinations of four groups of markers–age group, family history of breast cancer, hormone-related factors, precursor or precancerous changes in the breast are currently used to identify women at increased risk to breast cancer. Increased risk with advancing age probably reflects an increasing accumulation of chromosome damage as one gets older. A history of breast cancer in a mother or sister may reflect genetic susceptibility to breast cancer but could be due also to a shared environment. Childbearing or menstrual factors are likely to reflect hormone-related events which influence progression to invasive cancer. The presence of precursor or precancerous changes in breast tissue is evidence of progression towards cancer, although the final stage may be delayed for many years or may never manifest.

The various types of criteria are combined in order to define women at increased risk who are eligible for prevention trials. Thus, the Tamoxifen trial in the USA uses a formula which includes a woman's age, number of first degree relatives with breast cancer, history of previous biopsies (showing atypical hyperplasia or lobular cancer *in situ*) and ages at onset of menstruation and first childbirth [14]. However, there is little evidence about how to base a combination of criteria, and the above formula has not yet been validated [15].

It is clear from Table 2 that most Western women have at least one risk marker, and it is possible that having more than one combined in the same individual may multiply the risk. We therefore need to establish the relative strength of each marker – whether it is a strong or weak sign of risk for breast cancer. We also need to establish how closely one risk marker is related to another, because adding together two interrelated markers may give a false impression of higher risk. For example, Western women of a higher socio-economic status have a greater tendency to delay first childbirth, breast-feed for a shorter period, and eat a richer diet. Each may be associated with a greater risk of breast cancer.

To avoid arousing unnecessary alarm in women, it is useful to look at risk levels in perspective. A woman of 40 normally has an approximately 1 in 25 risk of developing breast cancer. If she shows a minor risk marker (Table 2) she multiplies her risk level by a factor of between 1 and 2, and this will lead to a risk level similar to that of a woman of 50 years of age. The psychologic impact of advancing a woman's risk level to that of a woman 10 years her senior will vary between women but generally will not cause excessive anxiety. However, evidence of a major risk marker (Table 1), which is fortunately much less common, is associated with a much greater risk and might justify some form of active intervention. The same might apply to a combination of several factors from Table 2 if one was sure that they were not interrelated. The woman at the highest risk of all might choose an operation to remove all breast tissue.

In adding risk markers together, it is important to emphasize that some markers apply mainly to breast cancer manifesting before the menopause while others apply mainly to older women. Thus, for premenopausal Western women, one would stress the relevance of a family history of the disease in a mother or sister, delayed or no childbirth, an onset of menstruation at a younger age and a short duration of breast feeding. For postmenopausal women on the other hand, one would stress the relevance of delayed onset of menopause or an abnormal degree of obesity. In particular, for older women, a family history of the disease is much less important than it is for younger women.

Conclusion

A new strategy is emerging in cancer control. Instead of aiming to destroy all potentially cancerous cells in the body, it may be possible to maintain them for a prolonged period in a state of dormancy. Recent research suggests that we may be able to control the genetic machinery of potentially cancerous cells.

References

1. Persson, J., Bergstrom, R., Sparen, P., Thorn, M., Adami, H.O. (1993). Trends in breast cancer incidence in Sweden 1958–1988 by time period and birth cohort. *Br. J. Cancer*, **68**, 1247–1253.
2. Parkin, D.M., Nectoux, J. (1991). Is female breast cancer increasing? In Stoll, B.A. (ed.), *Approaches to Breast Cancer Prevention*, Kluwer Academic Publishers, Dordrecht, 15–34.
3. Knudson, A.G., Strong, L.C. (1972). Mutation and cancer; a model for Wilm's tumor of the kidney. *J. Natl Cancer Inst.*, **48**, 313–324.
4. Tokunaga, M., Norman, J.E., Asano, M. *et al.* (1979). Malignant breast tumors among atomic bomb survivors. *J. Natl. Cancer Inst.*, **62**, 1347–1359.
5. Edwards, M., Hendee, W. (1989). How important is radiation in cancer risk? In Stoll, B.A. (ed.), *Social Dilemmas in Cancer Prevention*, Macmillan Press, London, 57–66.
6. MacKenzie, J. (1965). Breast cancer following multiple fluoroscopies. *Br. J. Cancer*, **19**, 1–7.
7. Wanebo, G.K., Johnson, K.G., Sato, K. *et al.* (1968). Breast cancer after exposure to the atomic bombings of Hiroshima and Nagasaki. *N. Engl. J. Med.*, **279**, 667–675.
8. Lynch, H.T., Marcus, J.N., Watson, P., Lynch, J.F. (1989). Familial and genetic factors; new evidence. In Stoll, B.A. (ed.), *Women at High Risk to Breast Cancer*, Kluwer Academic Publishers, Dordrecht, 27–40.
9. Mansfield, C.M. (1991). Motivating the public in cancer prevention. In Stoll, B.A. (ed.), *Approaches to Breast Cancer Prevention*, Kluwer Academic Publishers, Dordrecht, 221–228.
10. Trichopoulos, D. (1990). Hypothesis; does breast cancer originate in utero? *Lancet*, **335**, 939–940.
11. Hsieh, C.C., Trichopoulos, D. (1991). Breast size, handedness and breast cancer risk. *Eur. J. Cancer*, **27**, 131–135.
12. Le Marchand, L., Kolonel, L.N., Myers, B.C., Mi, M.P. (1988). Birth characteristics of premenopausal women with breast cancer. *Br. J. Cancer*, **57**, 437–439.
13. Janerich, D.T., Hayden, C.L., Thompson, W.D. *et al.* (1989). Epidemiologic evidence of perinatal influence in the etiology of adult cancers. *J. Clin. Epidemiol.*, **42**, 151–157.
14. Gail, M.H., Brinton, L.A., Byar, D.P. *et al.* (1989). Projecting individualized probabilities of developing breast cancer for white females who are being examined annually. *J. Natl. Cancer Inst.*, **81**, 1979–1886.
15. Bush, T.L., Helzlsouer, K.J. (1993). Tamoxifen for the primary prevention of breast cancer; a review and critique of the concept and trial. *Epidemiol. Rev.*, **15**, 233–243.

Chapter 2

Risk from Family History

BASIL A. STOLL

Women whose mothers or sisters have developed breast cancer are themselves at a two- or three-fold increased risk of manifesting breast cancer. Although shown by several studies in the USA and Europe, this observation does not necessarily mean that these women have a genetic susceptibility to the disease which will then be transmitted to their children. Their increased risk may be related to the lifestyle or environment which is shared within a family. In fact, recent research suggests that most familial breast cancer involves a combination of genetic susceptibility and lifestyle factors. Some members of the family inherit a genetic susceptibility to agents which favor the development of breast cancer. It is not clear whether these are chemicals in the environment or food, or the woman's own circulating hormones.

Pedigree studies have been used for many years to establish the existence of such hereditary influences. A widely quoted early study [1] found 13 breast cancers (one male) and 11 benign breast tumors, involving three generations in one family. Age at diagnosis of breast cancer was relatively early (average age 45) and both benign and malignant tumors of the breast occurred in the same branch of the pedigree. Another early study [2] found breast cancer in eight out of 35 women in one branch of a family, and seven of them died of their disease.

Vital progress was made about 25 years ago. It was noted that when women with a family history of breast cancer developed the disease, it was more likely to involve both breasts in younger women than in postmenopausal women [3]. In the first degree relatives (mother, daughter or offspring) of young women with cancer involving both breasts, the risk of developing breast cancer was 8.8 times as high as in the general population. There was a difference in risk according to whether a mother, sister or second-degree relatives was involved. Age at onset of the breast cancer varied between different family groups, but in a specific pedigree, there was a tendency for a similar age at onset. In some families, breast cancer was associated with other types of cancer, but in others, not. Some showed a higher

Basil A. Stoll (ed.), Reducing Breast Cancer Risk in Women, 11–18.
© 1995 *Kluwer Academic Publishers. Printed in the Netherlands.*

frequency of cancer affecting both breasts, but others not. All these observations suggested genetic heterogeneity between different pedigrees, that is, a variety of genetic mutations is likely to be involved [4].

The traditional approach of clinical geneticists is to collect information on families showing unusual clustering of breast cancer. Its frequency among first- and second-degree relatives is compared with that in the general population. Clustering may be due to the presence of a susceptibility gene, but since breast cancer is a common disease, some of the affected cases within a pedigree may be from chance occurrence and not gene carriers [5]. Thus a log of odds (LOD score) is required to calculate the probability that a chromosome marker is related to the type of disease seen in the family.

An extended pedigree study is used in order to identify individuals at risk to hereditary breast cancer. It is important to include second-degree relatives such as both sets of grandparents, aunts and uncles, because they are likely to have entered or passed through the age at which breast cancer usually appears. Both sets of grandparents must also be included because susceptibility may be transmitted through paternal as well as maternal lineage. Currently, increasing reliance is being placed on direct evidence of chromosome markers such as BRCA1, recently linked to hereditary breast cancer [6].

How Is Familial Risk Calculated?

Only a clinical geneticist can provide exact information on a woman's risk of developing breast cancer by examining an extended pedigree. Nevertheless, it is a generalization that the risk in women with affected relatives depends on: (a) The age at which the diagnosis was made in the affected relatives; (b) Whether the disease involved only one or both breasts; (c) The number of relatives affected and the genetic closeness of the relationship; (d) Whether one of the relatives was the woman's mother.

In general, having a mother or sister with breast cancer will approximately double or triple a woman's risk of developing the disease, but the risk can be expressed more exactly if the above knowledge is available. Thus, a woman's risk of breast cancer is increased by a factor of 3 if a first-degree relative developed the disease before the age of 45. It is increased by a factor of 5.5 if the disease involved both breasts in a first-degree relative. It is increased by a factor of 8.8 if the disease involved both breasts in a first-degree relative before the age of 45 [4].

In some families there is a tendency for the disease to appear at a more or less similar age in various members of the family, (Figure 1). Most occur at a premenopausal age but if different members of a family live under different conditions and have different lifestyles, these factors may either accelerate or decelerate the appearance of the tumor. Table 1 shows the risk of breast cancer appearing in relatives of breast cancer patients, expressing it as a lifetime risk rather than as a ratio. This analysis shows no evidence that *postmenopausal* breast

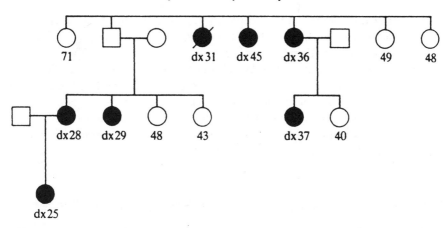

Figure 1. Typical family pedigree of breast cancer. Squares represent men, circles represent women and dark circles represent women with breast cancer. Ages represent age at diagnosis for women with breast cancer, age at death for family members who died without breast cancer, and age at last examination for living family members without breast cancer. (From [7] by permission.)

Table 1. Lifetime risk of developing breast cancer for relatives of breast cancer patient. Data from [4]

Family history of breast cancer	Lifetime risk for woman (%)
Premenopausal, both breasts, mother or sister	49
Premenopausal, one breast, mother or sister	33
Premenopausal, one breast, in sister	18
Postmenopausal, both breasts, in mother	28
Postmenopausal, one breast, in mother	16
Postmenopausal, one or both breasts, in sister	7
Postmenopausal, in second-degree relative	7

cancer, whether in one or both breasts, in a sister or second-degree relative, will increase a woman's risk beyond that of the general population.

Different figures have been suggested in the literature for the proportion of breast cancer cases in the population that is associated with a family predisposition in first-degree relatives. Based on recent reports, [8,9] the figure in the USA is likely to be 7 to 8%. This is assumed to be the percentage of cases associated with the dominant inheritance of a predisposing gene or genes. However, family clustering of breast cancer may also result from factors such as shared environment and lifestyle leading to exposure to similar factors which can cause genetic mutations. The availability of genetic screening will provide more accurate data.

Screening for the BRCA1 susceptibility gene is on the horizon. Its presence indicates an 85 to 90% lifetime breast cancer risk [10], but in families where it is recognized, it must be taken into account that each member of the family has a 50% chance of *not* carrying the gene. Women in this latter group have a lifetime risk of breast cancer similar to that of the general population. Until genetic screening is available, counseling of women must be guided by clinical factors. A history of even a single close relative who has developed cancer in both breasts at an early age is a clear indication of high risk. However, a history of even several relatives who have developed breast cancer in old age is probably of little significance.

Relation of Hereditary to Familial and Sporadic Breast Cancer

The current model for the origin of both hereditary and non-hereditary types of cancer [11] suggests that the majority of cancers derive from a single cell and that at least two separate mutations are required in order to initiate the cancer process. In hereditary cases, the individual inherits the first mutation from a parent and subsequently requires only a second mutation in the cell in order to initiate the cancer. In sporadic (non-hereditary) cases, two or more mutations are required in the same cell for the cancer to be initiated.

The development of hereditary breast cancer probably requires damage to several genes and it is this which probably accounts for the variations (heterogeneity) in the clinical characteristics of the disease. In addition, the disease may not be evident in some members of a family (incomplete penetrance) because the second mutation required for the development of the disease has not yet occurred. It is uncertain whether differences between members of the family in age at onset of breast cancer reflects a different combination of genetic mutations or whether it results from different hormonal or environmental stimulation. As noted above, sporadic cases may also arise within a family with hereditary susceptibility. Table 2 shows the distinctions made between sporadic, familial and hereditary types of breast cancer [12].

In clinical practice, a diagnosis of sporadic (non-hereditary) breast cancer is made if the patient shows no family history of the disease through two generations including grandparents, parents, aunts, uncles, siblings and offspring. Familial breast cancer is diagnosed if there is a record of breast cancer in one or more first- or second-degree relatives but the distribution does not fit with in Mendelian dominant gene inheritance. Hereditary breast cancer is diagnosed if the pedigree shows evidence in first- or second-degree relatives of an autosomal, dominant, highly penetrant, susceptibility gene. It is not infrequently associated with cancer of the ovary in the same individual, and rarely, may be associated with a specific pattern of tumor combinations at other sites, (Table 2).

Currently, the term hereditary breast cancer is applied to a group of conditions which all involve increased susceptibility to breast cancer. They differ in their age at onset, the tumors associated with them and in their associated genetic mutations.

Table 2. Definitions of hereditary, familial and sporadic breast cancers. From [12]

Hereditary breast cancer

Evidence of high incidence breast cancer in first- or second-degree relatives. Pedigree consistent with an autosomal dominant, highly penetrant, susceptibility gene.

Typically early age at onset and high proportion involves both breasts. Not infrequently associated with cancer of the ovary. Rarely associated with tumor combinations at other sites.

Familial breast cancer

Evidence of breast cancer involving one or more first- or second-degree relatives but does not fit definition of hereditary breast cancer.

Sporadic breast cancer

No family history of breast cancer through two generations including both sets of grandparents, parents, aunts, uncles, siblings and offspring.

Table 3. Classification of hereditary breast cancer. Data from [13]

Site-specific hereditary breast cancer
Predominantly breast involvement. Other tumors absent

Breast/ovarian syndrome
Association of breast and ovarian cancers

SBLA syndrome (Li–Fraumeni)
Association of breast cancer with sarcoma, brain tumor, leukemia and adrenocortical cancers

Cowden's syndrome
Association of breast cancer with mouth and skin lesions and thyroid tumors

Breast/gastrointesinal syndrome
Association of breast cancer with cancers of the stomach, colon and pancreas

There are predominantly five major types of hereditary breast cancers, and all involve premenopausal onset of the disease and a high likelihood of involvement of both breasts within a period of 5 years, (Table 3).

The most frequent variety is the breast-specific type carrying no association with other cancers or abnormalities. The breast/ovarian type carries an associated risk of ovarian cancer which may appear either before or after the breast cancer. These are the more common types and the other types are rare. The Li–Fraumeni (or SBLA) syndrome is associated with soft tissue or bone sarcoma, brain tumor, leukemia or adrenocortical cancer in addition to breast cancer. Cowden's syndrome is associated with thyroid tumors and lesions in the skin and mouth in addition to breast cancer. Breast/gastrointestinal syndrome involves cancers of the colon, stomach or pancreas in addition to breast cancer.

The possibility that the breast cancer characteristics differ between hereditary and sporadic types has been investigated. Most observers find a similar distribution of microscopic types of tumor although some have suggested that medullary type of cancer is more common in hereditary breast cancer. Again, the likelihood of recurrence and the prognosis are generally found to be similar in hereditary and sporadic types although aggressive tumors may be more common in hereditary breast cancer [13].

Apart from the specific syndromes of multiple cancers associated with hereditary breast cancer, endometrial cancer and malignant melanoma have been found to be more commonly associated with breast cancer and this may indicate a genetic association. The risk of breast cancer is also said to be increased in women whose pedigrees show an excess of prostate cancer in the family males as well as endometrial and ovarian cancer in the females [14].

Pedigree studies show the occasional involvement of males with breast cancer in susceptible families, but more important is the possible transmission of susceptibility through a male member of the family. Unaffected males may transmit the susceptibility gene to their daughters, (Figure 1). To recognize it may require extension of the pedigree to both sets of grandparents, aunts and cousins [12].

Combining Familial with Hormone-Related Risk Markers

Risk markers are commonly combined in order to identify women at increased risk of breast cancer eligible for trials of preventive agents such as Tamoxifen. A family history of breast cancer is usually combined with age group and childbirth/menstrual markers and this practice suggests that both independent and additive effects are proven. In fact, few studies have examined the relationship between a history of familial breast cancer and childbirth/menstrual factors in their effect on a woman's risk of breast cancer. A large case/control study [15] found no evidence of an additive effect between familial risk and that of age at first childbirth or early removal of the ovaries, but a slight *increase* in risk if there was later onset of menstruation.

It has been suggested that familial predisposition to breast cancer may be mediated through hormonal mechanisms, and abnormal hormonal profiles have been described in the daughters and sisters of women with breast cancer [16–18]. However, no consistent differences have been found between familial and sporadic breast cancer with respect to age at onset of menstruation, age at first childbirth and number of children [4].

In breast cancer presenting in premenopausal women, familial susceptibility is a relatively strong risk marker. This may explain why its effect on a woman's risk of developing breast cancer is little affected by minor risk markers such as age at onset of menstruation, age at first childbirth or even removal of the ovaries before the natural menopause [15]. Nevertheless, these hormone-related factors may influence the *age* at which breast cancer appears in different members of a family with hereditary susceptibility. This may be related to their effect on the development of precursor lesions in the breast of women with a genetic predisposition to breast cancer [19].

Conclusion

Familial breast cancer is likely in a woman if there is evidence of breast cancer occurring in her mother, sister or offspring. However, the lifetime risk of developing breast cancer in such a woman varies from 7% (equivalent to that of the general population) to 49% depending upon which relative is involved, the age at which cancer developed and whether one or both breasts were involved. Genetic screening for the BRCA1 gene will soon be available, and while positive testing in a breast cancer family indicates an 85–90% lifetime breast cancer risk, negative testing indicates a risk no higher than that of the general population.

References

1. Gardner, E.J., Stephens, F.E. (1950). Breast cancer in one family group. *Am.J.Hum.Genet.*, **2**, 30–40.
2. Woolf, C.M., Gardner, E.J. (1951). The familial distribution of breast cancer in a Utah kindred. *Cancer*, **4**, 515–520.
3. Anderson, D.E. (1971). Some characteristics of familial breast cancer. *Cancer*, **28**, 1500–1504.
4. Anderson, D.E. (1992). Familial versus sporadic breast cancer. *Cancer*, **70**, 1740–1746.
5. DeVilee, P., Cornelisse, C.J. (1990). Genetics of human breast cancer. *Cancer Surveys*, **9**, 605–630.
6. Easton, D.F., Bishop, D.T., Ford, D. *et al.* (1993). Genetic linkage analysis in familial breast and ovarian cancer; results from 214 families. *Am. J. Hum. Genet.*, **52**, 678–701.
7. King, M.C. (1990). Genetic analysis of cancer in families. *Cancer Surveys*, **9**, 417–435.
8. Colditz, G.A., Willett, W.C., Hunter, D.J. (1993). Family history, age and risk of breast cancer. *J.Am. Med. Assoc.*, **270**, 338–343.
9. Slattery, M.J., Kerber, R.A. (1993). A comprehensive evaluation of family history and breast cancer risk. *J. Am. Med. Assoc.*, **270**, 1563–1568.
10. King, M.C., Rowell, S., Love, S.M. (1993). Inherited breast and ovarian cancer. *J. Am. Med. Assoc.*, **269**, 1975–1980.
11. Knudson, A.G., Strong, L.C. (1972). Mutation and cancer; a model for Wilm's tumour of the kidney. *J. Natl. Cancer Inst.*, **48**, 313–324.
12. Lynch, H.F., Watson, P., Conway, T.A., Lynch, J.F. (1991). Monitoring high risk women. In Stoll, B.A. (ed.), *Approaches to Breast Cancer Prevention*, Kluwer Academic Publishers, Dordrecht, 191–206.
13. Lynch, H.T., Marcus, J.N., Watson, P., Lynch, J.F. (1989). Familial and genetic factors; new evidence. In Stoll, B.A. (ed.), *Women at High Risk to Breast Cancer*, Kluwer Academic Publishers, Dordrecht, 27–40.
14. Anderson, D.E., Badzioch, M.D. (1993). Familial breast cancer risks. *Cancer*, **72**, 114–119.

15. Brinton, L.A., Hoover, H., Fraumeni, J.F. (1982). Interaction of familial and hormonal risk factors for breast cancer. *J. Natl. Cancer Inst.*, **69**, 817–822.
16. Kwa, H.G., Cleton, F., De Jong–Bakker, M. *et al.* (1976). Plasma prolaetin and its relationship to risk factors in human breast cancer. *Int. J. Cancer*, **17**, 441–447.
17. Bulbrook, R.D., Moore, J.W., Clark, G.M. *et al.* (1978). Plasma oestradiol and progesterone levels in women with varying degrees of risk of breast cancer. *Eur. J. Cancer*, **14**, 1369–1375.
18. Fishman, J., Fukushima, D.K., O'Connor, J., Lynch, H.T. (1979). Low urinary estrogen glucuronides in women at risk for familial breast cancer. *Science*, **204**, 1089–1091.
19. Skolnick, M.H., Cannon–Albright, L.A. (1992). Genetic predisposition to breast cancer. *Cancer*, **70**, 1747–1754.

Chapter 3

Childbearing and Related Risk Factors

BASIL A. STOLL

A major influence on a woman's risk of developing breast cancer is the length
of her fertile life and her record of childbearing. Increased risk is associated with
either having had no children, or else with delay of the first childbirth until after
the age of 25. Risk is also increased if a woman shows evidence of prolonged
ovarian activity, such as onset of menstruation at a relatively early age (before
12 in Western countries) or delayed onset of menopause (after 49). These are the
classic risk indicators. Recent evidence shows that a woman's breast cancer risk is
influenced also by the age at which she has subsequent children after the first, by
her total number of children and the length of time for which she breast-feeds her
babies [1].

It is significant that most, if not all, of these risk indicators are related to a woman's lifestyle, and this in turn, is related to her social status. Most countries show a
correlation between high breast cancer risk in a woman and higher socio-economic
status. Higher social status is generally associated with a richer diet, fewer children, delayed first pregnancy and shorter duration of breast-feeding. International
surveys suggest that an overrich diet favors an earlier onset of menstruation and
that adult obesity in women favors a later onset of the menopause. Thus, the progressive increase in breast cancer that is being observed in Western countries may
be partly explained by improved socio-economic conditions allied with a Western
lifestyle and diet.

These factors influence the likelihood of breast cancer appearing either at a
younger or older age, although different risk indicators will predominate for each
of the age groups. Insufficient attention has been paid to this distinction. For breast
cancer diagnosed in women before the age of 45, the predominant risk markers
are those involved in early reproductive life, such as an onset of menstruation at
an early age, delayed first childbirth, a short duration of breast-feeding, a strong
family history of breast cancer and evidence of benign precursor lesions in the

Basil A. Stoll (ed.), Reducing Breast Cancer Risk in Women, 19–28.
© 1995 *Kluwer Academic Publishers. Printed in the Netherlands.*

breast. For breast cancer diagnosed after the age of 45, these markers are less likely to identify increased risk but instead, a late age at menopause and excessive obesity are the significant indicators [2].

Correlation with childbearing and menstrual indicators is found in most countries where breast cancer risk studies have been done including North America, Europe, Asia and South America. However, it should be pointed out that the degree of risk attached to each individual risk marker is not high. Most of them would increase a woman's risk to about 1.5 times that of the general population. This is small compared to the ratio of 5 to 10 which may be associated with a strong family history of breast cancer or the discovery of a benign precursor lesion in the breast.

Although individually small, childbearing and menstrual risk indicators may be additive in their effect on an individual woman's risk of developing breast cancer. In advising an individual woman, we need to concentrate on those markers relevant to her age group, as noted above.

A strong family history of breast cancer is more common in women developing breast cancer before the age of 45. A family history of breast cancer in a first-degree relative (mother, sister or daughter) is seen in over 10% of such cases. It is possible that genetic predisposition to breast cancer may involve a tendency towards abnormal hormone concentrations in breast tissue [3], but few studies have assessed how a family history of the disease interacts with reproductive risk factors in increasing risk. It is still uncertain to what degree they are additive because genetic risks are powerful risk indicators in premenopausal women and may dilute the impact of childbearing and menstrual factors [4].

Childbearing

It was established 25 years ago that childbearing protects a woman against the risk of breast cancer [5]. Women who have never had children are at greater risk to the disease than are women who have borne children. Only full-term pregnancies, but not miscarriages, are protective. The earlier the first childbirth, the greater the protection, (Table 1). In one study, the risk for women whose first delivery was after the age of 35 was three times as high as for women whose first delivery was before 20, and the risk persisted even in women aged over 75 [7].

The reasons for the above observations are uncertain. Either an early first birth protects the breasts from cancer-inducing factors or else a relatively low fertility is genetically associated with increased breast cancer risk, possibly through the presence of abnormal hormone concentrations in the breast. The first explanation is supported by the observation that only full-term births, but not miscarriages, are protective. While miscarriages are associated with proliferative changes in breast tissue, they may not progress to the full secretory pattern which occurs only in the last months of pregnancy [8]. The protective effect of an early first childbirth appears to be greater in breast cancer appearing in women before the age of 45 [2, 9, 10].

Table 1. Relative risk of developing breast cancer compared to controls; according to age of woman at birth of first child. Modified from [6]

Age at birth of first child (yrs)	Relative risk
Under 20	1.00
20–24	1.03
25–29	1.22
Over 30	1.33

Until recently, some Scandinavian studies had shown no clear association between age at first childbirth and breast cancer risk [11], but a recent combined analysis confirmed the correlation. It showed that women not bearing children were at 30% increased risk compared to those who had completed at least one pregnancy [9]. It is possible however, that fertility characteristics and family – planning habits may vary between populations and account for discrepancies in findings between one country and another [11].

While first childbirth before the age of 25 is protective, increasing evidence shows that any pregnancy after the age of 35 may increase a woman's risk of developing breast cancer. It has long been known that having one's first child after the age of 35 is associated with greater risk than having no children at all [5]. In one series it was related to a 40% greater risk than that associated with a first baby before the age of 20 [9]. There is now evidence that a mother's age at the time of childbirth influences breast cancer risk from subsequent childbirths after the first. They are protective if they occur before the age of 25 but are associated with an increased risk if they occur after the age of 30 [12]. Other studies also suggest that a woman's age at her last childbirth may be as important as her age at first childbirth in influencing breast cancer risk [7, 13]. It has led to the advice that a woman should complete her childbearing by the age of 35 [7].

The reasons for the increased cancer risk associated with late pregnancy are not clear. The aging process in the breasts, as judged by microscopic signs of involution, begins at the age of 35 or 40 in most Western women. Any factor which causes persistence of breast activity after that age may increase cancer risk [14]. During involution, breast tissue swings gradually from the influence of ovarian hormones to that of adrenal and pituitary gland hormones, and interruption of breast involution by pregnancy after the age of 30 or 35 may contribute to increased risk of breast cancer. Studies have shown that full-term birth is followed by a transient increase in breast cancer risk [15] and in the case of women over the age of 35, may stimulate the growth of an incipient breast cancer [16]. Overall,

Table 2. Relative risk of developing breast cancer compared to controls; according to number of children. Modified from [6]

Number of children	Relative risk
1	1.00
2	0.92
3	0.80
Over 4	0.76

therefore, women are advised to have their babies between teenage and the age of 35, if they aim to decrease their breast cancer risk.

Practically all studies confirm that a woman's breast cancer risk decreases with increasing numbers of children [5, 6, 9, 17], (Table 2). This protective effect is independent of the protective effect of an early first childbirth [7, 9]. A recent report suggests that a larger number of children protects only against the risk of breast cancer developing after the age of 45, but may increase the risk of it developing at an earlier age [1]. This observation awaits confirmation.

Breast-Feeding; Effect on Mother's Risk and Child's Risk

Compared to women in Western countries, more women in Japan and India breast-feed their children and do so for a more prolonged period. Since it suppresses ovarian activity (evidenced by cessation of menstruation) one might expect breast-feeding to protect women against breast cancer risk. Among Japanese and Indian women, the longer the duration of breast-feeding, the lower the breast cancer risk. Until recently, this correlation was not so clear among Western women.

Recent studies have shown that breast-feeding for relatively long periods is associated with a reduction in the risk of breast cancer in premenopausal women. It appears that earlier studies did not include a sufficient number of premenopausal women with breast cancer who had breast-fed for long periods. The longer the duration of breast-feeding, the greater the decrease in the risk of premenopausal breast cancer (Table 3), but there is no decrease in the risk of cancer appearing in older women. These observations have been confirmed not only in the USA [16, 18], but also in Canada [19], Britain [20] and Japan [21] although not all studies agree [22]. Women need to be questioned in greater detail about the reasons for stopping breast-feeding early, if we are to distinguish failure of milk production from social and other reasons.

Table 3. Relative risk of developing breast cancer compared to controls; according to duration of breast feeding by women with premenopausal breast cancer. Modified from [6]

Lifetime duration of breast-feeding (months)	Relative risk
0	1.00
Under 3	0.85
4–12	0.78
13–24	0.66
Over 24	0.72

The way in which prolonged breast-feeding decreases breast cancer risk is not known, but possible mechanisms include interruption of ovarian activity, an effect on pituitary hormone secretion or direct effect on breast cells. Full secretory activity in breast cells may lead to changes which protect them against cancer-promoting chemicals. Whatever the mechanism, prolonged breast-feeding should be encouraged.

This applies particularly to the prevention of breast cancer in younger women. Premenopausal breast cancer accounts for less than a quarter of all breast cancers, but has a worse prognosis than the postmenopausal disease. If women who breast-fed their children for less than three months were to do so for four to 12 months, it is calculated that their risk of premenopausal breast cancer might be reduced by 11%; if they did so for as long as 24 months, the incidence might be reduced by nearly 25% [6]. How many women would go to that length for protection?

About 50 years ago, it was shown that a factor present in mouse mother's milk was essential for the development of breast cancer in certain strains of mice. It was later shown that this was a retrovirus transmitted in breast milk from one generation to another. There is some evidence that a similar virus may be involved in humans, and suspect virus particles have been identified in breast milk both from breast cancer patients and normal women.

If such transmission applied to humans, one might expect a decreased risk of breast cancer in women who were never breast-fed. Studies have shown however no evidence that breast cancer patients and normal controls differ in their history of breast-feeding in infancy [23]. In the present state of knowledge, the role of a transmitted virus is unproven in the case of human breast cancer.

Table 4. Relative risk of developing breast cancer compared to controls; according to age of woman at menopause. Modified from [6]

Age at menopause (yrs)	Relative risk
Under 45	1.00
45–49	1.36
50–54	1.58
Over 55	1.43

Age at Onset of Menopause

It was observed about 40 years ago that women whose ovaries were removed before their natural menopause showed a reduced breast cancer risk compared to women whose menopause occurred naturally [24]. Subsequent studies showed that the protective effect was related to a woman's age at the time of the operation and that removal of the ovaries before the age of 35 reduced the breast cancer risk by about half [25]. The degree of protection is greater with the removal of both ovaries than the removal of only one, and a hysterectomy without removal of the ovaries also offers less protection.

A natural menopause at a relatively early age has a similar effect in reducing breast cancer risk, and numerous studies have shown that postmenopausal women with breast cancer show a higher mean age at the menopause than do the general population. The higher a woman's age at the natural menopause, the greater her risk of breast cancer, (Table 4). On the basis of a mathematical model, an age at menopause of 52 carries double the risk of an age at menopause of 42 [26].

These observations suggest that the development of postmenopausal breast cancer is stimulated by ovarian or related growth factors. There is evidence that removal of the ovaries reduces the incidence of precursor benign lesions in breast tissue [27]. This would presumably be associated with a reduced risk of developing breast cancer subsequently.

Age at Onset of Menstruation

Most studies report that the mean age at onset of menstruation is younger for breast cancer patients than for the general population. Although not all studies agree, the risk increases progressively with a decreasing age at first menstruation, (Table 5). Just as the protective effect of early first childbirth and prolonged breast feeding is greater for cancer appearing in younger women, so the risk associated with early onset of menstruation is increased for the same age group. On the basis of

Table 5. Relative risk of developing breast cancer compared to controls; according to age of woman at the onset of menstruation. Modified from [6]

Age at onset menstruation (yrs)	Relative risk
Under 11	1.00
12	0.98
14	0.83
Over 15	0.81

a mathematical model, it is found that an age at the onset of menstruation of 10 carries double the risk of an age at onset of over 16. This estimate corresponds to an increase in risk of 12% per year decrease in a woman's age at first menstruation [26].

Although the role of an earlier onset of menstruation may be less important than other reproductive factors in breast cancer risk, the observation supports the hypothesis that the longer a woman's fertile life span, the greater her risk of developing breast cancer. The total duration of menstrual activity can be calculated from age at onset of menstruation, age at menopause and duration of time spent in a pregnant or breast-feeding state. All these factors influence a woman's risk of breast cancer.

In Western countries, women are showing a trend towards achieving physical maturity at an ever younger age. Since the beginning of the century, the mean age of girls at the onset of menstruation has advanced from about 16 to 13 years. It is generally believed that the first effective promotion of breast cancer development begins at puberty in susceptible women, and that later steps are inhibited by an early first childbirth. The effect of earlier puberty on breast cancer risk may be reflected by the following observations among Japanese women.

Until 1960, the mortality rate from breast cancer among Japanese women was about one sixth of that among Western women. Their average age at onset of menstruation was 16 years, and it was estimated that the difference in age at puberty could account for half the difference in breast cancer mortality rates between Japan and the USA [28]. Since then, there has been a 35.5% increase in age-adjusted mortality from breast cancer in Japan – the highest increase in the world during that time [29]. It was associated with a fall to 14 years as the average age at onset of menstruation. Earlier puberty in Japanese girls is directly related to the intake of Western style foods, and inversely to the use of traditional Japanese food [30].

Relation to Other Factors

Tallness in Western women has recently been shown to be associated with an increased breast cancer risk. An earlier onset of menstruation is likely to be associated with an earlier growth spurt in adolescence, although not necessarily with being a tall adult because of 'catch-up' by the others. Nevertheless, the trend towards earlier puberty in Western girls has been associated not only with the achievement of final height at an earlier age, but also with increasing height among adults [31]. It has been suggested that an overrich Western nutrition stimulates earlier puberty, thus exposing breast tissue to a longer period when it may be damaged by cancer-promoting factors [32].

The relationship between the size of a woman's breasts and breast cancer risk is not clear but a recent study shows that women receiving cosmetic breast augmentation have only half the breast cancer risk which would be expected from women in their age group [33]. Women who have this operation generally have smaller than normal breasts to begin with. The size of the breast during fertile life reflects the number of cells which are potentially susceptible to cancer development. Breast tissue mass is influenced by childhood nutrition and may also be determined during fetal life [34].

The relationship between breast cancer and other aspects of menstrual activity has been investigated. No association has been found with menstrual irregularity, length of cycle, pain during menstruation or duration of flow. Most studies have shown no association with either a history of pain or swelling of the breasts at the time of menstruation.

It is currently assumed that breast tissue is most sensitive to cancer-promoting factors between the onset of puberty and first childbirth. On the basis that the most important of these factors are hormones from the ovary, it has been proposed that the number of ovulatory menstrual cycles before a woman's first childbirth are major determinants of risk, although subsequent pregnancies and the onset of the menopause will modify the time at which breast cancer manifests [35]. According to this concept, breast cancer incidence in a woman does not increase according to her calendar age but according to her 'breast tissue age'. This is closely associated with exposure of her breast tissue to sex hormones.

Conclusion

Conscious choices by women to delay pregnancy and to limit the number of their children are likely to be having a critical effect on breast cancer incidence in Western populations. Statistical studies suggest that in order to minimize breast cancer risk, women should have their babies between teenage and a maximum age of 35, and breast-feed them as long as possible. Overrich nutrition should be avoided in children because of its possible association with an earlier onset of menstruation, and in adults also because of its association with delayed menopause.

Individual childbearing or menstrual risk indicators may relate more particularly either to premenopausal or postmenopausal appearance of breast cancer. Surprisingly, a history of multiple childbirths is said to lessen the likelihood of breast cancer appearing after the age of 45 but to increase the likelihood before the age of 45. Thus, in calculating the risk for an individual woman, only those indicators relative to her age group need to be taken into consideration. This also applies to a family history of breast cancer which is more relevant to premenopausal breast cancer, and to obesity which is more relevant to postmenopausal breast cancer.

References

1. Kelsey, J.L., John, E.M. (1994). Lactation and the risk of breast cancer. *N. Engl. J. Med.*, **330**, 136–137.
2. Segala, C., Gerber, M., Richardson, S. (1991). The pattern of risk factors for breast cancer in a Southern France population. *Br. J. Cancer*, **64**, 919–925.
3. Fishman, J., Fukushima, D.K., O'Connor, J., Lynch, H.T. (1979). Low urinary estrogen glucuronides in women at risk for familial breast cancer. *Science*, **204**, 1089–1091.
4. Parazzini, F., La Vecchia, C., Negri, E., Franceschi, S., Boccilione, L. (1992). Menstrual and reproductive factors and breast cancer in women with family history of the disease. *Int. J. Cancer*, **51**, 677–681.
5. MacMahon, B., Cole, P., Lin, T.M. *et al.* (1970). Age at first birth and breast cancer risk. *Bull. WHO*, **43**, 209–221.
6. Newcomb, P.A., Storer, B.E., Longnecker, M.P. *et al.* (1994). Lactation and a reduced risk of premenopausal breast cancer. *N. Engl. J. Med.*, **330**, 81–87.
7. Kalache, A., Maguire, A., Thompson, S.G. (1993). Age at last full-term pregnancy and risk of breast cancer. *Lancet*, **341**, 33–36.
8. MacMahon, B. (1993). Reproduction and cancer of the breast. *Cancer*, **71**, 3185–3188.
9. Ewertz, M., Duffy, S.W., Adami, H.O. *et al.* (1990). Age at first birth, parity and risk of breast cancer; meta–analysis of 8 studies from the Nordic countries. *Int. J. Cancer*, **46**, 597–603.
10. Negri, E., La Vecchia, C., Duffy, S.W. *et al.* (1990). Age at first and second births and breast cancer risk in biparous women. *Int. J. Cancer*, **45**, 428–435.
11. Ewertz, M. (1988). Risk factors for breast cancer and their prognostic significance. *Acta Oncol.*, **27**, 733–737.
12. Trichopoulos, D., Hsieh, C.C., MacMahon, B. *et al.* (1983). Age at any birth and breast cancer risk. *Int. J. Cancer*, **31**, 701–704.
13. Kvale, G., Heuch, J. (1987). A prospective study of reproductive factors and breast cancer; age at first and last birth. *Am. J. Epidemiol.*, **126**, 842–850.
14. Henson, D.E., Tarone, R.E. (1993). On the possible role of involution in the natural history of breast cancer. *Cancer*, **71**, 2154–2156.
15. Bruzzi, P., Negri, E., La Vecchia, C. *et al.* (1988). Short term increase in risk of breast cancer after full term pregnancy. *Br. Med. J.*, **297**, 1096–1098.
16. Miller, W.R. (1993). Hormonal factors and risk of breast cancer. *Lancet*, **341**, 25–26.
17. Lipnick, R., Speizer, F.E., Bain, C. *et al.* (1984). A case–control study of risk indicators among women with premenopausal and early postmenopausal breast cancer. *Cancer*, **53**, 1020–1024.
18. Byers, T., Graham, S., Rzepka, T., Marshall, J. (1985). Breast cancer: evidence for a negative association in premenopausal women. *Am. J. Epidemiol.*, **121**, 664–674.
19. Yang, C.P., Weiss, N.S., Band, P.R. *et al.* (1993). History of lactation and breast cancer risk. *Am. J. Epidemiol.*, **138**, 1050–1056.
20. UK National Case – Control Study Group. (1993). Breast feeding and risk of breast cancer in young women. *Br. Med. J.*, **307**, 17–20.

21. Yoo, K.Y., Tajima, K., Kuroishi, T. *et al.* (1992). Independent protective effect of lactation against breast cancer; a case – control study in Japan. *Am. J. Epidemiol.*, **135**, 726–733.
22. London, S.J., Colditz, G.A., Stampfer, M.J. *et al.* (1990). Lactation and risk of breast cancer in a cohort of U.S. women. *Am. J. Epidemiol.*, **132**, 17–26.
23. Ekbom, A., Hsieh, C.C., Trichopoulos, D. *et al.* (1993). Breast feeding and breast cancer in the offspring. *Br. J. Cancer*, **67**, 842–845.
24. Lilienfeld, A.M. (1956). The relationship of cancer of the female breast to artificial menopause and marital status. *Cancer*, **9**, 927–934.
25. Trichopoulos, D., MacMahon, B., Cole, P. (1972). Menopause and breast cancer risk. *J. Natl. Cancer Inst.*, **48**, 604–613.
26. Moolgavkar, S.H., Day, N.E., Stevens, R.G. (1980). Two stage model for carcinogenesis; epidemiology of breast cancer in females. *J. Natl. Cancer Inst.*, **65**, 559–569.
27. Swerdlow, M., Humphrey, L.J. (1964). The relationship of breast disease to gynecologic disease. *Cancer*, **17**, 1165–1173.
28. Hoel, D.G., Wakabayashi, T., Pike, M.C. (1983). Secular trends in the distribution of the breast cancer risk factors; menarche, first birth, menopause and weight in Hiroshima and Nagasaki, Japan. *Am. J. Epidemiol.*, **118**, 78–89.
29. Kurihara, M., Aoki, K., Tominaga, S. (1984). *Cancer Mortality Statistics in the World*, University of Nagoya Press, Nagoya.
30. Kato, J., Tominaga, S., Suzuki, T. (1988). Factors related to late menopause and early menarche as risk factors for breast cancer. *Jpn. J. Cancer Res.*, **79**, 165–172.
31. Preece, M.A. (1989). The trend to greater height and earlier maturation. *Growth Matters*, 1, 3–4.
32. Stoll, B.A., Vatten, L.J., Kvinnsland, S. (1994). Hypothesis; early physical maturity does influence breast cancer risk. *Acta Oncol.*, **33**, 171–176.
33. Berkel, H., Bindsell, D.C., Jenkins, H. (1992). Breast augmentation; a risk factor for breast cancer? *N. Engl. J. Med.*, **326**, 1649–1653.
34. Trichopoulos, D. (1990). Hypothesis; does breast cancer originate in utero? *Lancet*, **335**, 939–940.
35. Henderson, B.E., Pike, M.C., Casagrande, J.T. (1981). Breast cancer and the oestrogen window hypothesis. *Lancet*, **2**, 363–364.

Chapter 4

Risk from Benign Breast Disease

BASIL A. STOLL

Biopsy evidence of a benign lump in the breast is one of the criteria of increased breast cancer risk used for entering women into clinical trials of Tamoxifen as a protective agent. It is currently being used both by the USA/Canada Breast Cancer Protection Trial and by the European/International Trial. Increasing numbers of women are having breast biopsies, particularly in the USA, and unnecessary anxiety may result if the prognostic significance of the pathologic report is not clear. In the past, the catch-all term 'fibrocystic disease' was used to describe normal physiologic as well as pathologic changes [1, 2], and uniform criteria for classification are still not agreed upon by all [3–7].

In the past 20 years, thousands of cases have been analyzed to determine the risk potential of various types of benign breast disease diagnosed from a biopsy of a persistent breast lump [8–16]. In order to keep the overall risk in perspective, it needs to be pointed out that: (i) less than 10% of women with benign breast disease go on to develop breast cancer; (ii) about half of all benign breast disease involves fibrocystic lesions and only 5–10% of these lesions (particularly those showing atypia) are associated with a relatively high risk of breast cancer; (iii) about 70% of women with fibrocystic lesions have no excess cancer risk at all after excision of the lump. On the other hand, *all* women need to be alerted to the risk of breast cancer because less than 20% of women diagnosed with breast cancer have a history of a biopsy for benign breast disease.

A different level of breast cancer risk is associated with each of the lesions lumped together as benign breast disease. However, the risk level associated with each lesion may need to be multiplied if a woman shows other characteristics known to increase risk. The strongest factor of this type is a history of breast cancer in a close relative, and in fact, inherited susceptibility may apply not only to some breast cancers but also to some benign lesions such as atypia [3, 5]. A woman's age at the time of biopsy, her childbearing history and her ethnic origin

Basil A. Stoll (ed.), Reducing Breast Cancer Risk in Women, 29–39.
© 1995 *Kluwer Academic Publishers. Printed in the Netherlands.*

are additional factors which influence her level of breast cancer risk following a biopsy diagnosis of benign breast disease.

Cancer Risk Associated with Benign Breast Disease

Cancer evolution in the human breast is likely to be influenced by both genetic and lifestyle factors [17]. Step-by-step progression from normal breast tissue to final invasive cancer probably always goes through precursor and preinvasive steps, but the duration of each stage may vary from months to many years. To assess the cancerous potential of benign breast lesions, they are mainly classified according to whether hyperplasia is present or not. Pathologists differ somewhat in their criteria [4], but moderate to severe hyperplasia is usually diagnosed in the presence of at least five cells thickness above the basement membrane, while atypia is diagnosed if in addition, highly abnormal-looking cells are grouped in highly abnormal patterns. Further progression is to *in situ* cancer, which shares some of the microscopic characteristics of atypia but is generally regarded as breast cancer in its preinvasive stage.

The serial progression described above suggests that hyperplasia is the first step in a pathologic sequence leading from normal tissue to *in situ* cancer. However, in an individual woman, the finding of hyperplasia, with or without atypia, does not necessarily identify a direct precursor of breast cancer. Its presence may reflect increased *susceptibility* to changes which favour the evolution of cancer [18]. Evidence for this is the observation that subsequent breast cancer may affect either breast after a report of hyperplasia. In one series, only 56% of subsequent breast cancers were in the same breast, although these appeared after an average of 11.2 years compared to 14 years for cancer appearing in the opposite breast [19]. Similar findings are noted in other reports.

The finding of hyperplasia with or without atypia (both being proliferative lesions) therefore indicates a more or less equal susceptibility to cancer in both breasts. This is in contrast to the finding of ductal cancer *in situ* (a later stage in the evolution towards invasive disease) where invasive cancer usually occurs in the same breast. In spite of this, it should be noted that neither atypia nor *in situ* cancer indicates a lesion which is inevitably committed to progress to invasive breast cancer. There is evidence that the foci of both may disappear at the time of the menopause, when stimulating factors such as estrogen or growth factors are withdrawn [20].

The frequency of proliferative and non-proliferative lesions in typical large series of cases is shown in Table 1. The frequency of breast cancer developing after these lesions at different periods of follow-up is shown in Table 2. As would be expected, the longer the follow-up, the greater the risk. Table 3 shows the relative risk (compared to the general population) of a woman developing breast cancer after various pathologic reports on a benign breast biopsy. For a non-proliferative lesion, the breast cancer risk for the patient is increased by a ratio of 1.6, in the

Table 1. Reported frequency of proliferative lesions in benign breast biopsies. (Modified from Rosen [3])

	Percentage of total patients showing:		
	Non-prolif. lesions	*Hyperplasia – no atypia*	*Hyperplasia with atypia*
	%	%	%
Carter (28)	40	52	8
Dupont (10)	42	51	7
Bodian (21)	20	61	15

Table 2. Reported frequency of breast cancer developing after benign breast biopsy in relation to the presence of proliferative lesions. (Modified from Rosen [3])

	Percentage of patients developing breast cancer after:			
	Non-prolif. lesions	*Hyperplasia – no atypia*	*Hyperplasia with atypia*	*Follow up*
	%	%	%	(years)
Carter (28)	2.2	3.1	5.1	8
Dupont (10)	2.2	4.3	12.9	17
Bodian (21)	8.2	8.6	9.1	21

presence of hyperplasia by a ratio of 2.1, and in the presence of atypia by a ratio of up to 3 [21].

In practice, these risk levels need to be taken in perspective. A woman aged 40 normally has a 1 in 25 chance of developing breast cancer [22]. The presence of hyperplasia will double her risk, approximately to the normal risk level of a 50 year

Table 3. Increase in relative risk of breast cancer according to microscopic report on benign breast biopsy. (Modified from Bodian [21])

Microscopic report	*Increase in relative risk*
Non-proliferative lesion	1.6
Hyperplasia – no atypia	2.1
Mild atypia	2.3
Moderate/severe atypia	3.0
Papilloma	2.9
Adenosis	3.7

old woman. This should not cause excessive alarm. However, a report of atypia, which is much less common (Table 1), is associated with a greater risk and might justify some form of active intervention.

There is wide variation in the rate at which progression to invasive cancer occurs subsequent to evidence of benign breast disease. The average interval between a biopsy report of hyperplasia and subsequent appearance of invasive cancer is 10 to 15 years. For atypia, the interval is shorter because it reflects a more advanced stage in progression. The interval is particularly short in women over 55 years of age [19]. One possible reason is that atypia lesions which persist after the menopause may be more aggressive in their growth, a result of the selective effect of the menopause [23].

Most observers agree that the breast cancer risk associated with proliferative lesions decreases as women get older [3]. The lesions themselves become less frequent after the age of 50 and while hyperplasia is common in cancerous breasts in premenopausal women, it almost disappears by the time of menopause [24]. Similarly, the frequency of *in situ* cancer and/or atypia decreases after the menopause [25], presumably because their growth is supported by estrogen. The implication is that the progression of such lesions to invasive cancer is not always inevitable and that it may be aborted by withdrawing or countering supportive hormones in premenopausal women.

In spite of the above evidence that atypia and *in situ* cancer are less evident after the menopause, it is well recognized that a woman's risk of developing breast cancer increases progressively after menopause. Morover, less than 10% of women having non-proliferative or proliferative lesions subsequently manifest breast cancer. These observations emphasize the inadequacy of using these lesions for selecting patients at risk to breast cancer. There is an urgent need for research directed at biochemical or genetic markers which will identify precursor lesions leading to invasive breast cancer.

Apart from the grouping of benign breast lesions by their proliferative activity, they are often classified by a combination of clinical and pathologic features. Thus, fibrocystic lesions account for about 50% of benign breast disease and fibroadenoma for about 30%, while papilloma, adenosis, mixed types and cysts account for most of the remainder [19]. Atypia is found in 37% of patients with adenosis and in 22% of those with papilloma, making both conditions markers of high risk for breast cancer, (Table 3). Although doubted at one time, it is now widely accepted that fibroadenoma is associated with a slightly increased risk of breast cancer [26]. Even the presence of cysts may elevate the risk of breast cancer if they are associated with proliferative activity or a family history of breast cancer [5].

Table 4. Increase in relative risk of breast cancer in women with previous benign biopsy, according to family history of breast cancer in first degree relative. (Modified from Dupont [27])

Microscopic report	No family history	Family history
Non-proliferative lesion	1.0	1.4
Hyperplasia but no atypia	1.9	2.7
Hyperplasia with atypia	4.3	11.0

Clinical Factors Which Multiply the Risk

Other risk markers used for selecting women for trials of protective agents may multiply the breast cancer risk associated with benign breast disease, and a history of breast cancer in a first degree relative (mother, sister or daughter) increases risk in this way. In the presence of hyperplasia, a family history increases the risk ratio from 1.9 to 2.7, and if atypia is present, the risk ratio is increased from 4.3 to 11.0, (Table 4). It is possible that hyperplasia is related to inherited susceptibility to breast cancer, and supporting this suggestion is the report that it was found in 35% of random biopsies taken from the breasts of first degree relatives of breast cancer patients compared with 13% in controls [17]. It has led to the suggestion that the same genes control susceptibility both to the precursor lesion and to breast cancer itself, even though sex hormones and other regulating factors may influence the rate of progression towards invasive cancer.

The younger a woman is at the time her breast biopsy shows atypia, the higher her risk of subsequently developing invasive breast cancer. Thus, the risk ratio is increased to 6 in women under 46, but to 3.7 in women aged 46–55, and to 2.3 in women over 55 [28]. However, another series has reported that the risk differential was greater when women were subdivided into premenopausal and postmenopausal groups than into younger and older age groups [29]. It suggests that menopause rather than age *per se* inhibits progression to invasive breast cancer in women with atypia, and this agrees with the conclusion in the previous section. On the other hand, the breast cancer risk following other benign breast lesions such as papilloma and adenosis appears to be higher in women over the age of 55 [19].

It is well recognized that the older a woman is at the time of her first baby, the greater her risk of breast cancer, and this risk is increased further in the presence of fibrocystic lesions which indicate increased susceptibility to breast cancer. Thus, the presence of hyperplasia without atypia increases the risk ratio in women having their first baby after 30 from 1.9 to 3.5, and in women having no children from 2.1 to 3.3. The risk ratio is increased to 10 and 11, respectively, in the presence of atypia, (Table 5).

The more risk factors a woman has, the greater her statistical risk of developing breast cancer. Thus, a history of breast cancer in a first degree relative increases the risk ratio for benign breast disease in women who have not had children from

Table 5. Increase in relative risk of breast cancer in women with previous benign biopsy, according to a woman's age at first childbirth. (Modified from Dupont [27])

Microscopic report	Age of woman at first childbirth		
	Under 20	Over 30	No children
Non-proliferative lesion	1.0	1.9	2.1
Hyperplasia but no atypia	2.2	3.5	3.3
Hyperplasia with atypia	3.6	10.0	11.0

1.7 to 3.4, and in those who delayed childbirth until after 30, from 1.2 to 5.1 [27]. As suggested above, inherited susceptibility in such cases may apply not only to breast cancer but also to precursor lesions.

The use of oral contraceptives has been shown in many studies to be associated with a reduced incidence of fibrocystic changes but not with a reduced risk of breast cancer [30]. There are conflicting reports on the effect of oral contraceptive use on the breast cancer risk associated with atypia. While disagreeing on whether the risk is decreased, none find it clearly increased [30]. It is suggested that while oral contraceptive use may decrease the symptoms of fibrocystic change in many women, it does not affect the microscopic precursors which may lead to invasive cancer [31].

The incidence of benign breast disease is affected by ethnic factors, and in the USA, there are marked differences between non-Hispanic whites, Hispanics and American Indians [32]. The incidence of hyperplasia and atypia in these populations parallel the incidence of breast cancer.

Women with larger breasts show a higher risk of developing breast cancer if they have evidence of hyperplasia. Their risk ratio is increased from 1.2 to 3.0 [27]. It may reflect the larger mass of glandular tissue at risk to cancer. Fat in the breast is known to convert circulating androgen into estrogen but the role of breast fat in increasing breast cancer is uncertain.

Since only about 5% of benign breast biopsies show the presence of atypia, attempts have been made to identify biochemical or genetic markers which may help to identify precursor lesions of breast cancer. Markers of this type include measurements of proliferative activity, levels of tissue growth factors and their receptors, and also evidence of the expression of oncogenes or loss of tumor-suppressor genes. When developed more fully, they should permit a more accurate risk level to be applied to biopsies of benign breast disease showing precursor and preinvasive lesions. At present, even expert pathologists have difficulty in distinguishing between some cases of atypia and *in situ* cancer; between *in situ* cancers of the ductal and lobular types; and between *in situ* cancers and invasive cancers [4, 33].

Risk from In Situ Cancer

In situ cancer is the transition stage to invasive cancer and although it resembles the latter microscopically, the abnormal cells have not broken through the basement membrane to invade the surrounding tissue. Most invasive breast cancers are likely to evolve through an *in situ* stage, but the process may be transitory or prolonged, or the patient may die of some other condition before invasive cancer manifests [34]. *In situ* cancer lesions show extreme proliferative activity similar to that in atypia and the dividing cells are grouped in bizarre patterns. Two types are identified by their cell structure – ductal cancer *in situ* (DCIS) and lobular cancer *in situ* (LCIS). Since most breast cancers arise in the terminal part of the duct system, the two types may co-exist in the same breast [35].

DCIS is seen in all age groups but is less common after the menopause. Before the wide use of mammography, DCIS represented less than 5% of new breast cancers and most were large tumors when diagnosed. Since the introduction of mammography screening, DCIS accounts for 10–20% of new breast cancers and they are often recognized when small because they frequently contain calcification. If excised with a small rim of normal tissue around, about 25% show invasive breast cancer at the same site within 15 years. The breast cancer risk associated with DCIS is about 10 times that of the general population of the same age group.

Because of its tendency to recur locally, there is uncertainty about the use of breast-conserving surgery in the case of DCIS. The lesion can be excised locally if it is small, but if it is large (or incomplete excision is reported by the pathologist) wide excision or even mastectomy may be indicated. Radiation therapy is being tested in the hope that breast-conserving surgery might be an effective alternative to mastectomy. A randomized clinical trial in the USA has recently reported that radiation therapy after complete excision of small DCIS lesions reduced subsequent incidence of invasive cancer in the same breast from 16.4% to 7.0% [33]. Similar trials are under way in Europe [36]. In the UK, a trial is currently evaluating the effect of adding either radiation therapy or Tamoxifen or both to wide excision [37].

DCIS is usually subdivided into comedo, cribriform, solid and papillary types by analysis of cell architecture, but mixed patterns are common and we need biologic markers of aggressiveness to provide additional information on the likelihood of recurrence [3]. Most surgeons agree that the most aggressive type, comedo carcinoma, has the highest risk of local recurrence and is unsuitable for breast-conserving surgery. Nevertheless, a survey of the results of treating DCIS by breas-conserving surgery and radiation at several hospitals found that the pathologic type did not affect survival rate or the incidence of distant metastases after a mean of 7 years follow-up [38].

The USA randomized trial mentioned above [33] on the addition of radiation to local surgery, has so far provided no evidence that survival was improved on distant metastases decreased. It has been emphasized [36] that we will not know whether the technique is an acceptable alternative to mastectomy until we have information about the survival of such patients after progression to invasive cancer has been treated by secondary mastectomy.

LCIS is more common in premenopausal women but is an uncommon lesion, representing only 1–3% of new breast cancers. It is found at several sites in the same breast in over two thirds of cases, and in both breasts in over one third of cases [35]. Following biopsy, invasive breast cancer appears in the same breast in about 30% of cases and in the opposite breast in about 15% of cases. The risk increases over the length of time the cases are followed up. The lifelong cumulative risk of developing invasive cancer after LCIS is about 1% per year, a risk similar to that of developing cancer in the second breast after primary breast cancer is treated.

It is customary to monitor the LCIS patient by regular clinical examination and mammograms, although a woman's anxiety may make her request more active treatment. Trials of Tamoxifen therapy are under way for LCIS in an attempt to decrease the risk of invasive breast cancer developing. Depending on the results of the current trials of Vitamin A analogues, this also may be given a trial in woman with a diagnosis of LCIS.

Mammographic Patterns Associated with Breast Cancer Risk

It has been claimed that a dense breast pattern in the mammogram, either prominence of the ducts (P2 pattern) or a dysplastic pattern over most of the breast (DY pattern), is associated with increased risk of developing breast cancer [39]. A recent analysis of 19 studies involving about 3,500 women [40] showed evidence of such association in 14 of them. Overall, women with dense breast patterns (P2 and DY) had double the risk of subsequent breast cancer compared to women with the diffuse fatty pattern and no visible ducts (N1). This increased risk translates into an incidence 1.3 times that of the general population. The risk is slightly higher in younger than in older women.

Some have questioned whether increased risk is directly associated with a dense breast pattern, on the basis that small breast cancers cannot be easily recognized in such mammograms and therefore cancer is more likely to grow between mammograms. This so-called 'masking' effect may account for a small part of the apparently increased risk but not for all of it [41]. It has been shown that a dense breast pattern is correlated with high risk pathologic features such as severe atypia [42, 43].

Investigation of a relationship between mammographic patterns and breast cancer risk is complicated by an effect on the former of a woman's age, weight, childbearing history and use of oral contraceptives. Combined estrogen/progestin oral contraceptives tend to decrease a prominent duct pattern (P2 pattern) and this effect becomes greater with lower estrogen levels in the pill [44]. With regard to the effect of pregnancy on the mammogram pattern, it is reported that delayed first childbirth or having no children is associated with a dense pattern [45, 46]. This observation has been related to well-established epidemiologic data showing that early first childbirth confers lasting protection against breast cancer.

Conclusion

What are the risk implications for the woman who has had a biopsy for a benign breast condition? It is generally agreed that women with no evidence of a proliferative lesion can be reassured that their risk is no greater than average. Significant elevation of breast cancer risk (a risk ratio of 3 or more) applies to women with severe degrees of atypia or a preinvasive lesion in the breast. Women whose findings lie between these extremes should be advised to be particularly careful about self-examination, regular mammograms and visits to their physician [21].

Such advice is based only on microscopic examination of biopsy specimens without benefit of information on familial or clinical factors which may multiply a woman's risk. There is a tendency to give undue weight to borderline breast pathology in the belief that such pathology represents disease, when a similar degree of risk due to childbirth, menstrual and family history of breast cancer may be ignored [47]. A strong family history of breast cancer in a mother, sister or daughter, allied with evidence of atypia can increase a woman's risk to 11 times that of women with no proliferative disease [27].

Atypia marks a relatively advanced precursor stage in the evolution of invasive breast cancer, and we need biochemical or genetic markers if we are to recognize early precursor lesions. When reliable markers of this type are available, they may identify women who might benefit from a trial of chemoprevention or hormonal manipulation. On the other hand, it must be taken into account that some atypia lesions and *in situ* cancers disappear spontaneously, suggesting that not all precursor or preinvasive lesions are irrevocably committed to progress towards invasive cancer.

References

1. Love, S.M., Gelman, R.S., Silen, W. (1982). Fibrocystic disease of the breast; a non-disease? *N. Engl. J. Med.*, **307**, 1010–1014.
2. Hutter, R.V.P. (1985). Goodbye to fibrocystic disease. *N. Engl. J. Med.*, **312**, 179–181.
3. Rosen, P.P. (1993). Proliferative breast disease – an unresolved diagnostic dilemma. *Cancer*, **71**, 3798–3807.
4. Bodian, C.A., Perzin, K.H., Lattes, R., Hoffman, P. (1993). Reproducibility and validity of pathologic classifications of benign breast disease and implications for clinical applications. *Cancer*, **71**, 3908–3913.
5. Dupont, W.D., Parl, F.F., Hartmann, W.H. *et al.* (1993). Breast cancer risk associated with proliferative breast disease and atypical hyperplasia. *Cancer*, **71**, 1258–1265.
6. Hughes, L.E., Mansel, R.E., Webster, D.J.T. (1987). Aberrations of normal development and involution; a new perspective on pathogenesis and nomenclature of benign breast disorders. *Lancet*, **2**, 1316–1319.

7. Black, M.M., Barclay, T.H.C., Cutler, S.J. Hankey, B.K., Asire, A.J. (1972). Association of atypical characteristics of benign breast lesions with subsequent risk of breast cancer. *Cancer*, **29**, 338–343.
8. Brinton, J. (1990). Relationship of benign breast disease to breast cancer. *Ann. N.Y. Acad. Sci.*, **586**, 266–271.
9. Tavassoli, F.A., Norris, H.F. (1990). A comparison of the results of long-term follow up for atypical intraductal hyperplasia and intraductal hyperplasia of the breast. *Cancer*, **65**, 518–529.
10. Dupont, W.D., Page, D.L. (1985). Risk factors for breast cancer in women with proliferative disease. *N. Engl. J. Med.*, **312**, 146–151.
11. Roberts, M.M., Jones, V., Elton, R.A. (1984). Risk of breast cancer in women with history of benign breast disease. *Br. Med. J.*, **2828**, 275–278.
12. Hutchinson, W.B., Thomas, D.B., Hamlin, W.B. (1980). Risk of breast cancer in women with benign breast disease. *J. Natl. Cancer Inst.*, **65**, 13–20.
13. Moskovitz, M., Gartside, P., Wirman, J.A., McLaughlin, C. (1980). Proliferative disorders of the breast as risk factors for breast cancer in a self-selected screened population; pathologic markers. *Radiology*, **134**, 289–291.
14. Cole, P.J., Elwood, J.M., Kaplan, S.D. (1978). Incidence rates and risk factors of benign breast neoplasms. *Am. J. Epidemiol.*, **108**, 112–120.
15. Kodlin, D., Winger, E.E., Morgenstern, N.L., Chen, V. (1977). Chronic mastopathy and breast cancer; a follow-up study. *Cancer*, **39**, 2603–2607.
16. Monson, R.R., Yen, S., MacMahon, B. (1976). Chronic mastitis and carcinoma of the breast. *Lancet*, **2**, 224–226.
17. Skolnick, M.H., Cannon-Albright, L.A. (1992). Genetic predisposition to breast cancer. *Cancer*, **70**, 1747–1754.
18. Anderson, T.J. (1991). Genesis and source of breast cancer. *Br. Med. Bull.*, **47**, 305–318.
19. Krieger, N., Hiatt, R.A. (1992). Risk of breast cancer after benign breast diseases. *Am. J. Epidemiol.*, **135**, 619–631.
20. Howell, A. (1989). Clinical evidence for the involvement of oestrogen in the development and progression of breast cancer. *Proc. Roy. Sco. Edin.*, **95B**, 49–57.
21. Bodian, C.A., Perzin, K.H., Lattes, R., Hoffman, P., Abernathy, T.G. (1993). Prognostic significance of benign proliferative disease. *Cancer*, **71**, 3896–3907.
22. Swanson, G.M. (1993). Breast cancer risk estimation; a translational statistic for communication to the public. *J. Natl. Cancer Inst.*, **85**, 948–849.
23. Stoll, B.A. (1994). Breast cancer; the obesity connection. *Br. J. Cancer*, **69**, 799–801.
24. Simpson, H.W., Mutch, F., Halberg, F., Griffiths, K., Wilson, D. (1982). Bimodal age-frequency distribution of epitheliosis in cancer mastectomies. *Cancer*, **50**, 2417–2422.
25. Nielsen, M., Thomsen, J.L., Primdahl, S., Dyreborg, U., Anderson, J.A. (1987). Breast cancer and atypia among young and middle aged women. A study of 110 medicolegal autopsies. *Br. J. Cancer*, **56**, 814–819.
26. McDivitt, R.W., Stevens, J.A., Lee, N.C. *et al.* and the CASH Group. (1992). Histologic types of benign breast disease and the risk for breast cancer. *Cancer*, **69**, 1408–1414.
27. Dupont, W.D., Page, D.L. (1989). Relationship to previous breast disease. In Stoll, B.A. (ed.), *Women at High Risk to Breast Cancer*, Kluwer Academic Publishers, Dordrecht, 47–56.
28. Carter, C.L., Corle, D.K., Micozzi, M.S., Schatzkin, A., Taylor, P.R. (1988). A prospective study of the development of breast cancer in 16,692 women with benign breast disease. *Am. J. Epidemiol.*, **128**, 467–477.
29. London, S.J., Connolly, J.L., Schnitt, S.J., Colditz, G.A. (1992). A prospective study of benign breast disease and the risk of breast cancer. *J. Am. Med. Assoc.*, **267**, 941–944.
30. Rohan, T.E., L'Abbé, K.A., Cook, M.G. (1992). Oral contraceptives and risk of benign proliferative epithelial disorders of the breast. *Intl. J. Cancer*, **50**, 891–894.

31. Hsieh, C.C., Crosson, A.W., Walker, A.M., Trapido, E.J., MacMahon, B. (1984). Oral contraceptive use and fibrocystic breast disease of different histologic classifications. *J. Natl. Cancer Inst.*, **72**, 285–290.
32. Bartow, S.A., Pathak, D.R., Black, W.C., Key, C.R., Reaf, S.R. (1987). Prevalence of benign, atypical and malignant breast lesions in populations at different risk for breast cancer. *Cancer*, **60**, 2751–2760.
33. Fisher, B., Costantino, J., Redmond, C. *et al.* (1993). Lumpectomy compared with lumpectomy and radiation therapy for the treatment of intraductal breast cancer. *N. Engl. J. Med.*, **328**, 1581–1586.
34. Ketcham, A.S., Moffat, F.L. (1990). Vexed surgeons, perplexed patients and cancers which may not be cancer. *Cancer*, **65**, 387–393.
35. Hermann, G., Keller, R., Tartter, P. *et al.* (1993). Labular carcinoma in situ as a non palpable breast lesion. Mammographic features and pathologic correlation. *Breast Dis.*, **6**, 269–276.
36. Van Dongen, J.A., Fentiman, J.S., Harris, J.R. *et al.* (1989). In situ breast cancer; the EORTC consensus meeting. *Lancet*, **2**, 25–27.
37. Spittle, M.F. (1990). The management of ductal carcinoma in situ of the breast. *Clin. Oncol.*, **2**, 63–64.
38. Solin, L.J., Tien Yeh, J., Kurtz, J. *et al.* (1993). Ductal carcinoma in situ of the breast treated by breast-conserving surgery and definitive irradiation. *Cancer*, **71**, 2532–2542.
39. Wolfe, J.N. (1976). Risk for breast cancer development determined by mammographic parenchymal pattern. *Cancer*, **37**, 2486–2492.
40. Funkhauser, E. Waterbor, F.W., Cole, P. (1993). Mammographic patterns and breast cancer risk; a meta-analysis. *Breast Dis.*, **6**, 277–284.
41. Whitehead, J., Carlile, T., Kopecky, K.J. (1985). Wolfe mammographic parenchymal patterns; a study of the masking hypothesis of Egan and Mosteller. *Cancer*, **56**, 1280–1286.
42. Wellings, S.R., Wolfe, J.N. (1978). Correlative studies of the histological and radiographic appearances of the breast parenchyma. *Radiology*, **129**, 299–306.
43. Bright, R.A., Morrison, A.S. Brisson, J. *et al.* (1988). Relationship between mammographic and histologic features of breast tissue in women with benign biopsies. *Cancer*, **61**, 266–271.
44. Leinster, S.J., Whitehouse, G.H. (1986). The mammographic breast pattern and oral contraception. *Br. J. Radiol.*, **59**, 237–239.
45. Bergkvist, L., Tabar, L., Bergström, R., Adami, H.O. (1987). Epidemiologic determinants of the mammographic patterns. *Am. J. Epidemiol.*, **126**, 1075–1081.
46. De Waard, F. (1992). Preventive intervention in breast cancer, but when? *Eur. J. Cancer Prev.*, **1**, 395–399.
47. Morrow, M. (1992). Precancerous breast lesions; implications for breast cancer prevention trials. *Int. J. Radiation Oncol. Biol. Phys.*, **23**, 1071–1078.

Chapter 5

Risk from Age, Race and Social Class

MARIANNE EWERTZ

Breast cancer is the most frequent cancer of women in all developed countries (except Japan), and in many developing areas such as Northern Africa,
the Caribbean, South America, Western Asia and Micronesia/Polynesia. It has
been estimated that some 719,000 new cases were diagnosed worldwide in 1985,
accounting for about 19% of all female cancers [1]. The annual incidence of breast
cancer worldwide will be more than one million cases by the year 2000 [2].

In the United States, 32% of all incident cancers in women are breast cancers,
corresponding to 180,000 new cases diagnosed in 1992 [3]. Based on current
incidence rates, one out of every nine women in the U.S. will develop breast cancer
at some time during her life. Over the past 30 years, breast cancer incidence has
been increasing worldwide, particularly in areas of low incidence, e.g. in Japan,
where incidence rates increased by 100% between 1968 and 1987 [4].

Effect of Age

The incidence of most adult solid cancers increases linearly with age (for example
in colon cancer), but the pattern is different for female breast cancer. The incidence
increases linearly up to around age 50, when the slope changes and resumes a
slower rate of increase with advancing age, (Figure 1). This shape of the age-
specific incidence curve was first described by Clemmesen (5) and the point of
changing slope is known as 'Clemmensen's hook'. It is unique for breast cancer in
females and is absent in male breast cancer, where the incidence increases linearly
with age like other solid tumours [6].

Apart from providing the information that cancer becomes more frequent with
age, age-specific incidence curves have given rise to hypotheses regarding cancer aetiology. The linear increase in most solid tumours has been interpreted as
the effect of continued exposure to carcinogenic agents [7]. This is also true for

41

Basil A. Stoll (ed.), Reducing Breast Cancer Risk in Women, 41–45.
© 1995 *Kluwer Academic Publishers. Printed in the Netherlands.*

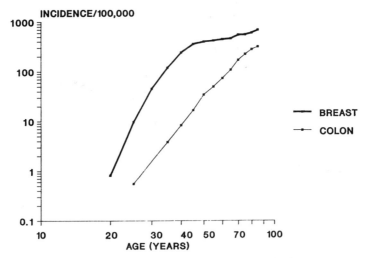

Figure 1. Age-specific incidence of cancer of the breast and colon among women in Denmark, 1983–1987.

female breast cancer up to around age 50, but thereafter the effect of exposure to carcinogenic agents seems to diminish.

Experimental, epidemiologic and clinical evidence indicates that estrogens are involved in breast cancer etiology, and this may relate 'Clemmesen's hook' to occurrence of the menopause. The exposure that diminishes around the menopause is that of ovarian production of estrogen and progestogen. These hormones are not carcinogenic by themselves, but may act to promote division and proliferation of cells which have already undergone malignant transformation [8]. Understanding age-effects in breast cancer incidence is essential to achieve insight into the biology of the disease.

Effect of Race

There is substantial international variation in breast cancer incidence. Figure 2 shows that the rates are highest in North America and Northern Europe, intermediate in Southern Europe and Latin America, and lowest in Asia [9]. Such variation may be due to genetic or environmental factors.

Studies of European migrants who have come from low incidence areas (e.g. Poland and Italy) to high incidence areas (e.g. the Unites States, Australia and Israel) show that the breast cancer rates approach those of a new host country within the life-span of the migrating women [10–12]. This points towards a role for environmental factors.

However, the speed with which the incidence among migrants approaches that of the adopted country varies from one ethnic group to another. Among

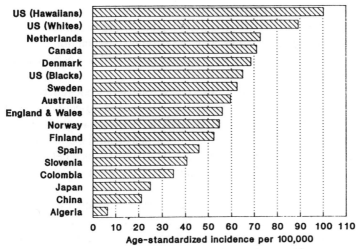

Figure 2. Age-standardized (World Population) incidence of female breast cancer [9].

Japanese migrating to the United States, first-generation migrants have breast cancer rates slightly higher than in Japan, while the incidence among second-generation migrants is even higher (although still lower than among US born women). The explanation may lie in the pace of acculturation, the Japanese adopting a US lifestyle more slowly than do Polish women for example [4]. It has also been suggested that environmental factors are more important early in life than later in determining breast cancer risk [13].

In the United States, age-adjusted incidence rates per 100,000 by race/ethnicity in California for 1988–1989 were 110.6 for white women, 96.3 for black women, 59.2 for Hispanic women and 52.8 for women of other races (mostly Asian-American). Among premenopausal women, blacks had slightly higher rates than whites, while the reverse was observed for postmenopausal women. These racial differences are thought to arise from differences in risk factors, e.g. socio–economic status, age at first childbirth, parity, age at menarche and menopause [4].

Effect of Social Class

Reports linking female breast cancer to affluence date back to the turn of the century [14] and since the 1950s, evidence confirms that breast cancer is associated with higher socio-economic status. The results appear consistent across study types (cross-sectional, case-control, cohort) and data sources (incidence, mortality, hospital-based series).

Several indicators of socio-economic status have been used, such as duration of schooling, employment of the patient and her husband, and social class indices. In the International Collaborative Study [15], the strongest association was observed for duration of schooling, and many later studies have used this as a measurement of socio-economic status.

The strength of the association has varied between studies but generally, relative risk estimates are from 1.3 to 2.0 for women of a higher socio-economic status.

Variation may arise from differences between the populations studied and study design. In the Scandinavian countries with populations of similar ethnic and cultural background, free access to medical care, and a smaller difference between rich and poor, women of higher socio-economic status have a 30% excess risk of breast cancer [16, 17].

There is no reason to believe that social class *per se* affects the risk of breast cancer. Social class can be regarded as an indicator of a high-risk lifestyle, reflecting a number of risk factors. Compared with women of low social class, women of high social class are likely to have their first child at a later age, to have fewer children, to use hormone replacement therapy during the menopause, and to have a higher alcohol consumption, all of which may increase the risk of breast cancer. The relation between social class and other risk factors, such as obesity, ages at menarche and menopause, may depend on cultural and behavioral patterns of the population studied.

Conclusion

International cancer statistics show that breast cancer is the most common cancer in women in much of the world. The disease is linked to affluence, with high incidence rates in Northern America and Northern Europe, high incidence rates among whites compared with Americans of other ethnicity, and is in all countries associated with higher socio-economic status.

The reason why breast cancer is more common in affluent women is probably related to their profile of high risk factors, notably those related to female sex hormones. The age-specific incidence curve of breast cancer (demonstrating 'Clemmesen's hook') supports the role of female sex hormones in breast cancer etiology.

References

1. Parkin, D.M., Pisani, P., Ferlay, J. (1993). Estimates of the worldwide incidence of eighteen major cancers in 1985. *Int. J. Cancer*, **54**, 594–606.
2. Miller, A.B., Bulbrook, R.D. (1986). UICC multi-disciplinary project on breast cancer: the epidemiology, aetiology and prevention of breast cancer. *Int. J. Cancer*, **37**, 173–177.
3. Boring, C.C., Squires, T.S., Tong, T. (1992). Cancer statistics 1992. *CA*, **42**, 19–38.
4. Kelsey, J.L., Horn–Ross, P.L. (1993). Breast cancer: magnitude of the problem and descriptive epidemiology. *Epidemiol Rev.*, **15**, 7–16.

5. Clemmesen, J. (1948). Carcinoma of the breast. I. Results from statistical research. *Brit. J. Radiol.*, **21**, 583–590.
6. Ewertz, M., Holmberg, L., Karjalainen, S., Tretli, S., Adami, H.-O. (1989). Incidence of male breast cancer in Scandinavia, 1943–1982. *Int. J. Cancer*, **43**, 27–31.
7. Cook, P.J., Doll, R., Fellingham, S.A. (1969). A mathematical model for the age distribution of cancer in man. *Int. J. Cancer*, **4**, 93–112.
8. Pike, M.C., Spicer, D.V., Dahmoush, L., Press, M.F. (1993). Estrogens, progestogens, normal breast cell proliferation, and breast cancer risk. *Epidemiol. Rev.*, **15**, 17–35.
9. Parkin, D.M., Muir, C.S., Whelan, S.L. *et al.* (1992). *Cancer Incidence in Five Continents*, Vol. VI. IARC Scientific Publications No. 120, Lyon.
10. Nasca, P.C., Greenwald, P., Burnett, W.S., Chorost, S., Schmidt, W. (1981). Cancer among the foreign-born in New York State. *Cancer*, **48**, 2323–2328.
11. McMichael, A.J., Giles, G.G. (1988). Cancer in migrants to Australia: Extending the descriptive epidemiological data. *Cancer Res.*, **48**, 751–756.
12. Parkin, D.M., Steinits, R., Khlat, M. *et al.* (1990). Cancer in Jewish migrants to Israel. *Int. J. Cancer*, **45**, 614–621.
13. Shimizu, H., Ross, R.K., Bernstein, L. *et al.* (1991). Cancers of the prostate and breast among Japanese and white immigrants in Los Angeles County. *Br. J. Cancer*, **63**, 963–966.
14. Clemmesen, J. (1965). *Statistical Studies in the Aetiology of Malignant Neoplasms*, Vol. I. Review and results. Munksgaard, Copenhagen.
15. MacMahon, B., Lin, T.M., Lowe, C.R. *et al.* (1970). Lactation and cancer of the breast. *Bull. WHO*, **42**, 185–194.
16. Ewertz, M. (1988). Risk of breast cancer in relation to social factors in Demark. *Acta Oncol.*, **27**, 787–792.
17. Vågerö, D., Persson, G. (1986). Occurence of cancer in socio-economic groups in Sweden. *Scand. J. Soc. Med.*, **14**, 151–160.

Chapter 6

Assessing a Woman's Genetic Risk

DAVID E. GOLDGAR and CONSTANCE M. GOLDGAR

Because of the increased risk of breast cancer in relatives of breast cancer cases and the existence of families with unusual clusters of breast cancer cases, genes have been recognized as playing an important role in breast cancer etiology. Lynch and co-workers [1, 2] recognized a subset of breast cancer that appeared to be transmitted as an autosomal dominant trait and also families where breast cancer is associated with cancer at several other sites. They suggested that 5% of all breast cancer is autosomal dominant in origin, 82% is sporadic and 13% polygenic or multifactorial.

This hypothesis of a breast cancer susceptibility that is dominantly inherited has been supported by several groups [3–7]. These investigators have examined the evidence for genetic inheritance in breast cancer families ascertained from a variety of sources. The data were most consistent with autosomal dominant inheritance for a major susceptibility locus with high, but not complete, lifetime penetrance in genetically susceptible women. In addition, it was concluded that because the risk to gene carriers was not 100%, there must be other genetic or environmental effects which influence risk.

In the analysis of the CASH data of 4,730 breast cancer cases and matched controls, Claus *et al.* [7] provided evidence for the existence of a rare, dominant allele with a frequency of 0.003 linked to an increased susceptibility to breast cancer, implying a carrier rate of 6/1000 in the general population. Carriers of the allele appeared to be at greater risk than non-carriers at all ages, with the ratio of age-specific risks at younger ages and declining steadily thereafter. For example, the estimated increased risk due to this susceptibility allele ranged from almost 100-fold in women in their twenties to a modest two-fold increase in women in their eighties. The cumulative lifetime risk of breast cancer for women carrying the susceptibility allele was predicted to be approximately 92%; the risk for non-carriers was estimated to be around 10%.

Basil A. Stoll (ed.), Reducing Breast Cancer Risk in Women, 47–54.
© 1995 *Kluwer Academic Publishers. Printed in the Netherlands.*

Approximately 1 in 200 to 400 women in the general population are said to have inherited susceptibility to breast cancer [5, 7]. Although segregation analysis has supported the hypothesis that the genetic predisposition to breast cancer may be due to a single major gene, this is extremely unlikely. When interpreting data from such analyses, it is important to recognize that estimates of a gene frequency actually represents the sum of allele frequencies of a number of probable susceptibility loci. Likewise, estimates of penetrance (or the degree to which the susceptibility is expressed as breast cancer) are an average of the effects of each locus. Confirmation of the existence of several loci which contribute to familial breast cancer can come only through localization of such genes to specific chromosomal regions by linkage analysis of breast cancer families, or through identification of germ-line mutations of specific candidate loci in familial breast cancer patients.

Mapping of breast cancer susceptibility genes is complicated by the heterogeneity of the disease. Over the past five years, however, a number of genes responsible for inherited predisposition to breast and/or ovarian cancer have been identified or localized. In particular, BRCA1, the p53 gene, the ataxia-telangiectasia gene and the androgen receptor are now known to increase susceptibility to breast cancer. These genes differ in terms of the risks of cancer which they confer, the cancer phenotypes with which they are associated, and their gene frequencies. However, it is also known that these genes alone do not account for all, or perhaps even most, of the families with early-onset breast cancer. It is unlikely, as well, that these loci account for a high proportion of familial clustering of postmenopausal breast cancer.

BRCA1

The existence of a specific gene, referred to as BRCA1, conferring an increased susceptibility to breast cancer, was confirmed in late 1990 with the finding of linkage between early-onset breast cancer and a specific marker on the long arm of chromosome 17 [8]. Shortly thereafter it was recognized that families with inherited susceptibility to ovarian cancer as well as breast cancer were due to this gene [9]. A large study conducted by the Breast Cancer Linkage Consortium (BCLC) analyzed data from 214 families collected in Europe and North America. This analysis localized BRCA1 to an estimated 14 centimorgan interval flanked by the markers D17S250 and D17S588 [10]. Subsequently, the BRCA1 locus has been further localized to a narrower interval flanked by D17S776 and D17S78 [11–13].

Based on genotypings at a series of marker loci surrounding the BRCA1 locus, the BCLC estimated that 45% of families with a high risk of breast cancer alone, and virtually 100% of breast cancer families who have one individual case of ovarian cancer, are linked to the 17q site. The penetrance for breast cancer in gene carriers in the BCLC families was estimated to be 38% by age 40, and 66% by age 60 [10]. As detailed in the upcoming sections, these preliminary estimates have been refined using a broader-based set of families and more informative genetic markers.

Risks of Cancer in BRCA1 Mutation Carriers

Once BRCA1 has been cloned and specific mutations can be identified in individual women, more realistic estimates of the penetrance will be obtained from population-based studies of mutations. While the BRCA1 gene has yet to be identified, genetic markers that are tightly linked to the gene have been found, making it feasible to do genetic testing and counseling for the gene in some high-risk families. At present, we can only determine an individual woman's inherited risk in the context of a BRCA1-linked family from linkage studies. The family must be sufficiently informative for linkage study, and several affected living family members who are closely related to the person whose risk is being evaluated must participate. However, given these limitations, it is possible to identify gene carriers in these families with a reasonable degree of confidence.

Easton *et al.* [10], in the original analysis of the BCLC data, estimated an 85% lifetime risk of developing breast and/or ovarian cancer, an overall risk for breast and ovarian cancer of 59% by age 50, with more than 50% of the breast cancers occurring before age 50. At the few research centers where such testing may be done, the risks in BRCA1-linked families will most likely vary from these figures, within the context of the pedigree analyzed [12].

More recently, Easton *et al.* [14] reported an analysis of a subset of families submitted to the BCLC; these families contained at least 4 cases of breast or ovarian cancer diagnosed before age 60. The estimated cancer risk for breast cancer conferred by BRCA1 in these families was estimated to be 51% by age 50 and 85% by age 70. For ovarian cancer, estimates were 23% by age 50 and 63% by age 70. The age-specific incidence of breast cancer in BRCA1 mutation carriers follows a very different pattern from that seen in the general population: relative risks decline significantly with age from over 200-fold in the age group under 40 years to 15-fold in the 60–69 year age group [14]. Ford *et al.* [15], utilizing the updated set of BCLC families above and more informative markers, re-estimated cumulative risks of breast cancer by age in unaffected BRCA1 carriers.

One caveat in interpreting the risks of BRCA1 carriers is that the families participating in the BCLC consortium data were selected because multiple relatives developed breast cancer. Other families with breast cancer linked to less severe mutations in BRCA1 most likely exist. Women carrying less severe BRCA1 mutations might be at increased risk, but perhaps not so dramatically high as is seen in the BCLC families. It has been estimated that approximately 2–4% of breast cancer cases in the general population are associated with BRCA1 germline mutations [16]. Ford *et al.* [15] estimated proportions of breast cancer in the general population due to BRCA1 stratifying for age. According to their estimates, for ages 40 and under, BRCA1 would account for approximately 7.8% of breast cancer cases;

for ages 40–49 and 50 or over, BRCA1 would be responsible for 3.7% and 0.9% respectively. There is potential observational evidence from tumor deletion studies that somatically acquired abnormalities of the BRCA1 locus may also play a role in the development of sporadic cases of breast cancer [17, 18].

The risks associated with the BRCA1 gene are obviously much greater than the relative risks of 2 to 3 commonly quoted for positive family history in first degree relatives. However, it must be noted that even in dramatically affected families demonstrating dominant inheritance, each individual has a 50% probability of *not* carrying the susceptibility allele. The lifetime risks of breast cancer for non-carriers would be estimated as that of a woman in the general population – approximately 7% to the age of 70 years [19]. It is therefore important to be able to distinguish women carrying mutations in breast cancer susceptibility gene(s) from women who have not inherited the susceptibility gene(s).

Accurate estimates of the proportion of familial breast cancer due to BRCA1 must await the isolation of the BRCA1 gene. For most women we are still far from being able to accurately predict individual risk.

Non-BRCA1 Genes Which May Increase Breast Cancer Risk

Although great excitement has been generated over the localization of the BRCA1 locus and great effort is underway to isolate this gene, it is likely that the BRCA1 locus is responsible for only a minority of breast cancer cases due to inherited susceptibilities. There are a number of specific genes which have been associated with an increased risk of breast cancer.

P53

The first gene to have been implicated in the genesis of breast cancer is the p53 gene on chromosome 17p [20]. Germline p53 mutations are most often associated with the Li–Fraumeni syndrome in which families typically exhibit multiple affected members with childhood cancers, primarily sarcomas and brain tumors [21]. Another hallmark of this syndrome is the presence in the family of cases of very early-onset breast cancer, with age at onset usually before age 30. It has been estimated that 60% of Li–Fraumeni families are due to germline p53 mutations. However, in Li–Fraumeni-like families, i.e., families which have some of these characteristics but not the defining childhood cancers, a recent study found 10% were attributable to germline p53 mutations [22]. Overall, it is thought, however, that germline p53 mutations account for only a small (>5%) proportion of very early-onset breast cancers and a negligible fraction of familial breast cancer in general [23].

Ataxia–Telangiectasia

Ataxia-telangiectasia (A–T) is a progressive neurological disorder which appears to be inherited in an autosomal recessive fashion. It is associated with a high incidence of cancer (<61-fold), particularly lymphomas and leukemias, but also primary carcinomas of other organs, including the breast [24]. Patients with the disease are homozygous for a mutant gene, the A–T gene, assigned to the chromosomal region 11q23 [25]. It has been suggested that the high incidence of cancers associated with this disorder may be due to 'fragile' chromosomes; the chromosomes of affected individuals seem particularly susceptible to damage from ionizing radiation, as well as specific cytotoxic drugs.

It has been reported that about 1% of the population carry the A–T gene [26] and that individuals who carry one abnormal copy of the A–T gene are also at an increased risk of cancer of any type, approximately twice that of the population at large for men, and 3-fold for women carriers [26]. The heterozygote relative risk for breast cancer in women carriers was estimated to be significantly higher, with a relative risk of 6.8 [25]. The gene frequency for A–T has been estimated as 1–3%; if this is true, the A–T locus could then account for up to 20% of breast cancers from woman heterozygotes. It should be noted that this paper generated a great deal of controversy; the results were questioned on the basis of methodological issues of control groups as well as radiation exposure assessment which could reduce the risk reported [27–29].

In addition, in a recent examination of a number of early-onset non-BRCA1-linked breast cancer families, no evidence of linkage to the A–T region of chromosome 11 was found [30]. The importance of this gene in breast cancer remains to be verified.

The Search for Additional Breast Cancer-Causing Genes

It is clear that BRCA1 does not account for the majority of the observed familial clustering of breast cancer. In fact, as noted above, BRCA1 probably only accounts for about half of the striking families with many cases of early-onset breast cancer. Mapping of breast cancer susceptibility genes is complicated by the heterogeneity of the disease. In addition, the disease is not completely penetrant among susceptible individuals, with expression depending on age, gender and environmental factors.

Since the Breast Cancer Linkage Consortium (BCLC) data were submitted, at least 10 breast/ovarian cancer families have been identified which appear to be unlinked to BRCA1. In order to better assess the relationship of ovarian cancer to BRCA1, members of the BCLC were invited to send updated 17q marker typing data on each of their breast cancer families which contained at least one case of ovarian cancer. Analysis of these 165 breast/ovarian families showed that, overall, the best estimate of the proportion linked to BRCA1 was 75% [31]. Interestingly, in families of breast cancer or breast/ovarian cancer studied thus far, which also include one or more cases of male breast cancer, all have proved to be unlinked to the BRCA1 region of 17q [32].

When one considers families with female breast cancer only, and at least one ovarian cancer, the BCLC estimated that approximately 79% were due to BRCA1; when the criterion is tightened to only include families with two or more cases of ovarian cancer case, an even higher proportion (93%) were attributable to BRCA1. This is of importance in assessing risk since a family with many cases of ovarian cancer has a high chance of being suitable for genetic counseling based on linkage analysis of genetic markers in the BRCA1 region; conversely, a woman whose family history includes only site-specific breast cancer would require a great deal more linkage evidence before being amenable to BRCA1 counseling, since perhaps only 25% of such family histories are due to BRCA1.

The classification of unlinked families into three phenotypic groups based upon the presence of ovarian cancer and male breast cancer could reduce further antici-pated genetic heterogeneity, thus reducing the complexity of the task of finding these additional loci. A collaborative effort to perform a total genomic search using a set of extended families from North America and Europe is currently underway. Preliminary examination of linkage in a subset of these families to a set of candidate loci or regions, including those described above, have thus far found no evidence of linkage to any of the selected regions or genes. Other subsets of breast cancer will likely be described.

Conclusion

It is relatively well-established that a positive family history is the strongest epi-demiologic risk factor known for breast cancer, stronger than any known reproduc-tive, hormonal, or dietary factors. Although correlated family environment could account for some portion of the observed familiality, there is substantial evidence that the majority of this familial effect is due to the action of a number of specific genes.

This evidence comes from several sources: the observation that there is an increased risk to more distant relatives of breast cancer probands who do not share common environments; the results of segregation analyses which show that the pattern of familiality is consistent with the actions of dominant highly-penetrant susceptibility loci; and, most convincingly, the mapping of one such susceptibility gene, BRCA1, to the long arm of chromosome 17. However, it has become increas-ingly clear that BRCA1 does not account for the majority of the observed familial clustering of breast cancer. In fact, BRCA1 probably only accounts for about half of the striking families with many cases of early-onset breast cancer, and only a minority of those without ovarian cancer.

It is likely that in the near future, a number of other highly-penetrant suscepti-bility loci for breast cancer will be identified through genetic linkage studies, and that the role of specific known genes which seem to be associated with increased breast cancer risk will be clarified.

References

1. Lynch, H.T., Krush, A.J., Giurgis, H. (1973). Genetic factors in families with combined gastrointestinal and breast cancer. *Am. J. Gastroent.*, **59**, 31–40.
2. Lynch, H.T., Guirgis, H.A., Albert, S. *et al.* (1974). Familial association of carcinoma of the breast and ovary. *Surgery*, **138**, 717–724.
3. Hill, J.R., Carmelli, D., Gardner, E.J., Skolnick, M.H. (1978). Likelihood analysis of breast cancer predisposition in a Mormon pedigree. In Morton, N.E., Chung, C.S. (eds.), *Genetic Epidemiology*, Academic Press, New York.
4. Go, R.C.P., King, M.C., Bailey-Wilson, J., Elston, R.C., Lynch, H.T. (1983). Genetic epidemiology of breast cancer and associated cancers in high-risk families. I. Segregation analysis. *J. Natl. Cancer Inst.*, **71**, 455–461.
5. Newman, B., Austin, M.A., Lee, M., King, M.-C. (1988). Inheritance of human breast cancer: evidence for autosomal dominant transmission in high risk families. *Proc. Natl. Acad. Sci. USA*, **85**, 3044–3048.
6. Bishop, D.T., Albright, L.C., McClellan, T., Gardner, E.J., Skolnick, M.H. (1988). Segregation and linkage analysis of nine Utah breast cancer pedigrees. *Genetic Epidem.*, **5**, 151–169.
7. Claus, E.B., Risch, N., Thompson, W.D. (1991). Genetic analysis of breast cancer in the Cancer and Steroid Hormone study. *Am. J. Hum. Genet.*, **48**, 232–242.
8. Hall, J.M., Lee, M.K., Newman, B. *et al.* (1990). Linkage of early-onset familial breast cancer to chromosome 17q21. *Science*, **250**, 1684–1689.
9. Narod, S.A., Feunteun, J., Lynch, H.T. *et al.* (1991). Familial breast-ovarian cancer locus on chromosome 17q12–q23. *Lancet*, **338**; 82–83.
10. Easton, D.F., Bishop, D.T., Ford, D., Crockford, G.P. (1993). Genetic linkage analysis in familial breast and ovarian cancer: results from 214 families. *Am. J. Hum. Genet.*, **52**, 678–701.
11. Chamberlain, J.S., Boehnke, M., Frank, T.S. *et al.* (1993) BRCA1 maps proximal to D17S579 on chromosome 17q21 by genetic analysis. *Am. J. Hum. Genet.*, **52**, 792–798.
12. Goldgar, D.E., Cannon-Albright, L.A. Oliphant, A.R., *et al.* (1993). Chromosome 17q linkage studies of 18 Utah breast cancer kindreds. *Am. J. Hum. Genet.*, **52**, 743–748.
13. Simard, J., Feunteun, J., Lenoir, G. *et al.* (1993). Genetic mapping of the breast-ovarian cancer syndrome to a small interval on chromosome 17q12–21: exclusion of candidate genes EDH17B2 and RARA. *Hum. Molec. Genet.*, **2**, 1193–1199.
14. Easton, D.F., Ford, D., Bishop, D.T. and the Breast Cancer Linkage Consortium *et al.* Breast and ovarian cancer incidence in BRCA1 carriers, (Submitted).
15. Ford, D., Easton, D.F., Bishop, D.T. *et al.* (1994). Risks of cancer in BRCA1–mutation carriers. *Lancet*, **343**, 692–695.
16. Biesecker, B.B., Boehnke, M., Calzone, K. *et al.* (1993) Genetic counseling for families with inherited susceptibility to breast and ovarian cancer. *J. Am. Med. Assn.*, **269**, 1970–1974.
17. Cornelis, R.S., Devilee, P., Van Vliet, M. *et al.* (1993) Allele loss patterns on chromosome 17q in 109 breast carcinoma indicate at least two distinct target regions. *Oncogene*, **8**, 781–785.
18. Jacobs, I.J., Smith, S.A., Wiseman, R.W. *et al.* (1993) A deletion unit on chromosome 17q in epithelial ovarian tumours distal to the familial breast/ovarian cancer locus. *Cancer Res.*, **53**, 1218–1221.
19. Weber, B.L., Garber, J.E. (1993). Family history and breast cancer: probabilities and possibilities. *J. Am. Med. Assn.* **270**, 1602–1603.
20. Malkin, D., Li, F.P., Strong, L.C. *et al.* (1990) Germ line p53 mutations in a familial syndrome of breast cancer, sarcomas, and other neoplasms. *Science*, **250**, 1233–1238.

21. Li, F.P., Fraumeni, J.F. (1969). Soft tissue sarcomas, breast cancer and other neoplasms: a familial syndrome? *Ann. Intern. Med.*, **71**, 747–760.
22. Warren, W., Eeles, R.A., Ponder, B.A.J. *et al.* (1992). No evidence for germline mutations in exons 5–9 of the p53 gene in 25 breast cancer families. *Oncogene*, **7**, 1043–1046.
23. Borreson, A.L., Anderson, T.I., Garber, J. *et al.* (1992). Screening for germ line TP 53 mutations in breast cancer patients. *Cancer Res.*, **52**, 3234–3236.
24. Swift, M., Reitnauer, P.J., Morrell, D. Chase, C.L. (1991). Incidence of cancer in 161 families affected by ataxia telangiectasia. *N. Engl. J. Med.*, **325**, 1831–1836.
25. Gatti, R.A., Berkel, I., Boder, E. *et al.* (1988). Localization of the ataxia–telangiectasia gene to chromosome 11q22–23. *Nature*, **336**, 577–580.
26. Swift, M., Reitnauer, P.J., Morrell, D., Chase, C.L. (1987). Breast and other cancers in families with ataxia–telangiectasia. *N. Engl. J. Med.*, **316**, 1289–1294.
27. Wagner, L.K. (1992). Correspondence: risk of breast cancer in ataxia–telangiectasia. *N. Engl. J. Med.*, **326**, 1359–1360.
28. Hall, E.J., Geard, C.R., Brenner, D.J. (1992) Correspondence: Risk of breast cancer in ataxia–telangiectasia. *N. Engl. J. Med.*, **326**, 1359–1360.
29. Land, C.E. (1992) Correspondence: Risk of breast cancer in ataxia–telangiectasia. *N. Engl. J. Med.*, **326**, 1359–1360.
30. Wooster, R., Mangion, J., Eeles, R. *et al.* (1992). A germline mutation in the androgen receptor gene in two brothers with breast cancer and Reifenstein syndrome. *Nat. Genet.*, **2**, 132–134.
31. Narod, S.A., Easton, D.F., Lynch, H.T. *et al.* A Number of Breast-Ovarian Cancer Families Appear to be Unlinked to the BRCA1 Locus on Chromosome 17q, (Submitted).
32. Stratton, M.R., Ford, D., Seal, S. *et al.* (1994). Familial male breast cancer is not linked to the BRCA1 locus on chromosome 17q. *Nat. Genet.*, **7**, 103–107.

Chapter 7

Ethics and Economics of Genetic Testing for Breast Cancer

ROBERT A. HIATT

The primary gene responsible for the heritable form of breast cancer (BRCAI) is discussed in Chapter 6 and it is expected that the test for the presence of the gene will be available shortly [1, 2]. Approximately 1 in 200, or 600,000 women in the United States may carry a gene that increases their susceptibility to breast cancer [1, 3–6]. Inheritance follows the patterns of autosomal dominant transmission and is associated with as high as an 85% lifetime risk of either breast or ovarian cancer [7,8]. Breast cancer that develops in association with BRCAI primarily strikes younger women and it has been estimated that as many as half of the women who develop breast cancer under 50 years of age may carry the gene [7].

Because of the number of people at risk, and the fears generated by breast cancer, interest in genetic testing for this cancer will be high. It is essential that medical providers prepare themselves to meet these needs. Furthermore, locating such a gene will eventually lead not only to an understanding of the genetic aspects of inheritable breast cancer but will also provide insights into the development of breast cancer through somatic mutation. There is the possibility that breast cancer incidence and mortality could be reduced by preventive strategies that either replace the products of the faulty gene or replace the faulty genetic material itself [1, 9].

But before such therapies are available, and indeed before widespread testing can be recommended, there is much work that needs to be done to answer the scientific, technical, cost and ethical issues raised [2, 9]. All these innovations will undoubtably generate enormous new demands on the medical system. The response to these demands will require a multidisciplined effort that should include primary care practitioners, geneticists, genetic counsellors, oncologists, psychologists, medical ethicists, other medical specialists, and policy makers. The type of care and services being called for, although not new, are because of their magnitude, an essentially new problem for health care providers. Meanwhile, commercial com-

Basil A. Stoll (ed.), Reducing Breast Cancer Risk in Women, 55–65.
© 1995 *Kluwer Academic Publishers. Printed in the Netherlands.*

panies are unlikely to wait for technologically feasible approaches to prevention and are announcing plans to offer testing for genetic cancer risk [2].

Ethical Questions

The kinds of ethical questions raised by cancer genetic screening in general, and breast cancer screening in particular, have already been suggested by the experience with Huntington's Disease [10–13]. Ethical questions can be considered in three broad categories: individual rights, the potential conflict between individual rights and those of others, and the obligations and concerns of health care providers [3].

Individual Rights

It is clear that a woman has a right to have the nature of the test and the implications of its results explained and to give informed consent to be tested. Information should be provided on what risk of breast cancer is associated with a positive result. The risk of false positives and false negatives should be fully explained. The individual should be prepared as well as possible for the impact the results may have on his or her psychological well-being [8, 14, 15]. A discussion of confidentiality and the possible consequences associated with the intentional or unintentional revelation of a positive result to family members and interested third parties needs to be discussed.

Currently, the risk associated with a positive result is unclear because investigators expect to find several mutations of BRCA1. Genotyping analyses in high-risk families have shown the risk to be extremely high, reaching over 50% by age 50 years and 86% by age 80 years [1, 7]. However, these families probably represent the upper end of a spectrum and other families may carry a gene mutation with a lesser risk. When the BRCA1 gene is cloned and all its various mutations can be sequenced, then risk associated with each variant can be determined. Until that time, informed consent can only be based on the assumption that all women are in the highest risk category.

A woman has the right to know the likelihood of a false positive as well as a false negative, although the precise operational characteristics of the test are not yet known. False positive tests could lead to substantial psychosocial stress [14], and in some cases, unnecessarily drastic preventive measures, such as prophylactic mastectomies. False negatives could lead to an unwarranted sense of security and mean that opportunities for early detection or prevention will be lost.

Once she is fully informed of the nature and implications of the test, for reasons of her own a woman may not wish to be tested [16]. A woman, who because of family history has already undergone prophylactic bilateral mastectomy may be more comfortable assuming she is a carrier. However, early experience of groups counseling families with inherited breast cancer found that almost all families want to know their status [8].

While individuals have the right to be fully informed and to confidentiality regarding the results, any test that holds the possibility of serious illness resulting from genetic factors places the individual's right to confidentiality in potential conflict with the legitimate rights of other individuals and groups.

Rights of Other Individuals

While breast and other cancers are unlike other genetic conditions such as Huntington's Disease, where the safety of others could be at stake if the affected individual's performance were to falter [12], the psychologic and economic consequences to family and friends are substantial when a woman develops and dies from breast cancer. In other words, there may be some limits on the right to the privacy of the individual where emotional harm, genetic risk, or fiduciary responsibility could fall to others close to the affected individual.

Should a woman be obligated to tell her family if she learns she has a BRCA1 mutation? Should she be required to divulge this information to her spouse or prospective spouse? Clearly there are major consequences to the family in terms of financial obligations, the emotional burdens of a serious illness, and the implications of risk for all first-degree female relatives. Furthermore, the significance of the results may not be limited to the female relatives since there is also some evidence that men who carry the BRCA1 gene may be susceptible to an increased incidence of prostate cancer [17] and may pass the gene on to offspring.

Under what conditions should a physician consider releasing results of genetic testing to others without a patient's consent? From a legal standpoint there has been some reluctance to interfere with the time-honored professional confidentiality of the doctor-patient relationship, except in extreme cases where clear harm may come to other parties from the actions of the patient. Examples include threats of murder by psychiatric patients or child abuse [18]. On the other hand, in the United States the President's Commission for the Study of Ethical Problems in Medical and Biomedical and Behavioral Research took the position that a physician could release genetic information to relatives without the consent of patient, if a good faith effort to obtain voluntary consent had already been sought; if harm would probably occur to the relative; if the harm to identifiable persons was likely to be serious; and that only the minimal amount of genetic information was released [19].

The individual's right to the confidentiality of test results may conflict with the interests of employers and either health or life insurance carriers. If prospective employers have access to test results, they might be motivated to refuse employment on that basis in order to keep insurance costs down [3, 18]. Some companies already refuse employment for smokers, raising public fears about what other grounds will be used to deny employment to individuals known to be at risk of serious medical illness. A logical and worrisome extension of such practices could be large numbers of unemployable citizens whose health care and well-being will fall to the public's responsibility [18].

Early experience with the counseling of high risk women has found that many fear having the test results disclosed even to their personal physicians because the medical record containing genetic test results may be seen by the insurance companies [20]. In the United States, life insurance companies function on the basis of actuarial probabilities assigned to the risk of death. If a woman were known to have a mutation of BRCA1 and the associated risk of early mortality, a life insurance company could either refuse to insure her or charge prohibitively high premiums [18]. More importantly, health insurance would likely be unobtainable by a woman with a known BRCA1 mutation. In an effort to avoid 'adverse selection', companies would refuse to offer health insurance and in the case of illness, a large portion of our population's health care could become a matter of public responsibility [18]. In those countries with universal health coverage this should not present a serious problem and it is unknown at the time of this writing what kinds of protections the changes being considered in the United States health care system will provide to individuals with genetic diseases. Where universal coverage does not exist, legislation may be needed to resolve the conflicts of both employers and insurers with those of the individual.

The Obligations of Health Care Providers

There are also important ethical obligations for health care providers and policy-makers with regard to the criteria for testing, identifying those eligible for testing, deciding on the appropriate options for those who test positive, and providing systems, personnel, and training.

General agreement on the criteria for testing will have to be developed by national professional societies, policymakers, and providers. This must take into consideration factors such as a personal history of premenopausal breast or ovarian cancer, or a family history of a first degree relative with premenopausal breast cancer or ovarian cancer. In setting these criteria, however, some care will be required so as not to make them either too broad or too narrow. If the criteria are broad, more women are going to be unnecessarily subjected to the psychosocial consequences of the testing process and the demand on the medical care system to provide testing services will be greater. If the criteria are too narrow, fewer women with the gene will be identified.

One of the principles of an appropriate screening test is that an effective preventive strategy exists for those testing positive for the condition. It can be argued that it is unethical to test for a gene if nothing can be done about it. Yet that is what is happening with Huntington's Disease, where the only benefit is knowing whether the individual will be affected later in life. With breast cancer, although there are no proven preventive measures, there are at least the imperfect options of early and repeated mammography, clinical breast examination, prophylactic mastectomy and/or oophorectomy, and the use of Tamoxifen [1, 21–23].

Another decision that will involve institutional providers at a policy level is the age at which testing should begin [24]. Unfortunately, guidelines for screening children for late-onset disorders do not currently exist [25]. Some might argue that genetic testing of the fetus is appropriate in the same way that they are now tested for cystic fibrosis, Down's Syndrome and hemophilia [18]. Voluntary testing could be performed along with a battery of other tests following amniocentesis or chorionic villus sampling and the option of abortion considered. However, the impact of the distant possibility of cancer in later life is substantially different from the impact of birth defects immediately manifest in children, and the perceived threat will depend on the type of cancer, how easily it can be treated, and the expected age of onset. The knowledge of the more distant liability posed by genetic testing for cancer and the emotional and legal issues surrounding the option of therapeutic abortion suggest that genetic testing of a fetus for BRCA1 or other cancer gene is unlikely to gain wide support.

Screening could also be performed in the neonatal period in the manner in which phenylketonuria (PKU) is tested for currently. Here too the question of available therapy or prevention procedures comes into play. With PKU a low phenylalanine diet instituted during infancy can prevent mental retardation. There is nothing, however, that can be done currently for an infant with BRCA1 and this mitigates against testing in the neonatal period. This may change when effective gene therapies become available, but for now, testing in the neonatal period cannot be recommended.

When then should genetic testing be undertaken? The age of consent (18 years in the United States) seems most appropriate because the woman herself is then legally responsible for the decision. It is also a time when the option of instituting regular mammography could be begun and not too long before a women might consider prophylactic mastectomy. Just how women at this age might be identified and offered genetic testing is another question.

When a health care organization has records that would allow it to identify women at high risk of breast cancer and likely to benefit from testing, what is its obligations to actively contact these women and inform them of their options? In addition, when it is decided who should be tested on the basis of risk profiles based on personal and family histories of breast and ovarian cancer, what obligations does the provider or health care organization have to women who are not eligible by these criteria? It may be an obligation for the provider to counsel these women as well, in order both to explain why they are not eligible and to use the opportunity to remind them of their normal level of risk and what appropriate early detection procedures are available to them.

If genetic testing is made available, then genetic counseling must also be provided. In most health care settings it may be not be feasible for the provider to spend an adequate amount of time with a patient both before and after genetic testing. Furthermore, most providers do not have the training in genetics and genetic counseling to properly assist their patients. Thus, in most medical care settings and within most larger health care organizations, genetic counselors and other medical personnel will have this responsibility. However, the overall task will clearly be a multidisciplinary endeavor [8], especially since there are only approximately 1000 clinical geneticists in the United States and the needs go far beyond their capabilities [18]. Primary care providers will still need to provide the initial screening to determine who is appropriate to refer for genetic counseling and testing. Primary care providers are currently unprepared to provide even this initial screening and there are training needs that need to be addressed promptly by provider organizations and professional societies as part of continuing medical education as well as earlier training in medical schools [20].

A special case where ethical considerations arise for institutions is in the question of stored biologic specimens used in medical research. If a researcher wants to test these specimens and they were obtained without specific informed consent, what obligation is there to contact the individual and obtain consent? Is there a time limit on how far back a specimen was collected before notification is no longer necessary and what level of effort is required to make contact? For instance, if a paraffin block exists from a specimen collected 40 years ago, does the researcher still have to attempt to locate the individual and/or her relatives? Although the question of elapsed time has not been addressed, some commentators believe that individuals should be asked for permission before performing genetic test on such stored specimens [13]. If the specimen has already been tested as a result of a survey, the individual should be told that a test has been done and asked whether they want to know the result [13].

Clearly the ethical challenges raised by genetic testing have formidable implications for the medical profession. Technology will continue to advance and require constant modifications of guidelines and policies. It will be important for the practitioner to remain informed of the technologic possibilities and to integrate these with a knowledge of the natural history of breast cancer, the available methods of prevention and treatment, available genetic counseling capabilities, and the individual personality of the patient.

Economic Questions

Like most new technologies, genetic testing is unlikely to save anyone money, at least in the short term. The savings achieved by identifying a small number of women with a genetic predisposition to breast cancer and minimizing treatment by early intervention are likely to be far outweighed by the costs of testing, training, and counseling for the large number of women eligible for screening, and the prevention procedures required by the women who test positive. What will these costs be and who will pay for them? A formal assessment of cost and effectiveness for BRCA1 testing or for almost any other application of genetic screening has not yet been performed and may even be beyond our current capability [3]. Clearly the costs will be substantial and some thought must be given to quantifying them for the purposes of policy decisions and allocation of resources. The elements of the medical care delivery process that will be included in programs testing for BRCA1 or other inherited genes will include the following:

Public education

The public must be informed as to the nature and meaning of genetic testing and what are the risks and benefits. Those who are potential carriers should be encouraged to seek testing. Undoubtably there will be extensive coverage of the issues raised by the availability of genetic testing in woman's magazines, newspapers, and other general media that will inform as well as raise questions and anxiety about personal risks. Where possible, providers might work with the local media to enhance the accuracy and appropriateness of the information being broadcast and it would behoove responsible practitioners to provide reliable, useful, and easily understood educational messages to allay people's anxieties and satisfy the need for more information. There will, therefore, be some costs associated with the development, production, and dissemination of health education materials (e.g. brochures, videos) designed to meet this need.

Identification of high risk women

Health plans or other organized systems of medical care with a defined and listed population base may be able to use computer-stored information to assist in identifying women at potentially high risk (e.g. women with a record of breast cancer treatment and their first degree relatives). In other practice settings, providers will need to rely on more general information provided to the public and on their own inquiries into their patient's family histories. As this pool of potentially high risk women is identified, some sort of systematic questioning of these women will be necessary to determine the actual level of risk. This may be done either through mailed questionnaires or personal interviews conducted by either primary care providers, genetic counselors, or medical assistants. The development of questionnaires, the training and support for those who conduct the interviews, and the analysis of data will contribute to costs.

Pre-test counseling

For women identified at high risk, genetic counseling should be delivered following the principles of informed consent, non-directiveness, and patient advocacy [8]. Specific pre-test counseling is needed because, analogous to testing for the human immunodeficiency virus (HIV), a person may not fully appreciate the serious implications of allowing themselves to be tested and the possible consequences of either a positive or a negative result need to be discussed. This role is probably best played by trained genetic counselors whose expertise includes an understanding of the genetics of the disease, the technologic aspects of the test, and the psychosocial issues raised by testing and the possible results.

Testing

The cost of the test is currently unknown, although a reasonable estimate would be around $150. In addition there will be the cost of the visit and phlebotomy.

Post-test counseling

Perhaps the most critical interaction is during the post-test counseling when the results are available. Again this function is probably best carried out by trained genetic counselors who can disclose results, the possibilities for error, and present the management options for women who test positive in a sensitive manner. Women who test negative also need counseling to understand the possibility of test error and the need to adopt or maintain the recommended early detection practices for women at normal risk. It must not be forgotten that the lifetime risk for women without a genetic predisposition is still around one in nine [22]. Also women in a high risk family who test negative for the gene may find it hard to accept a negative result after harboring the expectation that they share the risk of other family members. Counseling may have to focus on dissuading such women *not* to have prophylactic mastectomies [20].

For women who have tested positive, the psychosocial impact is likely to be substantial and skilled counseling will be required to help women make decisions on which, if any, preventive options they wish to follow. Again the principles of non-directiveness and patient advocacy are critical in this process. Informational needs about treatment options are best supplied by a clinician, if possible, an oncologist. Some research groups dealing with small numbers of women in a teaching hospital setting have used a three-person team including a geneticist, an oncologist, and a genetic counselor [8]. Psychological counseling may also be required to alleviate anxiety and fear that could adversely affect decisions about prevention and management [16]. However, this approach may turn out to be too labor intensive in practice as the number of women needing such counseling increases and other less costly alternatives will need to be explored. The experience with Huntington's Disease has been that comprehensive guidelines have not actually been adhered to in practice because of time and cost considerations [8].

Preventive options

The most expensive part of the process for women who test positive will be the cost of whatever preventive options are selected. However, the costs of pre-test counseling and testing could turn out to contribute more to the overall costs of genetic testing if the specificity of the process to identify candidates for testing is not high. Currently, the options are regular mammography begun at an early age, say 20 years, prophylactic bilateral mastectomy and/or oophorectomy, and the preventive use of Tamoxifen, the efficacy of which is currently under investigation in large-scale clinical trials. In the not to distant future, it is quite possible that technology will offer other options, such as laser surgery of early breast cancer and various forms of gene therapy [9].

Monitoring system

Providers need to consider their obligation to follow women who have tested positive in order to ensure that they have every opportunity to carry out whatever preventive options are appropriate. If annual mammograms are elected, for example, the provider should monitor the woman's screening practices and provide reminders if appointments are missed. The development of such a system, or the modification of existing tracking systems, needs to be considered in any cost equation.

Training

Finally, because the challenge of genetic testing is so new and because the integration of genetic counseling into primary care practice has to date been minimal, much training is required. Clearly, with only approximately 1000 clinical geneticists in practice in the United States [18] more will be needed. Even so, geneticists and genetic counselors will not, and probably should not be expected to perform all the steps outlined above. Primary care providers (family practitioners, internists, and obstetrician/gynecologists) are likely to be the first level of contact, in making appropriate referrals, and, if properly trained, can provide the initial assessment of risk and advice necessary to select women in need of genetic counseling and make appropriate refferals. For health plans and large practices, medical assistants can be used to perform various tasks such as general education, standardized risk assessment, and follow-up. The proper place for training is in programs of medical education [20], but before that can be accomplished, training of our current practitioners at each level (medical assistant, primary care practitioner, and genetic counselor) will be required.

Only very crude estimates for the magnitude of costs is currently possible. On the basis of BRCA1 being present in approximately 1 in 200 women in the United States, approximately 600,000 women may be carriers in this country alone [1]. The cost of the test alone (at $150) would amount to $90 million, if all were to be tested. This does not even consider the additional cost of testing for men from families with inherited breast and ovarian cancer who could also carry BRCA1 with the same frequency [17]. Add to that the costs of general education and identification, pre- and post-test counseling, preventive treatments, and training; and the costs could rise into the billions of dollars.

Guidelines on the Use of Genetic Testing

To help providers, scientists, policymakers, and the public in understanding where we are now and the questions that still need to be answered, the National Advisory Council for Human Genome Research in the United States has issued a statement on the use of DNA testing for cancer risk which says that despite the promising nature of the discovery of BRCA–1, 'it is premature to offer testing of either high-risk families or the general population as part of general medical practice until a series of crucial questions has been addressed' [2]. The questions they pose are:

1. How many different mutations of BRCA1 will be found, what are their actual frequencies, and what is the risk of cancer associated with each?
2. What are the technical and laboratory issues associated with detection of mutations in these genes, what frequency of false-positive and false-negative results will occur, and how can quality control of testing be assured?
3. How effective are interventions to prevent cancer morbidity and mortality in high-risk families and in the general population?
4. How can education about the complexities of DNA testing be provided to large numbers of potentially at-risk individuals, how can informed consent be ensured, and how can effective, culturally sensitive, nondirective genetic counseling be offered about such profoundly wrenching issues?
5. How will the possibility of genetic discrimination against those found to be at high risk be avoided?

Policy statements such as this serve to focus the systematic clinical research needed to establish programs of testing and may help provider organizations in responding to premature demands for testing. Each of these questions relate to the critical ethical issues in genetic testing covered in this chapter. The Statement clearly sets out the scope of work required in this field at the current time.

Conclusion

The introduction of genetic testing, and testing for BRCA1 in particular, will have a major impact on the practice of medicine and will raise many difficult ethical and economic issues. The questions raised by genetic cancer screening will require a substantial amount of thoughtful discussion, consensus building, and the establishment of standards of practice and codes of conduct. They are unlikely to be resolved quickly, but will need to be formulated both on the basis of the limited experience with other genetic disorders and through experience. This chapter has briefly outlined some of the ethical and economic questions that will provide challenges for primary care providers and other health professionals for some time to come.

References

1. King, M.C., Rowell, S., Love, S. (1993). Inherited breast and ovarian cancer: what are the risks? what are the choices? *J. Am. Med. Assoc.*, **269**, 1975–1980.
2. National Advisory Council for Human Genome Research (1994). Statement on use of DNA testing for presymptomatic identification of cancer risk. *J. Am. Med. Assoc.*, **271**, 785.
3. Blumenthal, D., Zeckhauser, R. (1989). Genetic diagnosis. Implications for medical practice. *Int. J. Technol. Assess. Health Care*, **5**, 579–600.

4. Newman, B., Austin, M.A., Lee, M.A., King, M.-C. (1988). Inheritance of human breast cancer: evidence for autosomal dominant transmission in high-risk families. *Proc. Natl. Acad. Sci. U.S.A.*, **85**, 3044–3048.

5. Hall, J.M., Lee, M.K., Newman, B. *et al.* (1990). Linkage of early-onset familial breast cancer to chromosome 17q21. *Science*, **250**, 1684–1689.

6. Narod, S.A., Feunteun, J., Lynch, H.T. *et al.* (1991). Familial breast-ovarian cancer locus on chromosome 17q12–23. *Lancet*, **338**, 82–83.

7. Easton, D.F., Bishop, D.T., Ford, D., Crockford, G.P. (1993). Breast Cancer Linkage Consortium. Genetic linkage analysis in familial breast and ovarian cancer: results from 214 families. *Am. J. Hum. Genet.*, **52**, 678–701.

8. Biesecker, B., Boehnke, M., Calzone, K. *et al.* (1993). Genetic counseling for families with inherited susceptibility to breast and ovarian cancer. *J. Am. Med. Assoc.*, **269**, 1970–1974.

9. Wivel, N.A., Walters, L. (1992). Germ-line gene modification and disease prevention: some medical and ethical perspectives. *Science*, **262**, 533–538.

10. Shaw, M.W. (1987). Testing for the Huntington gene: a right to know, a right not to know, or a duty to know. *Am. J. Med. Genet.*, **26**, 243–246.

11. Smurl, J.F., Weaver, D.D. (1987). Presymptomatic testing for Huntington's Chorea: guidelines for moral and social accountability. *Am. J. Med. Genet.*, **26**, 247–257.

12. Harper, P. (1992). Ethical issues in genetic testing for Huntington's Disease: lessons for the study of familial cancers. *Dis. Markers*, **10**, 189–193.

13. Bobrow, M., Harper, P., Harris, J., Evans, G., Hunt, A. (1992). Seminar on ethical issues arising from molecular studies in human genetic disease: held under the auspices of the UK Cancer Family Study Group in Manchester, 21st May 1992. *Dis. Markers*, **10**, 185–187.

14. Lerman, C., Rimer, B.K., Engstrom, P.F. (1991). Cancer risk notification: psychosocial and ethical implication. *J. Clin. Oncol.*, **9**, 1275–1282.

15. Thirlaway, K., Fallowfield, L. (1993). The psychological consequences of being at risk of developing breast cancer. *Eur. J. Cancer Prev.*, **2**, 467–471.

16. Bobrow, M., Harper, P., Harris, J., Evans, G., Hunt, A. (1992). Ethical issues: the geneticist's view point. Panel discussion. *Dis. Markers*, **10**, 211–228.

17. Arason, A., Barkardottir, R.B., Egilsson, V. (1993). Linkage analysis of chromosome 17 markers and breast-ovarian cancer in Icelandic families and possible relationship to prostatic cancer. *Am. J. Hum. Genet.*, **52**, 711–717.

18. Rothstein, M.A. (1990). Legal and ethical issues in the laboratory assessment of genetic susceptibility to cancer. *Birth Defects*, **26**, 179–190.

19. President's Commission for the Study of Ethical Problems in Medicine and Biomedical and Behavioral Research, Screening, and Counseling for Genetic Conditions (1983). *The Ethical, Social, and Legal Implications of Genetic Screening, Counseling, and Educational Programs.* United States Government Printing Office, Washington, D.C.

20. Lynch, H.T., Watson. P. (1992). Genetic counseling and hereditary breast/ovarian cancer. *Lancet*, **339**, (letter), 1181.

21. Lynch, H.T., Watson, P., Conway, T.A. *et al.* (1993). DNA screening for breast/ovarian cancer susceptibility based on linked markers. *Arch. Intern. Med.*, **153**, 1979–1987.

22. Fletcher, S.W., Black, W., Harris, R., Rimer, B.K., Shapiro, S. (1993). Report of the International Workshop on Screening for Breast Cancer. *J. Natl. Cancer Inst.*, **85**, 1644–1656.

23. Lynch, H.T., Conway, T., Watson, P., Schreiman, J., Fitzgibbons, R.J. (1988). Extremely early onset hereditary breast cancer (HBC): surveillance/management implications. *Nebr. Med. J.*, **73**, 97–100.

24. Harper, P.S., Clarke, A. (1990). Should we test children for 'adult' genetic diseases? *Lancet*, **355**, 1205–1206.

25. Chapman, M.A., (1990). Predictive testing for adult-onset genetic disease: ethical and legal implications for the use of linkage analysis for Huntington disease. *Am. J. Hum. Genet.*, **47**, 1–3.

PART TWO

ADVISING THE HIGH-RISK WOMAN

Chapter 8

Counseling the High-Risk Woman

VICTOR G. VOGEL

The four major steps in the assessment and counseling of women at increased risk
for breast cancer are the collection of family history data, calculation of cancer
risk, communication of risk status, and education to reduce the risk [1]. Women at
increased risk for breast cancer are often misinformed about their risks and are not
screened adequately [2]. There is an obvious need for increased counseling, but
adverse effects may result from communicating such knowledge. These include
psychological and emotional consequences, risks of breaches in confidentiality as
well as adverse economic and social consequences. Upon learning of their increased
risk, women may experience feelings of denial, low self-esteem, anxiety or guilt
[3]. Thus, both the patient's desire for information and the level at which the patient
chooses to control decision-making, must be considered in the counseling process.

The Clinical Counseling Encounter

Women who seek accurate and valid information about their risk of breast cancer
often harbor fears and anxieties as well as possible misinformation about risk
factors.

Mood disorders such as anxiety, depression, energy level and sleep disturbances,
are as common and severe in women at risk for breast cancer as they are in women
with breast cancer [4]. Because of these disorders, the counselor must be skilled
at dealing with psychological distress and must provide ample opportunity for the
patient to express her concerns and fears. As these issues emerge, the counselor
should respond with accurate, factual information and make sure that the patient is
doing everything possible to understand her fears and and manage her risk.

It is appropriate for physicians who treat breast cancer patients to offer risk
assessment and counseling also to patients' relatives who live nearby. If a clinician

69

Basil A. Stoll (ed.), Reducing Breast Cancer Risk in Women, 69–80.
© 1995 *Kluwer Academic Publishers. Printed in the Netherlands.*

is unable or unwilling to provide counseling for women at increased risk, the women should be referred to competent counselors.

When family members live at a distance and cannot visit the clinic for personalized counseling, informational letters can be an effective mechanism for educating family members. It is important also to notify the family members' physicians with recommendations for appropriate screening interventions. When family members live in close proximity to one another, family counseling is an effective means for transmitting information about risks and for outlining possible preventive interventions.

Women who learn that their risk is low may express disbelief [5] or a troubling emotion called 'survivor guilt'. This is experienced by those who live through a disaster (e.g. war, plane crash, earthquake) in which others, including loved ones, suffer or die. A woman comes finally to understand that she is not responsible for the illness of her relatives and her fears about her own risk may lessen in response to education and information. The overriding and guiding requirement is that the counselor identify for the patient the potential benefits to be derived from obtaining additional information. Information-seeking by some women at risk is an attempt to control and manage anxiety [6] and information delivered in a supportive environment should lessen, rather than heighten, anxiety in subjects at risk. The greater danger lies in clinicians not delivering information to patients who need it, either because the clinician is not informed about the factors that contribute to breast cancer risk or else does not recognize the need to deliver the information.

Patients frequently present a list of questions about which they are seeking answers or additional information. Competent counseling consists of attentive listening and the provision of the most informed responses to the patients' queries. Women will often bring friends or family members for emotional support and subsequent clarification of the information delivered. If written material pertaining to breast cancer risk factors is available, this should be provided to the patient. Many women choose to take notes or tape record the counseling session; this should be both encouraged and allowed. The patient should have as much time as is reasonable to ask her questions. Most visits require one hour, and a return visit in three to six months is advised for clarification of information and behavioral reinforcement of preventive strategies.

One strategy to control costs is to have a nurse practitioner or other physician extender to do risk evaluations, and have the physician respond to more specific medical questions such as the implications of benign breast pathology, indications for prophylactic mastectomy, or the advisability of using hormone replacement therapy. The session should end with specific recommendations including management of symptomatic benign breast disease and a mammographic screening prescription based on the patient's individual risk profile. All visits should include a comprehensive physical examination in addition to breast examination with the patient both seated and supine.

Instructions in breast self-examination (BSE) technique should be supplemented with silicone teaching models and video tapes whenever possible. The clinician must never assume that the patient knows the technique of BSE, and an evaluation of the patient's technique is necessary after the training. The counselor should advise the patient that the desired frequency for BSE is only once monthly at a time in the menstrual cycle when the breasts are least tender, recognizing that some patients, due to their anxiety, examine their breasts as often as daily.

Women at increased risk for breast cancer tend to overestimate that risk [7]. Providing them with accurate information about their risk should heighten awareness while reducing anxiety. Although information about *relative risk* is useful to epidemiologists, formulating risk information in this way may be ambiguous for the public which does not routinely deal with comparative risk assessments [8]. A more useful strategy is to use *lifetime probability* of disease, expressing risk as that proportion of women likely to be affected among a group at similar risk, over a period of 10 or 20 years. In addition, clinicians must use caution in generalizing the results of mathematical models for women seeking risk information because the data used to develop the models are derived from case-control or screening studies, and inherent selection biases in the populations studied must be recognized. Validation studies of risk assessment models are needed before any model is applied widely in clinical counseling [9].

Counseling about risk may have unwanted psychological effects [3]. A substantial proportion of women with abnormal mammograms but no evidence of cancer reported significant impairments in mood and daily functioning [10, 11]. Similarly, in a study of first-degree relatives of breast cancer patients, 53% reported intrusive thoughts about breast cancer and 33% reported impairment in daily functioning due to breast cancer worries [12]. For first-degree relatives of newly diagnosed breast cancer patients, the process of psychological adjustment may be especially complex, as these women must cope both with concerns about their own breast cancer risk and also with concerns about the welfare of loved ones [13, 14]. More than one-fourth of high-risk women may show clinically elevated levels of psychological distress [15].

Because family members often accompany their relatives during visits for treatment, clinicians should consider the possibility of offering counseling to anxious relatives during these times. Relatives of breast cancer patients report frequent 'waves of feelings' and 'thinking about it when (they) didn't want to', and in many, these thoughts and feelings are associated with sleep disturbance and impairment in daily functioning. These are more prevalent among first-degree relatives who are older and less educated. There is also a significant association between the time since diagnosis of a woman's breast cancer and psychological difficulties reported by first-degree relatives.

Daughters and sisters of breast cancer patients perceive their risk of developing breast cancer to be high [2, 7], and they are the women most likely to request risk assessment, predictive testing, and counseling [16, 17]. Having had a mammogram done leads one to a higher perceived risk of developing breast cancer, while a woman's age is inversely related to her perceived risk [18]. Younger women with more worries about cancer and more overall mood disturbances are more likely to seek genetic testing [17], especially if they have an information-seeking, coping style for dealing with stress [6]. The observation that a history of mood disturbance is more likely in those seeking information, indicates the need for the inclusion of psychological expertise in the counseling team, with referrals for psychiatric counseling when appropriate.

Notification of increased cancer risk can have negative consequences on women, including persistent worry, intrusive thoughts, depression, confusion, sleep distur- bance and avoidance of cancer-screening examinations [3, 12, 17]. The impact on the family of the woman at risk can be equally severe, leading to a collective sense of powerlessness, ambivalence, interdependence, role restructuring and uncertain- ty [19]. These adverse consequences may be minimized if standard psychological tests or structured interviews to assess depression, suicide potential and life stres- sors are used in preparatory counseling sessions [20]. Poor coping strategies can be replaced through retraining, reassurance and structured counseling. Evidence from breast cancer patients suggests that improving communication between women and their medical advisers may also help to improve patients' ability to cope with the stress of their illnesses [21]. Communication is improved by spending more time with patients, by encouraging them to ask questions and express concerns, and by coaching them to increase their information-seeking behaviors.

Mammography in Monitoring High-Risk Women

Women who have one first-degree relative affected with premenopausal breast cancer or who have two affected first-degree relatives of any age are clearly at increased risk. Similar degrees of risk exist for women whose multivariate risk scores are five or greater [22]. For example, a 30-year-old woman whose relative risk for breast cancer is greater than 5 has an annual risk of breast cancer approx- imately equal to that of a woman age 45, and relative risk can be thought of as a multiplier of the annual incidence of breast cancer. Among women who are no longer actively attempting to conceive children, annual mammographic screening should begin at age 30 if their relative risk for breast cancer is 5 or greater, or if they have at least two affected first-degree relatives.

Two-thirds of young women who are at increased risk for breast cancer have mammographic images of normal density that are amenable to usual radiologic interpretation (Vogel and Higginbotham, unpublished data). However, there is no clear evidence that mammographic screening can decrease mortality from breast cancer in women younger than 50 years [23]. Only a prospective study of screening mammography in young women at increased risk will resolve the existing uncer- tainty, but until the issue is resolved, annual screening of high-risk women offers the *potential* of decreased mortality. Mammographic screening should of course, be suspended during pregnancy and lactation in women at increased risk, both to protect the fetus and to eliminate the false-positive lesions identified in the breast during pregnancy.

Because adequate mammographic visualization can be very difficult in young women with dense breasts [24], ultrasonography should accompany screening mammography to distinguish cystic lesions that occur frequently in young women, from the solid lesions that require biopsy for diagnosis. This strategy will minimize the number of biopsies performed in young women who receive regular screening.

Mammographic screening offers several benefits as well as potential risks. The benefits include a demonstrated decrease in mortality for breast cancer diagnosed in women older than 50 years, the ability to use conservative surgery for smaller, less advanced lesions, and the psychologic reassurance gained by a woman after a negative mammogram [25]. However, it increases the likelihood of women having to undergo additional investigations such as breast ultrasound, fine needle aspiration, needle biopsy, or open biopsy. In addition, there is the possibility of over-treating lesions that are actually benign and would not have come to clinical attention in the absence of screening [26].

Screening mammography has inherent limitations in its sensitivity, and as many as 15% of negative mammograms may be false-negative [27]. The false reassurance that follows a negative mammogram may lead to decreased compliance with attendance for scheduled screenings. There is also some psychologic morbidity associated with undergoing mammographic screening and some women experience an increase in measured anxiety and psychologic distress immediately following mammographic screening [10, 11].

Counselors must explain to anxious, young women that controversy surrounds the assessment of benefit attributed to mammographic screening in women younger than 50 years, but that in women whose breast cancer is not detected by screening, half will die from the disease. In women older than 50, screening mammography reduces breast cancer mortality by 30% [25], and if screening in younger women were to reduce mortality from breast cancer by the same proportion, lives would be saved. This remains unproved to date.

It is possible to make calculations on the benefits of screening only those women younger than 50 who have risk factors making them more susceptible to the disease [23]. Risk factor profiles can identify a 3-fold increase in risk in approximately 20% of women between the ages of 30 and 49 years. In this author's opinion however, if mammography can detect breast cancer in young women, the opportunity should be offered to all young women and not merely to those at increased risk.

Thus, there are both potential benefits and risks from screening younger women with annual or less frequent mammography. With the increasing emphasis on containment of rising health care costs, regular mammographic screening in younger women may require that they forgo other health care services, some of which may be of greater demonstrated benefit than screening mammography [28].

Screening at Other Sites in High-Risk Women

Patients at highest risk for breast cancer are women with a prior diagnosis of breast, colon, endometrial, or ovarian carcinomas [29, 30]. The risk for development of second breast cancers among women with a primary breast cancer is up to 0.75% annually [31], leading to a 15% cumulative risk at 20 years for the development of a second breast primary tumor. Women from families with inherited multi-site cancers, those with prior colon, endometrial, or ovarian cancer are at an increased risk for breast cancer [32,33]. These families often contain a number of individuals affected with a single site-specific malignancy, suggesting an increased risk for breast cancer among all women in the family. It is desirable that clinicians convey the information to all family members who are at risk, either in groups, individual counseling sessions or in writing.

Several genetic syndromes place women at risk for malignancy at multiple anatomic sites (including breast, colon, endometrium, and ovary) [29, 30, 33, 34], but the ability of screening tests to reduce cancer mortality at sites other than the breast is less certain. Patients often ask clinicians to make recommendations about screening at other sites, and the following screening strategies are for ovarian, colon, and endometrial cancers [1].

Screening for ovarian cancer can be attempted with transvaginal Doppler flow pelvic ultrasound or CA–125 antigen testing. CA–125, a marker widely used for monitoring the progress of epithelial ovarian malignancy [35], has not yet been incorporated into population screening for ovarian malignancy [36] and its sensitivity is poor for each stage of disease [37]. False-positive elevations occur in a variety of gynecological conditions, especially uterine leiomyomata and endometriosis [38, 39]. The sensitivity and specificity of ultrasound examination as a screening procedure in healthy women, are uncertain.

Although the risks for developing ovarian cancer can be considerable among women from affected families, the lack of specificity of CA–125 levels and pelvic ultrasound examination may result in unnecessary invasive procedures in a group of screened women [40]. A difficult clinical situation arises when a woman at increased risk is screened with an imperfect screening test. A questionable mass noted on a vaginal ultrasound or an elevated level of CA–125 obligates the clinician to investigate the abnormality further, particularly in the setting of increased risk. Because benign ovarian cysts, endometriosis, and other gynecologic abnormalities can lead to spurious elevations in the CA–125 level, and because vaginal ultrasound cannot distinguish between benign and malignant ovarian cysts, caution must be used in the broad application of a screening strategy that incorporates these tests. Clinicians should divulge these uncertainties *before* applying the tests.

There is no consensus regarding colon screening for those with a previous diagnosis of breast cancer. Few epidemiologic studies have investigated the effect of a breast cancer diagnosis on the subsequent risk of colon cancer, although one study suggested a 3-fold increase in that risk among Israeli women [41]. Because the risk of colon cancer increases among women age 50 years and older who have never had breast cancer, it is reasonable to recommend sigmoidoscopic or colonoscopic screening examination for asymptomatic women with a history of breast cancer [42]. Indeed, recent studies indicate mortality reduction from colorectal cancer using either fecal occult blood testing [43] or sigmoidoscopy [44] in individuals at usual risk for colorectal malignancy.

A more difficult dilemma applies to colon cancer screening in women whose relatives have had breast cancer but not colon cancer. In families with a history of Lynch Type II disease, regular colonoscopic screenings should begin at an early age in all members at risk [33]. Patients from families with familial clustering of breast cancer but no definite genetic syndromes that include colon cancer, should be screened at least annually by sigmoidoscopy, beginning at age 40.

The risk of endometrial malignancy increases in women with a history of breast cancer [45]. Few published studies address the appropriate screening strategy for women at increased risk for endometrial cancer. Annual endometrial biopsy is indicated for women who have received or are receiving adjuvant Tamoxifen therapy [46] and for women receiving estrogen replacement therapy [47]. Using available techniques, endometrial samples can be obtained with minimal discomfort to the patient [48]. An endometrial screening strategy for women who have no prior diagnosis of malignancy but whose genetic histories place them at increased risk is not well defined, but women from Lynch Type II families should have annual endometrial screening beginning at age 35, if they are no longer actively attempting to conceive.

Management after Genetic Testing

The gene known as BRCA1 appears to be associated with the syndrome of familial breast and ovarian cancer, and if present, a woman's chance of developing breast cancer increases to more than 80 percent by age 60. The gene has been cloned [49] and the specific mutations associated with breast cancer are identified. Many women in the population (especially those with mothers and sisters with breast or ovarian cancer) will demand testing. Published experience from individuals at risk for Huntington's disease indicate, however, that not all who are at risk will choose to be tested [50].

Genetic testing has its risks as discussed in Chapter 7. The US Committee on Assessing Genetic Risks recommends caution in the use of predictive tests because the predictions will be probabilistic rather than deterministic, and the dangers of stigmatization and discrimination are real and profound [51]. A positive predictive genetic test is likely to cause psychological disturbances in the tested subjects, and the possibility of a loss of employment and insurance, the creation of family discord, and social stigmatization are quite real [52].

Research in predictive testing for Huntington's disease suggests that the severity of psychological distress decreases over time following delivery of test results [53]. Paradoxically, some individuals who expected positive results with predictive testing but received news of negative tests occasionally suffered adverse consequences [54]. It is not known whether predictive testing for breast cancer will cause similar effects. Persons declining the opportunity for predictive testing cite the absence of therapy for the disease as a major reason for their decision [50], and this has important implications for breast cancer testing.

Only three management options are available to women who carry BRCA1 or other genes that increase the risk of developing breast cancer. The first option is regular breast screening by physical examination, breast self-examination (BSE) and mammography. This approach is not ideal for a number of reasons:

1. The ability of screening mammography to identify early breast cancer in young women is not proven [23], and we do not know whether mammographic screening has the same sensitivity, specificity, or predictive value in women at genetic risk for breast cancer as it does in women over age 50. Most women who desire genetic testing and screening will be younger than 50 years and there are no data about the optimal screening frequency in young women at increased risk.

2. While there are suggestive data on the benefit of BSE, there is no completed study that proves its efficacy in familial breast cancer. Although there is no reason to believe that monthly BSE will not detect rapidly growing breast cancer, women at increased risk should be aware of the limitations of the available evidence.

3. The best schedule for physical examination of the breast by a health professional is not yet determined. Annual examination may not be frequent enough, while examination at 3 to 6-month intervals may be too frequent. The clinician must explain these limitations of our knowledge, offer a definite screening plan with appropriate cautions, and advise the patient when new information requires modification of the initial schedule.

The second management option is prophylactic mastectomy. Some investigators quote that breast cancer can occur after prophylactic surgery [55], but this is most often seen with subcutaneous mastectomy [56] and should be rare following total mastectomy. The clinician should discuss this possibility with the patient, along with the very real possibility that prophylactic surgery will be done in some women who never will develop breast cancer, even among carriers of BRCA1 [49]. The impact of bilateral total mastectomy on both self-esteem and self-image is profound, and sexual response is altered after mastectomy. The clinician must discuss these consequences of prophylactic surgery with the patient and her husband, sexual partner, or significant other persons. Some patients will weigh the evidence to be in favor of prophylactic surgery as a means both to manage risk and relieve anxiety.

The third management option is Tamoxifen prophylaxis. This is problematic because it has not yet been demonstrated to prevent breast cancer in a prospective clinical trial; it may not be as effective in women who are genetically predisposed to the disease; it carries significant (at least 3-fold) risk of endometrial cancer; and it can sometimes induce troublesome hot flashes. For these reasons, it is inappropriate to recommend Tamoxifen for primary prevention of breast cancer outside the context of a clinical trial.

Many investigators advocate individual counseling for predictive genetic testing, largely to preserve confidentiality. Many women derive emotional and psychological support, however, from the presence of relatives in the counseling session. The patient should indicate whether her desire for confidentiality is greater than her need for support from the presence of family members of her choosing at the counseling sessions, and the counselor should accommodate these wishes.

While we occasionally counsel women younger than 30 years, we believe that beginning counseling for breast cancer risk management is problematic for women younger than 30 for several reasons. While some counselors would now say that predictive genetic testing could influence the decision by younger women to bear children our understanding of the implications of single genes involved in breast cancer risk (e.g. BRCA1) is incomplete, and the most predictive gene mutations remain to be identified. Many younger women will choose to have children in the absence of definitive predictive testing. In such cases, prophylactic mastectomy or early initiation of mammographic screening are not relevant while agents such as Tamoxifen are contraindicated in a woman who might become pregnant. We provide information to young women if they seek it, but we do not initiate active interventions until a woman completes childbearing or, at age 30, indicates that she is not actively attempting to conceive.

For the woman at increased risk for breast cancer, the presence of genetic or other predisposition towards the development of breast cancer will likely outweigh any effects of lifestyle on breast carcinogenesis. Thus, if a woman is a member of a family in which the predisposition towards breast cancer is transmitted as an autosomal dominant trait, dietary fat modification or increased consumption of antioxidant vitamins may have no impact upon her risk of developing breast cancer.

Conclusion

Counseling women who are anxious about their risk of developing breast cancer is a challenge because of the complexity of the issues and the uncertainty about outcomes. Using the accumulating data, the concerned clinician can guide the woman at increased risk through her maze of choices and allow her to adopt strategies that are most beneficial to herself (Table 1). Both the counselor and patient must recognize that the ideal management prescription has not been defined, and the counselor must assure the patient that new options will be presented as they become available. Such partnerships will allay anxiety and maximize the potential for benefit while preserving the relationship between the counselor and the woman at risk.

Table 1. Counseling strategies for women at increased risk for breast cancer

1.	Quantify risk in terms of the probability that an individual will develop breast cancer in a given interval (e.g. 10, 20, or 30 years) using a validated risk assessment model.
2.	Incorporate histologic information from breast biopsy into the risk assessment and discuss the implications with the patient.
3.	Review the limitations and uncertainties of mammographic screening in younger women, including its risks and benefits, and recommend a specific screening schedule.
4.	Review the risks and benefits of estrogen replacement therapy for women approaching or post-menopause and facilitate the process of deciding whether to accept or forgo replacement therapy.
5.	Explore the risk for cancer at other sites and make a specific recommendation for a screening strategy.
6.	Assist in the interpretation of results from predictive genetic testing and review options for management in the face of uncertainty.
7.	Attend to the psychological needs of the woman at risk and her family.
8.	Adhere to ethical principles throughout the counseling process.

Acknowledgement

The expert secretarial assistance of Mrs. Wilda Baker is greatly appreciated.

References

1. Vogel, V.G., Yeomans, A., Higginbotham, E. (1993). Clinical management of women at increased risk for breast cancer. *Breast Cancer Research Treat.*, **28**, 195–210.
2. Vogel, V.G., Graves, D.S., Vernon, S.W. *et al.* (1990). Mammographic screening of women with increased risk of breast cancer. *Cancer*, **66**, 1613–1620.
3. Lerman, C. Rimer, B.K., Engstrom, P.F. (1991). Cancer risk notification: Psychosocial and ethical implications. *J. Clin. Oncol.*, **9**, 1275–1282.
4. Lerman, C., Schwartz, M. (1993). Adherence and psychological adjustment among women at high risk for breast cancer. *Breast Cancer Research Treat.*, **28**, 145–155.
5. Lynch, H.T., Watson, P. (1992). Genetic counseling and hereditary breast/ovarian cancer. *Lancet.*, **339**, 1181.
6. Miller, S.M. (1980). When is a little knowledge a dangerous thing? Coping with stressful events by monitoring versus blunting. In Levine, S. Ursin, H. (eds.), *Coping and Health: Proceedings of a NATO Conference*, Plenum, New York, 145–169.
7. Bondy, M.L., Vogel, V.G., Halabi, S. *et al.* (1992). Identification of women at increased risk for breast cancer in a population-based screening program. *Cancer Epidemiol Biomark Prevent.*, **1**, 143–147.
8. Newell, G.R., Vogel, V.G. (1988). Personal risk factors – What do they mean? *Cancer*, **62**, 1695–1701.
9. Bondy, M.L., Lustbader, E.D., Halabi, S. *et al.* (1994). Validation of a breast cancer risk assessment model in women with a positive family history. *J. Natl. Cancer. Inst.*, **86**, 620–625.
10. Lerman, C., Rimer, B., Trock, B. *et al.* (1991). Psychological and behavioral implications of abnormal mammograms. *Ann. Intern. Med.*, **114**, 657–661.

11. Lerman, C., Trock, B., Rimer, B. *et al.* (1991). Psychological side-effects of breast cancer screening. *Health Psychol.*, **10**, 259–267.
12. Lerman, C., Daly, M., Sands, C. *et al.* (1993). Mammography adherence and psychological distress among women at risk for breast cancer. *J. Natl. Cancer Inst.*, **85**, 1074–1080.
13. Lewis, F., Ellison, E.S., Woods, N. (1985). The impact of breast cancer on the family. *Semin. Oncol. Nurs.*, **1**, 206–213.
14. Northouse, L.L., Cracchiolo–Caraway, Pappas A.C. (1991). Psychologic consequences of breast cancer on partner and family. *Semin. Oncol. Nurs.*, **7**, 216–223.
15. Kash, J.M., Holland, J.C., Halper, M.S. *et al.* (1992). Psychological distress and surveillance behaviors of women with a family history of breast cancer. *J. Natl. Cancer Inst.*, **84**, 24–30.
16. Lynch, H.T., Watson, P., Conway, T.A. *et al.* (1993). DNA screening for breast/ovarian susceptibility based on linked markers. *Arch Intern Med.*, **153**, 1979–1987.
17. Lerman, C., Daly, M., Mosny, A. *et al.* (1994). Attitudes about genetic testing for breast-ovarian cancer susceptibility. *J. Clin. Oncol.*, **12**, 843–850.
18. Vernon, S.W., Vogel, V.G., Halabi, S. *et al.* (1993). Factors associated with perceived risk of breast cancer among women attending a screening program. *Breast Cancer Research Treat.*, **28**, 137–144.
19. Lewis, F.M., Ellison, E.S., Woods, N.F. (1985). The impact of breast cancer on the family. *Semin Oncol Nursing*, **1**, 206–213.
20. Lerman, C., Croyle, R. (1994). Psychological issues in genetic testing for breast cancer susceptibility. *Arch Intern Med.*, **154**, 609–616.
21. Lerman, C., Daly, M., Walsh, W.P. (1993). Communication between patients with breast cancer and health care providers. *Cancer*, **72**, 2612–2620.
22. Gail, M.H., Brinton, L.A., Byar, D.P. *et al.* (1989). Projecting individualized probabilities of developing breast cancer for white females who are being examined annually. *J. Natl. Cancer Inst.*, **81**, 1879–1886.
23. Vogel, V.G. (1994). Screening younger women at risk for breast cancer. *Monographs J. Natl. Cancer Inst.*, **16**, 55–60.
24. Meyer, J.E., Kopans, D.B., Oot, R. (1983). Breast cancer visualized by mammography in patients under 35. *Radiology*, **147**, 93–94.
25. Hurley, S.F., Kaldor, J.M. (1992). The benefits and risk of mammographic screening for breast cancer. *Epidemiol. Reviews*, **14**, 101–130.
26. Lantz, P.M., Remington, P.L., Newcomb, P.A. (1991). Mammography screening and increased incidence of breast cancer in Wisconsin. *J. Natl. Cancer Inst.*, **83**, 1540–1546.
27. Svane, G., Potchen, E.J., Siena, A. *et al.* (1993). How to interpret a mammogram. In *Screening Mammography – Breast Cancer Diagnosis in Asymptomatic Women*, Mosby, St Louis, 148–201.
28. Mushlin, A.I., Fintor, L. (1992). Is screening breast cancer cost-effective? *Cancer*, **69**, 1957–1962.
29. Lynch, H.T., Watson, P., Bewtra, C. *et al.* (1991). Hereditary ovarian cancer: Heterogeneity in age at diagnosis. *Cancer*, **67**, 1460–1466.
30. Muller, H., Weber, W., Kuttapa, T. (1985). *Familial Cancer*, Karger, New York.
31. Donovan, A.J. (1991). Bilateral breast carcinoma. In Bland, K.I., Copeland, E.M., III, (eds.), *The Breast – Comprehensive Management of Benign and Malignant Disease*, W.B. Saunders, Philadelphia, 1021–1029.
32. Lynch, H.T., Krush, A.J., Guirgis, H. (1973). Genetic factors in families with combined gastrointestinal and breast cancer. *Am. J. Gastroenterol.*, **1**, 31–40.
33. Lynch, H.T., Albano, W.A., Lynch, J.F. *et al.* (1983). Recognition of the cancer family syndrome. *Gastroenterol.*, **84**, 672–673.
34. Claus, E.B., Risch, N., Thompson, W.D. (1993). The calculation of breast cancer risk for women with a first degree family history of ovarian cancer. *Breast Cancer Res. Treat.*, **28**, 115–120.
35. Bast, R.C. Jr., Klug, T.L., St. John, E. *et al.* (1983). A radioimmuno-assay using a monoclonal antibody to monitor the course of epithelial ovarian cancer. *N. Engl. J. Med.*, **309**, 883–887.

36. Jacobs, I., Stabile, I., Bridges, J. *et al.* (1988). Multimodal approach to screening for ovarian cancer. *Lancet*, **i**, 268–271.

37. Van Nagell, J.R., Jr. (1991). Ovarian cancer screening. *Cancer*, **68**, 679–680.

38. Einhorn, N., Knapp, R.C., Bast, R.C. *et al.* (1989). CA–125 assay used in conjunction with CA 15–3 and TAG–72 assays for discrimination between malignant and non-malignant disease of the ovary. *Acta Oncol.*, **28**, 655–657.

39. MacKay, E.V., Khoo, S.K., Daunter, B. (1992). Tumor markers. In Coppleson, M. (ed.), *Gynecologic Oncology*, Churchill Livingston, Edinburgh, 405–415.

40. Bourne, T.H., Whitehead, M.I., Campbell, S. *et al.* (1991). Ultrasound screening for familial ovarian cancer. *Gynecol Oncol.*, **43**, 92–97.

41. Rosen, P., Fireman, Z., Figer, A. *et al.* (1986). Colorectal tumor screening in women with a past history of breast, uterine, and ovarian malignancies. *Cancer*, **57**, 1235–1239.

42. Eddy, D.M. (1990). Screening for colorectal cancer. *Ann. Intern. Med.*, **113**, 373–384.

43. Mandel, J.S., Bond, J.H., Church, T.R. *et al.* (1993). Reducing mortality from colorectal cancer by screening for fecal occult blood. Minnesota Colon Cancer Control Study. *N. Engl. J. Med.*, **328**, 1365–1371.

44. Newcomb, P.A., Norfleet, R.G., Storer, B.E. *et al.* (1992). Screening sigmoidoscopy and colorectal cancer mortality. *J. Natl. Cancer Inst.*, **84**, 1572–1575.

45. MacMahon, B., Austin, J.H. (1969). Associations of carcinomas of the breast and corpus uteri. *Cancer*, **23**, 275–280.

46. Fornander, T., Rutqvist, L.E., Wilking, N. (1991). Effects of tamoxifen on the female genital tract. *Ann. N. Y. Acad. Sci.*, **622**, 469–476.

47. Kaunnitz, A.M., Masciello, A., Ostrowski, M. *et al.* (1988). Comparison of endometrial biopsy with endometrial Pipelle and Vabra aspirator. *J. Reprod. Med.*, **33**, 427–431.

48. Henig, I., Chan, P., Tredway, D.R. *et al.* (1989). Evaluation of the Pipelle curette for endometrial biopsy. *J. Reprod. Med.*, **34**, 786–789.

49. Miki, S., Swenson, J., Shattuck-Eidens, D. *et al.* (1994). A strong candidate for the breast and ovarian cancer susceptibility gene BRCA1. *Science*, **266**, 66–71.

50. Babul, R., Adam, S., Kremer, B. *et al.* (1993). Attitudes toward direct predictive testing for the Hungtington disease gene. *J. Am. Med. Assoc.*, **270**, 2321–2325.

51. Committee on Assessing Genetic Risks. (1994). Executive Summary. In Andrews, L.B., Fullerton, J.E., Holtzman, N.A., Motulsby, A.G. (eds.), *Assessing Genetic Risks – Implications for Health and Social Policy*, National Academy Press, Washington, D.C., 1–28.

52. Li, F.P., Fraumeni, J.F., Jr. (1992). Predictive testing for inherited mutations in cancer-susceptibility genes. *J. Clin. Oncol.*, **10**, 1203–1204.

53. Wiggins, S., Whyte, P., Huggins, M. *et al.* (1992). The psychological consequences of predictive testing for Huntington's disease. *N. Engl. J. Med.*, **327**, 1401–1405.

54. Huggins, M., Block, B., Wiggins, S. *et al.* (1992). Predictive testing for Huntington disease in Canada: adverse effects and unexpected results in those receiving a decreased risk. *Am. J. Med. Genet.*, **423**, 508–515.

55. King, M.-C., Rowell, S., Love, S.M. (1993). Inherited breast and ovarian cancer. What are the risks? What are the choices? *J. Am. Med. Assoc.*, **269**, 1975–1980.

56. Eldar, S., Meguid, M.M., Beatty, J.D. (1984). Cancer of the breast after prophylactic subcutaneous mastectomy. *Am. J. Surg.*, **148**, 691–693.

Chapter 9

Mastectomy for Cancer Prevention

MARY JANE HOULIHAN and ROBERT M. GOLDWYN

At present, we are unable to identify which women will inevitably develop breast cancer, but factors associated with an increased risk include a history of a previous breast cancer, a strong family history of breast cancer, and previous breast biopsies which demonstrated *in situ* breast cancer or atypical proliferative lesions.

Mastectomy for Second Breast

The risk of cancer in the contralateral breast of a woman who has had one breast cancer is estimated to be 1% per year during her remaining lifetime [1, 2], a risk five times greater than the general population. Within this group, women with multiple foci of cancer in their first breast, a positive family history, or lobular carcinoma *in situ* may be more likely to develop a second breast cancer, (Table 1).

However, only a small proportion of women who have had breast cancer are likely to consider contralateral prophylactic mastectomy. Many women's initial cancers have been treated with breast-conserving surgery (excision of the tumor and axillary dissection) and post-operative radiotherapy. These women are not likely to choose a more aggressive option for prophylaxis than for the treatment of their breast cancer. Women with Stage II, III, or IV breast cancer are not good candidates for prophylactic mastectomy since the risk of dying from their first breast cancer outweighs the risk of dying from a subsequent breast cancer. This leaves only a small percentage of women with Stage I breast cancer treated by mastectomy to be considered for contralateral prophylactic mastectomy [3].

Basil A. Stoll (ed.), Reducing Breast Cancer Risk in Women, 81–89.
© 1995 *Kluwer Academic Publishers. Printed in the Netherlands.*

Table 1. Factor's influencing risk of developing a second breasst cancer. Adapted from [2]

	Incidence of second breast cancer %
Age	
– less than 40 years	12.2
– 60–70 years	2.2
Pre-menopausal	8.3
Post-menopausal	2.4
Lobular carcinoma *in situ*	23.0
Infiltrating breast cancer	
Stage 1 (survived 15 years)	7.0
Multicentric first cancer	20.0

Family History as Basis

A positive family history is a significant risk factor for the development of breast cancer, and the genetic studies of Anderson [4,5] have established which relationships are associated with the greatest risk. A significant increase was observed in first-order relatives (mother, sister) of women with pre-menopausal or bilateral breast cancer compared with relatives of women who had post-menopausal or unilateral breast cancer. Early and bilateral breast cancer in two first-order relatives was associated with a 30% risk of developing breast cancer before the age of 40.

In contrast, the relative risk of breast cancer in women with a single first-degree relative with pre-menopausal or post-menopausal unilateral breast cancer is 1.8 and 1.2, respectively (1.0 being 2.3%) [4]. These data suggest that most cases of breast cancer involve genetic interaction with environmental factors. However, a strong genetic effect is seen in the case of Cowden's disease, Muir's syndrome, and Li–Fraumeni (SBLA) syndrome [6–9].

Perhaps the most important genetic marker for familial breast cancer will be the BRCA1 gene. This gene, located on chromosome 17q, is an autosomal dominant gene with incomplete penetrance. Women with the BRCA1 gene will have near a 90% chance of developing breast cancer. On the other hand, those women in a breast cancer-laden family who do not carry this gene will likely have a risk similar to the general population, which should be comforting. Hopefully, within 10 years, a blood test should be available to determine the presence or absence of the BRCA1 gene.

When considering a prophylactic mastectomy for a woman with a strong family history, the family history should be carefully confirmed. In the past, mastectomies were frequently performed for benign processes suspected of being malignant at the time. If a woman has a number of relatives who had mastectomies performed who then went on to live to an old age, the diagnosis of breast cancer should be questioned. Also, there have been reports of women with fictitious family histories who may request prophylactic mastectomy. For these reasons, either the medical records of the relatives with breast cancer or the histology of the specimens should be examined in order to validate the family history prior to performing prophylactic mastectomy.

Microscopic Pattern as Basis

Certain benign histological patterns found on biopsy are associated with an increased risk of subsequent breast cancer development. These are carcinoma *in situ* and atypical proliferative processes (atypical ductal and lobular hyperplasia).

In carcinoma *in situ* (ductal carcinoma *in situ* and lobular carcinoma *in situ*), ductal and lobular elements undergo malignant degeneration but do not cross the basement membrane. Ductal carcinoma *in situ* (DCIS) [10–12] may be considered a pre-malignant lesion whose biological behavior is not well understood. Left untreated, the risk of subsequent breast cancer development varies. The subsequent cancer occurs in the vicinity of the biopsy site. Management of DCIS ranges from wide excision with or without radiation therapy to total mastectomy with the intent being to remove all involved breast tissue [13–20]. Because we know little about the natural history of DCIS, it is important to discuss the controversies about the treatment of DCIS with the patient and to respect a patient's individual feelings about cosmesis and breast cancer risk [21]. Although the degree of risk to the contralateral breast remains unclear, most would feel that the risk is not great enough to consider prophylactic contralateral mastectomy.

Lobular carcinoma *in situ* (LCIS), which is an incidental pathologic finding at biopsy, is now regarded as a histological marker for increased susceptibility to breast cancer rather than a pre-malignant lesion in itself [22, 23]. Subsequent cancers are more likely to be ductal and may occur in either breast. The incidence of subsequent breast cancer development after a biopsy demonstrating LCIS is about 16% over a 15-year period (about 1% per year). Current management options include: (i) close observation with semi-annual physical examination and annual mammogram or (ii) bilateral mastectomy.

Atypical ductal hyperplasia (ADH) and atypical lobular hyperplasia (ALH) are histological diagnoses being made increasingly [24], and now represent about 15% of all pathologic lesions reported on mammographic abnormalities in our institution. DuPont and Page [10] have reported that ADH is associated with an increased risk of subsequent breast cancer, the relative risk being 5.3 compared to non-proliferative lesions and as high as 11 when a woman has both ADH and a first-degree relative with breast cancer.

Thus, in women with ductal carcinoma *in situ*, lobular carcinoma *in situ*, or atypical ductal hyperplasia, prophylactic mastectomy is an option to be considered. However, since 70–85% of all breast biopsies for benign lesions suggest no increased breast cancer risk, most women should be reassured. For the small group of women with atypical proliferative lesions, especially with a positive family history, careful follow up with regular mammograms and breast exams should be utilized rather than prophylactic mastectomies.

What Type of Mastectomy?

We believe that if a prophylactic mastectomy is to be done, it should be a total mastectomy. In other words, the procedure should remove all the breast tissue. The procedure may be performed through a skin-sparing incision, but the skin flaps should be thin, leaving only the thin layer of subcutaneous fat beneath the skin, and the pectoralis major fascia should be removed. Subcutaneous mastectomy or partial mastectomy with irradiation is inadequate. Subcutaneous mastectomy preserves the skin of the breast and the areola and nipple [25], and breast tissue is regularly left under the nipple-areola and often elsewhere [26]. Another disadvantage of subcutaneous mastectomy is that reconstruction afterwards is no easier than after a more definitive mastectomy, and the results of reconstruction following subcutaneous mastectomy are generally displeasing, even if the patient has had an expander as a prelude to a prosthesis. The resultant breast has a greater likelihood of being abnormally firm and occasionally painful. It almost never has normal sensation, and the nipple is generally numb.

Additional support for total mastectomy comes from laboratory animal studies. Two groups [27, 28] have investigated whether risk reduction in breast cancer is proportionate to the amount of breast tissue removed in rats subjected to mammary cancer induction by dimethylbenzanthracene. In mice liable to spontaneous mammary tumors, the same question was studied [29]. In both animal models, the risk of breast tumor development was not found to be related to the amount of breast tissue removed, and these studies raise concerns about the efficacy of subcutaneous mastectomy as prophylaxis for breast cancer.

If the patient has lobular carcinoma *in situ*, a case can be made for bilateral mastectomy because of the multicentricity and bilateral risk of subsequent invasive cancer. Prophylactic mastectomy of the contralateral breast is advised for: (i) pre-cancerous microscopic findings of intraductal carcinoma; (ii) atypical ductal hyperplasia with a positive family history (first-order blood relative with pre-menopausal cancer); and (iii) invasive breast cancer in the ipsilateral breast.

What Type of Reconstruction?

We need to decide first whether reconstruction should be done at the time of the mastectomy or delayed. The advantages of immediate reconstruction include sparing the patient another hospitalization, another anaesthetic, and another disruption in her life. Several studies have shown that women who did not delay their resonstruction were more content [30, 31] and did not experience as much depression post-operatively as those whose reconstructions were postponed.

The disadvantages of immediate reconstruction are the presence of an open wound and the shortage of tissue, which would be avoided if the wound were allowed to heal and the skin permitted to stretch. However, with the increasing use of skin-sparing mastectomies, the removal of the nipple-areolar complex with a 5–8 mm rim of surrounding skin, skin shortage is less of a problem. Our experience has shown a slightly increased incidence of wound complications, primarily infection, after immediate reconstruction, especially when the patient has been irradiated and if a foreign body such as an implant or an expander is used [32, 33].

A determining factor in the choice of type of reconstruction is the appearance of the opposite breast aside from its cancer potential [34]. Frequently, the opposite breast is extremely large and even with the use of a sizeable flap combined with an implant, may be impossible to match. The patient may then be advised to have a reduction of that breast, but we generally prefer to do the reduction at a later stage, commonly when we rebuild the nipple and areola for the reconstructed breast. Delaying the reduction allows the rebuilt breast to assume its final contour and position, thus facilitating the surgeon's aim to attain symmetry.

The patient who is already bewildered by the decision of submitting to a mastectomy will not find it easy to make a further decision about the type of reconstruction [34]. The most common types of breast reconstruction are by a prosthesis alone (perhaps with an expander initially) or by a flap.

Almost all implants used today for breast reconstruction contain saline within a silicone envelope. In recent years, polyurethane has been used as a coating on the outer shell in order to reduce fibrosis and consequent capsular contracture, which the patient feels as an abnormal firmness of her reconstructed breast [35].

An alternative means of overcoming capsular contracture is the use of an expander. It takes advantage of the elastic properties of skin which allow it to be slowly distended through serial percutaneous fillings, usually with saline, over weeks or months. A relatively new advance is an expander that allows the filling port to be removed, leaving the expander as the permanent prosthesis. In the presence of an open wound, which is the case after a mastectomy, the incidence of complications with an expander or implant is greater in terms of infection, flap ischemia, and subsequent implant extrusion than if either of those foreign bodies had been inserted after the wound had completely healed [33].

Even when an expander is used, it is difficult to achieve a natural-looking and permanently soft breast, particularly one that is ptotic and pendulous. Only autogenous tissue in the form of a flap seems able to accomplish these objectives, particularly the absence of abnormal firmness. The flaps most commonly used for breast reconstruction consist of skin and underlying muscle either from the back (latissimus dorsi musculocutaneous flap) or from the abdomen (rectus abdominis flap). Most of these flaps are transferred leaving their vascular pedicle undivided, but 'free flaps' are becoming more popular. The advantages are that a larger amount of tissue can be used without fear of necrosis and the donor tissue can be obtained from well-hidden areas of the body, such as the buttocks. However, even in the most skilled hands [36], the microsurgical transfers of tissue have a failure rate of 2–8%.

In general, the latissimus dorsi flap is particularly useful for building a small or medium-size breast [37] and, in order to make a larger breast, it can be combined with an implant. The advantages of the latissimus dorsi flap are its excellent vascularity [38] and the fact that the donor-site scar is on the back, where most of it can be hidden under a brassiere. Some women, however, object to this location for a scar because they may wish to wear clothing that exposes the back.

The rectus abdominis musculocutaneous flap consistently furnishes enough tissue to match a large opposite breast without the need for an implant [39, 40]. However, for a very large breast, an implant may be necessary. A disadvantage of the rectus abdominis flap is the abdominal scar, which may be less prominent if the flap is taken lower in the abdomen. However, the lower one takes the flap, the greater the likelihood of ischemia and necrosis. The mid-abdominal flap is safer from the point of vascularity, but the scar running across the abdomen and intersecting with the umbilicus is readily visible.

Recently, the rectus abdominis musculocutaneous flap has been taken as a free flap. If the microsurgical anastomosis is successful, a larger amount of the flap can be utilized without fear of necrosis than if it remained attached by its pedicle. An important consideration in using the rectus abdominis flap is that it may weaken the abdomen and a hernia may develop [41]. To prevent this occurring, synthetic material such as Prolene mesh or Marlex is used over the donor site to reinforce the abdomen.

Other types of flaps of skin and muscle from the upper chest or upper abdomen, either with an implant or an expander, have been used [42, 43]. However, these techniques are less common than the use of the latissimus dorsi and rectus abdominis musculocutaneous flaps. Transplanting fat from elsewhere in the body to reconstruct the breast is unpredictable [44, 45] because of absorption and liquefaction.

Most patients, particularly if they are younger, request nipple and areola reconstruction, and this is usually postponed until three months after the time of breast reconstruction. We prefer a quadropod flap, based on the tissue of the chest wall or on the tissue of a flap. The areola is simulated by tattooing the skin.

The women for whom mastectomy is being proposed as prophylaxis against breast cancer must understand that breast reconstruction, even at its best, is merely an approximation of the normal breast. Therefore, the more the patient regards her mastectomy and reconstruction as a potential improvement in survival, the greater the likelihood of her satisfaction. If a woman intellectually understands the rationale for her treatment but emotionally expects the new breast to look and feel as normal as her previous one, she will be seriously disappointed and most likely angry. The patient must be adequately informed, and it is useful to give her written material so that she and her family can read it at home [46].

We show patients photographs of results from breast reconstruction by the various methods. The purpose of these slides is not to urge the patient into an operation but to present realistically the results that she may expect from the procedure. Patients are shown slides that illustrate an average result, a superior result, and a poor result. Patients frequently request to speak to others who have undergone the same procedure. While this can help a patient, we warn her that the patient to whom she will speak is very likely to be someone very satisfied with the procedure and therefore may give her an overly optimistic view of the operation.

Any patient who is to have immediate reconstruction is shown a photograph of the usual defect that is encountered immediately after mastectomy. The purpose here is to let the patient know that we are trying to create something literally from nothing, so that she will understand the surgical problems that must be resolved in order to give her a semblance of a breast.

Conclusion

Deciding which patient should have a prophylactic mastectomy and when it should be performed is difficult. While treatment must be tailored to the physical and emotional needs of the patient, the personal experience of the surgeon (and perhaps of the oncologist also) tends to sway the patient's decision.

We believe that the mastectomy should be as total as possible, although we realize that others might differ in their opinion. It would seem logical that if one is trying to give the patient protection, one should give her as much protection as possible without going as far as radical mastectomy.

Breast reconstruction is more successful today than it was a decade ago, but even now results fall short of the surgeon's desires and, quite often, the patient's expectations. For that reason, the surgeon must discuss in detail not only the mechanics of the reconstruction but also its limitations.

References

1. Fisher, B., Gebhardt, M.C. (1978). The evolution of breast cancer surgery: past, present, and future. *Semin. Oncol.*, **5**, 385–394.
2. Robbins, G.F., Berg, J.W. (1964). Bilateral primary breast cancers: a prospective clinico-pathological study. *Cancer*, **17**, 1501–1525.
3. Leis, H.P., Jr. (1971). Selective, elective prophylactic contralateral mastectomy. *Cancer*, **28**, 956–961.
4. Anderson, D.E. (1974) Genetic study of breast cancer: identification of a high risk group. *Cancer*, **34**, 1090–1097.
5. Anderson, D.E. (1974). Breast cancer in families. *Cancer*, **40**, 1855–1860.
6. Walton, B.J., Morain, W.D., Baughman, R.D. Cowden's disease: a further indication for pro-phylactic mastectomy. *Surgery*, **99**, 82–85.

7. Muir, E.G., Yates-Bell, A.J., Barlow, K.A. (1966). Multiple primary carcinomata of the colon, duodenum, larynx associated with keratatocanthomata of the face. *Br. J. Surg.*, **54**, 191–195.
8. Li, F.P., Fraumeni, J.F., Jr. (1969). Soft tissue sarcomas, breast cancer and other neoplasms: a familial syndrome. *Ann. Int. Med.*, **71**, 747–751.
9. Williams, W.R., Osborne, M.P. (1978). Familial aspects of breast cancer: an overview. In Harris, J.R., Hellman, S., Henderson, I.C., Kinne, D.W. (eds.), *Breast Diseases*, J.B. Lippincott Co., Philadelphia, 109–120.
10. DuPont, W.D., Page, D.L. (1985). Risk factors for breast cancer in women with proliferative breast disease. *N. Engl. J. Med.*, **312**, 146–151.
11. Rosen, P.P., Braun, D.W., Jr., Kinne, D.E. (1980). The clinical significance of preinvasive breast carcinomas. *Cancer*, **46**, 919–925.
12. Farrow, J.H. (1970). Current concepts in detection and treatment of the earliest of the early breast cancers. *Cancer*, **25**, 468–477.
13. Lagios, M.D., Margolin, F.R., Westdahl, P.R., Rose, M.R. (1989). Mammographically detected duct carcinoma *in situ*: frequency of local recurrence following tylectomy and prognostic effect of nuclear on local recurrence. *Cancer*, **63**, 618–624.
14. Gump, F.E., Jicha, D.L., Ozello, L. (1987). Ductal carcinoma *in situ* (DCIS). A revised concept. *Surgery*, **102**, 790–795.
15. Zafrani, B., Fourquet, A., Vilcoq, J.R. *et al.* (1986). Conservative management of intraductal breast carcinoma with tumorectomy and radiation therapy. *Cancer*, **57**, 1299–1301.
16. Recht, A., Danoff, B.S., Solin, L.J. *et al.* (1985). Intraductal carcinoma of the breast: results of treatment with breast biopsy and irradiation. *J. Clin. Oncol.*, **3**, 1339–1343.
17. Montague, E.D. (1984). Conservation surgery and radiation therapy in the treatment of operable breast cancer. *Cancer*, **53**, (Suppl. 3), 700–704.
18. Rosner, D., Bedwani, R.N., Vana, J. *et al.* (1980). Noninvasive breast carcinoma: results of a national survey by the American College of Surgeons. *Ann. Surg.*, 192, 139–147.
19. Ashikari, R., Hajdu, S.I., Robbins, G.F. (1971). Intraductal carcinoma of the breast (1960–1969). *Cancer*, **28**, 1182–1187.
20. Fisher, E.R., Sass, R., Fisher, B. *et al.* (1986). Pathologic findings from the National Surgical Adjuvant Breast Project (Protocol No. 6). I. Intraductal carcinoma (DCIS). *Cancer*, **57**, 197–208.
21. Ketcham, A.S., Moffat, R.L. (1990). Vexed surgeons, perplexed patients, and breast cancers which may not be breast cancers. *Cancer*, **65**, 387–393.
22. Haagensen, C.D., Lane, N., Lattes, R. *et al.* (1978). Lobular neoplasia (so-called lobular carcinoma *in situ*) of the breast. *Cancer*, **42**, 737–769.
23. Wheeler, J.E., Enterline, H.T., Roseman, J.M. *et al.* Lobular carcinoma *in situ* of the breasts: long-term follow-up. *Cancer*, **34**, 554–569.
24. Rubin, E., Visscher, D.W., Alexander, R.W. (1988) *et al.* Proliferative disease and atypia in biopsies performed for nonpalpable lesions detected mammographically. *Cancer*, **61**, 2077–2082.
25. Goldwyn, R.M., Goldman, L.D. (1976). Subcutaneous mastectomy and breast replacement. In Goldwyn, R.M., (ed.), *Plastic and Reconstructive Surgery of the Breast*, Little, Brown, Boston, 441–454.
26. Menon, R.S., van Geel, A.N. (1989). Cancer of the breast with nipple involvement. *Br. J. Cancer*, **59**, 81–84.
27. Jackson, C.F., Palmquist, M., Swanson, J. *et al.* (1984). The effectiveness of prophylactic subcutaneous mastectomy in Sprague-Dawley rats induced with 7,12-dimethylbenzanthracene. *Plast. Reconstr. Surg.* **73**, 249–255.
28. Wong, J.H., Jackson, C.F., Swanson, J.S., *et al.* (1986) Analysis of the risk reduction of prophylactic partial mastectomy in Sprague-Dawley rats with 7,12-dimethylbenzanthracene-induced breast cancer. *Surgery*, **99**, 67–71.

29. Nelson, H., Miller, S.H., Buck, D. (1989). Effectiveness of prophylactic mastectomy in the prevention of breast tumurs in C_3H mice. *Plast. Reconstr. Surg.* **83**, 662–669.
30. Stevens, L.A., McGrath, M.H., Druss, R.G. *et al.* (1984) The psychological impact of immediate breast reconstruction for women with early breast cancer. *Plast. Reconstr. Surg.*, **73**, 619–626, (discussed in Ref. 31).
31. Goin, M.K. (1989) The psychological impact of immediate breast reconstruction for women with early breast cancer. *Plast. Reconstr. Surg.*, **73**, 627–628.
32. Bailey, M.H., Smith, J.W., Casas, L. *et al.* (1989) Immediate breast reconstruction: reducing the risk. *Plast. Reconstr. Surg.*, **83**, 845–851.
33. Armstrong, R.W., Berkowitz, R.L., Bolding, F. (1989). Infection following breast reconstruction. *Ann. Plast. Surg.*, **23**, 284–288.
34. Goldwyn, R.M. (1987). Breast reconstruction after mastectomy. *N. Engl. J. Med.*, **317**, 1711–1714.
35. Kerrigan, C.L. (1989). *Report on the membrane breast implant.* Prepared for the Minister of Health and Welfare, Canada. i–51.
36. Shaw, W.W. (1984). Microvascular free flap breast reconstruction. *Clin. Plast. Surg.*, **11**, 333–341.
37. Bostwick, J., III, Nahai, F., Wallace, J.G. *et al.* (1982). Sixty latissimus dorsi flaps. *Plast. Reconstr. Surg.*, **63**, 31–41.
38. Maxwell, G.P., McGibbon, B.M., Hoopes, J.E. (1979). Vascular considerations in the use of a latissimus dorsi myocutaneous flap after mastectomy with an axillary dissection. *Plast. Reconstr. Surg.*, **64**, 771–780.
39. Hartrampf, C.R., Scheflan, M., Black, P.W. (1982). Breast reconstruction with a transverse abdominal island flap. *Plast. Reconstr. Surg.*, **69**, 216–224.
40. Vasconez, L.O., Psillakis, J., Johnson-Glebeik, R. (1983). Breast reconstruction with contralateral rectus abdominis myocutaneous flap. *Plast. Reconstr. Surg.*, **71**, 668–675.
41. Hartrampf, C.R., Jr., Bennett, K.G. (1987). Autogenous tissue reconstruction in the mastectomy patient: a critical review of 300 patients. *Ann. Surg.*, **205**, 508–519.
42. Ryan, J.J. (1982). A lower thoracic advancement flap in breast reconstruction after mastectomy. *Plast. Reconstr. Surg.*, **70**, 153–158.
43. May, J.W., Jr., Atwood. J., Bartlett, S. (1987). Staged use of soft tissue expansion and lower thoracic advancement flaps in breast reconstruction. *Plast. Reconstr. Surg.*, **79**, 272–277.
44. Bircoll, M., Novack, B.H. (1987). Autologous fat transplantation employing liposuction techniques. *Ann. Plast. Surg.*, **18**, 327–329.
45. Czerny, V. (1987). Plasticher ersatz Brustdruse der durch ein Lipoma. *Verh. Dtsch. Ges. Chir.*, **24**, 216.
46. Goldwyn, R.M. (1984). Consultation for breast reconstruction. *Plast. Reconstr. Surg.*, **73**, 818–819.

Chapter 10

Trial of Tamoxifen Therapy for Protection

BASIL A. STOLL

The evolution of breast cancer is likely to be promoted by estrogen acting together with other hormones [1]. Since promotion steps in cancer development are often reversible, it has been proposed that the progression of breast cancer may be suppressed by giving an antiestrogen for a prolonged period.

Tamoxifen is an antiestrogen which is one of the most effective and least toxic treatments known for any form of cancer [2]. It is widely used in the treatment of both advanced and early breast cancer and during its clinical trials was found to reduce the number of new cancers appearing in the second breast of women receiving treatment. It is the latter observation which has led to world-wide trials to assess its effectiveness in reducing the incidence of breast cancer in women who are at high risk to the disease.

A randomized trial of Tamoxifen as preventive treatment was launched in 1992 in the USA under the aegis of the US National Cancer Institute. The trial will examine the effect of Tamoxifen in women identified as being at increased risk to breast cancer, but misgivings of the National Women's Health Network in the USA were voiced when the trial was launched [3]. They argued that uncertainties about the long-term safety of Tamoxifen made it difficult to justify its use in healthy women. They also questioned whether the ability to reduce the incidence of second breast cancers was relevant to the prevention of breast cancer in healthy women. The following discussion therefore traces the evolution of current Tamoxifen prevention trials, the safety record of the agent and the ethics of the current trials.

Rationale Underlying Tamoxifen Preventive Therapy

Tamoxifen has been used for 25 years to control the growth of advanced breast cancer in women, and is currently the recommended treatment for postmenopausal patients if a tumor shows specific receptors for estrogen. It causes shrinkage or

Basil A. Stoll (ed.), Reducing Breast Cancer Risk in Women, 91–101.
© 1995 *Kluwer Academic Publishers. Printed in the Netherlands.*

disappearance of a tumor for an average of 1 to 2 years in more than half of such patients. Control may be prolonged for up to 10 years if Tamoxifen is given in intermittent courses [4].

It is less widely known that Tamoxifen is also effective against advanced disease in *premenopausal* women. In such cases, response rates are similar to those achieved by removing a patient's ovaries. Thus, for premenopausal women with advancing receptor-positive tumors, Tamoxifen is recommended as an alternative to suppressing ovarian hormone secretion either by surgery or radiation treatment [5].

Following the successful use of Tamoxifen therapy in advanced breast cancer, it was tested for its ability to delay recurrence or prolong life after the surgical removal of early breast cancers, particularly in cases where the disease had spread to the axilla. Analysis of 69 randomized trials involving 28,896 women [6] reported a 17% reduction in the annual rate of death among the women receiving adjuvant Tamoxifen treatment for 1 to 2 years. The survival advantage became apparent 1 to 2 years after treatment was begun and persisted even after the treatment was stopped. Benefit was found to be more significant for women over the age of 50 and for tumors showing estrogen receptors, but a more prolonged disease-free survival was shown also for premenopausal women and in tumors not showing estrogen receptors.

An important observation was made in a trial which compared survival in women given adjuvant Tamoxifen at the time of primary surgery with that in women given the agent at the time the disease first relapsed [7]. Survival was found to be longer in patients given Tamoxifen early, suggesting that the suppressing effect of the agent on breast cancer growth was greater if it was given earlier in the evolution of the tumor. This possibility received support from the observation of a decreased incidence of cancer in the second breast after women had received adjuvant Tamoxifen following primary surgery. Out of eight trials involving almost 5000 premenopausal and postmenopausal patients, seven reported a decreased incidence of second breast cancers [7–14]. Only 1.6% of patients on Tamoxifen developed second breast cancers compared to 2.4% of those not receiving the agent. The annual odds of developing a second breast cancer were reduced by 26% when Tamoxifen was given for less than 2 years and by 53% when given for longer than 2 years [15].

In decreasing the incidence of second breast cancers, two possible mechanisms are suggested. First, Tamoxifen may suppress the growth of microscopic metastases spreading across the midline from the first breast cancer. Second, it may stop precursor on precancerous lesions in the second breast from developing into invasive cancer by suppressing their proliferative activity [16]. The second hypothesis is the basis of current trials of Tamoxifen therapy in women who are identified as being at increased risk to breast cancer.

Reports of experimental studies may be relevant to understanding the suppressive effect of Tamoxifen in these circumstances. Human breast cancer cells which have been transplanted into the breast pad of castrated immune – deficient mice, show long-term suppression of their growth following administration of Tamoxifen to the mice. However, the growth reactivates when the agent is withdrawn and estrogen substituted, showing that the effect of Tamoxifen is suppressive, but not lethal to the cells [17]. A second experimental model is the hormone-responsive breast cancer which develops in some rat strains after treatment by cancer-stimulating chemicals. The tumors are prevented by castrating the rats, while short term Tamoxifen administration delays the appearance of the tumors even if the rats are not castrated. Continuous low daily doses of Tamoxifen will suppress the appearance of the tumors for as long as the agent is continued [18].

In the rat therefore, cancer cells on their precursors can be held in a state of dormancy by Tamoxifen, and there is evidence to suggest that in the human, an estrogen antagonist could act in the same way. It is observed that at the time of the menopause, many precursor and precancerous lesions disappear spontaneously from breast tissue [1], possibly as a result of the fall in the circulating estrogen level. A similar mechanism has been suggested to explain the marked decrease in breast cancer risk found in women whose ovaries have been removed before the age of 45.

Safety Record of Tamoxifen

Although Tamoxifen is usually classified as an antiestrogen, its administration may also lead to partial estrogenic effects on some tissues. The net estrogenic/antiestrogenic balance in an individual will depend on the circulating levels of the agent and its breakdown products, and also upon their effects on the woman's own hormone secretion. Obvious differences are seen between circulating hormone levels in postmenopausal and premenopausal women who are given Tamoxifen therapy. In postmenopausal women, total circulating levels of estrogen are unchanged, while pituitary gonadotropin and prolactin levels are reduced to the lower limits of normal. In premenopausal women on the other hand, Tamoxifen may increase the circulating estrogen level up to five times normal although it returns to baseline levels when therapy is stopped. Both estrogenic and antiestrogenic side effects may therefore result from Tamoxifen and these have considerable relevance to the use of the agent in trials aiming to prevent breast cancer.

It is estimated that about three million women worldwide have taken Tamoxifen over the past 25 years, and that currently about 1 million women are taking adjuvant Tamoxifen to reduce the risk of recurrence after primary surgery for early breast cancer [2]. Observations have been made on many thousands of women in adjuvant trials where they have received 20 to 30 mg daily for at least 2 years, and a minority has been observed for up to five years. About 5% left the trials because of symptoms which they attributed to Tamoxifen. The majority of these symptoms were probably unrelated to the agent because the recorded incidence of these symptoms was almost as high in women taking the placebo tablets [19], (Table 1).

Table   1. Incidence of symptoms from
Tamoxifen compared to placebo in adjuvant
trial involving 2861 patients. Table modified
from [19]

Symptoms	Placebo (%)	Tamoxifen (%)
Hot flushes	3	4
Fluid retention	2	2
Vaginal discharge	1	2
Nausea	1.5	1.5
Skin rash	1	1

Side-effects which can be related to Tamoxifen are seen in about 20% of cases
and are usually mild. Most are related to the antiestrogenic effects of the agent.
Hot flushes may be noted in both premenopausal and postmenopausal women, and
other gynecologic symptoms include irregular menstruation, vaginal discharge or
dryness, and occasional bleeding from the uterus. Nausea is seen only occasionally
while skin rashes, depression or headache are rare side-effects.

Thrombosis and thrombophlebitis are said to be more common in women taking
Tamoxifen but it is well recognized that all cancer patients have an increased risk
of these conditions. Recent reports on adjuvant trials of Tamoxifen do not show
an increased incidence of thrombosis [20, 21]. Liver cancers have been reported in
rats given Tamoxifen dosage which is proportionally 6 times higher than the 20 mg
daily dose given in the preventive trials [22]. Among 4028 women given adjuvant
Tamoxifen at a dose of 40 mg daily, 2 cases of liver cancer were reported [15].
This dosage is twice the level recommended in the prevention trials.

Eye symptoms recorded in women receiving Tamoxifen therapy at 20 mg daily
include occasional retinal, lens or corneal changes which disappear when treatment
is stopped [23]. A total of 4 cases were recorded among 2375 women receiving
adjuvant Tamoxifen therapy [15].

The risk of uterine endometrial cancer in Tamoxifen-treated women has received
the greatest publicity and 59 cases from 9 reports have recently been reviewed
[24]. It has been recognized for many years that women with breast cancer are at
increased risk to endometrial cancer, but the frequency of endometrial cancer in
women receiving 20 mg Tamoxifen daily in adjuvant trials is reported to be 0.3%
compared to 0.1% in the control group [15]. Most developed in women taking the
agent for a prolonged period. Characteristic effects of Tamoxifen on the uterine
lining are now recognized, including thickening and polyp formation, but it varies
between individuals as well as on the dose and duration of Tamoxifen therapy
[25, 26]. Present knowledge suggests that women taking Tamoxifen for 5 years or
longer may increase their risk of developing endometrial cancer by a factor of 2 to
3.

A pilot trial of Tamoxifen in healthy women [27, 28] unexpectedly showed that 20 mg Tamoxifen daily lowered blood cholesterol levels by 20%. This developed within a few months of starting therapy and was maintained throughout treatment.

The principal change was in low density lipoprotein cholesterol (the 'bad' type). The finding has since been confirmed by several reports. One might therefore expect Tamoxifen administration to reduce the incidence of coronary heart disease and strokes when taken by older women, but so far, the evidence is still inconclusive. The overview analysis of almost 30,000 women showed a borderline–significant reduction in deaths from coronary heart disease in Tamoxifen-treated cases [6]. The Scottish trial showed a 67% reduction in heart attacks in postmenopausal patients receiving 20 mg Tamoxifen daily for 5 years, compared to controls [15]. The Swedish trial showed less frequent diagnosis of heart disease in women taking Tamoxifen for five years compared to those treated for only two years [21].

There is also evidence that the partial estrogenic activity of Tamoxifen may help to increase bone mineral density in postmenopausal women and thus decrease the risk of fractures associated with osteoporosis. Studies have shown that bone mineral density in the lumbar spine may be slightly increased, but the effect on the neck of the femur (where fractures are common) has not been studied. In general, it is likely that Tamoxifen stabilises bone loss in postmenopausal women to a degree comparable with that of estrogen replacement therapy [19].

Review of Current Prevention Trials

Tamoxifen is the first chemopreventive agent to undergo world-wide trials in breast cancer. In the USA, the Breast Cancer Prevention Trial was launched in 1992, enrolling women between 35 and 78 years of age, whose risk of developing breast cancer was considered to be greater than 1 in 10 [29,30]. The women are randomized into two groups, one to receive 20 mg Tamoxifen daily for five years, the others a placebo.

Every woman over the age of 60 is considered to carry a risk greater than 1 in 10, but women are excluded from the trial if they have taken hormone replacement therapy, have a previous history of cancer or thrombosis or have a life expectancy of less than 10 years. Women aged 35–59 are eligible if their degree of risk is similar to that of a 60 year old. The calculation is based on a formula which multiplies the risks associated with age group, family history of breast cancer, number of breast biopsies, pathologic findings, age at first childbirth, number of pregnancies and age at onset of menstruation [31]. An example of such a risk profile is shown in Table 2.

Although younger women with lobular cancer *in situ* are eligible for admission to the trial, women with ductal cancer *in situ* are not. Younger women in the trial must take steps to avoid pregnancy. The outcome to be measured by the trial will be not only the appearance of breast cancer, but also the incidence of coronary

Table 2. Examples of risk indicators which may make a woman eligible for participation in the North American Breast Cancer Prevention Trial. Women with such profiles are not necessarily eligible and eligibility is determined from a risk profile formula [31]. Table modified from [37]

Age group	Risk profile
35–39	One or more first degree relatives with breast cancer
	and
	History of benign breast biopsy at least twice
40–44	Two or more first degree relatives with breast cancer
	or
	History of benign breast biopsy at least twice
45–54	One or more first degree relatives with breast cancer
	or
	History of benign breast biopsy at least twice
50–59	One or more first degree relatives with breast cancer
	or
	First live birth at age 30 or older
Over 60	All women

artery disease, stroke, osteoporosis, other cancers and deaths from other causes. It is estimated that it will take 5 to 10 years to evaluate the first results.

A similar comparison of 20 mg Tamoxifen daily for five years, with a placebo, was launched in Italy in 1992 [32, 33]. It is restricted to women between the ages of 35 and 70 whose uterus has been removed thus avoiding any risk of endometrial cancer. In order to focus on women at average or higher risk of breast cancer, it excludes women at below average risk, as defined by a history of childbirth before the age of 20 or a history of more than four children.

The UK/International Trials involve women in the UK, Australia, New Zealand and various European countries, and were launched in 1992 and 1993 [34, 35]. They use similar dosage and duration of Tamoxifen to the previously launched trials, but the criteria for admission are somewhat different. Women aged 45–65 are eligible if their breast cancer risk is twice that of the general population, while women between 35 and 44 can enter if their risk is ten times that of the general population in their age group. This distinction takes into account the greater concern about the safety of long-term Tamoxifen in younger women [36]. Calculations of a woman's risk are based on a formula involving family history of breast cancer, history of breast biopsies, age at first childbirth, number of pregnancies and presence of density in the mammogram [34].

Why was five years selected as the duration for Tamoxifen treatment in all the trials? It was noted above that in experimental studies Tamoxifen administration suppresses tumor development, but growth is renewed when treatment is stopped.

In the human, an attempt has been made to use reduction of cancer in the second breast as a guide to the duration of Tamoxifen preventive treatment [2]. Two studies showed no reduction in second breast cancer from one year of Tamoxifen administration while two years of treatment reduced risk by one third in both premenopausal and postmenopausal cases. A direct comparison of two and five years duration of Tamoxifen showed no significant difference, and both groups demonstrated a risk reduction maintained for one to two years after Tamoxifen was stopped. In one trial of two years adjuvant Tamoxifen, risk reduction was beginning to fade in postmenopausal women after a median duration of 7.8 years and had disappeared completely in premenopausal women.

Currently, more than 15 studies are comparing different durations of adjuvant Tamoxifen treatment in randomized trials, some comparing two years with longer durations and some comparing five years with indefinite treatment. Much more evidence is needed before we can conclude that giving adjuvant Tamoxifen for an indefinite period is both beneficial and safe. In the future, the duration of adjuvant Tamoxifen therapy might depend on a woman's age group and the estrogen receptor level of her tumor. Such knowledge may help to determine the optimal duration of protection therapy, but meanwhile, a five year trial appears to be a relatively safe and logical choice.

A second question is, why there are differences in selection criteria between the various preventive trials in different parts of the world? All agree that women under the age of 35 should not be included in trials. The Italian trial is the only one that enrols women who are at an average risk to breast cancer, but excludes those with a below-average risk and those whose uterus has not been removed. The other trials concentrate on women whose risk of developing breast cancer is greater than one in ten. This degree of risk has been chosen both to justify any potential adverse effects from treatment and also to yield a significant result from the trial in a reasonable time.

The Breast Cancer Prevention Trial in the USA has recognized the need to represent ethnic minority populations in the trials in order to allow the results to be generalized to the whole population. A problem arises however, from the inclusion of poor and disadvantaged participants in the trial, because of the difficulties of long-term follow up of such women. In a pilot study, 25% of patients at a regional county hospital were lost to follow-up two years after the diagnosis of breast cancer [19]. It is clear that the prolonged duration of the prevention trial will involve problems of patient compliance apart from emotional and economic considerations. Also, since dietary fat levels may effect the risk of breast cancer, variations in a woman's fat intake during the five years of Tamoxifen administration might possibly influence the results of the trial [19].

Ethics of Tamoxifen Trials

No woman can be assured that by taking Tamoxifen she is likely to be protected against the risk of breast cancer. Otherwise, it would be unethical to enrol women into a randomized research trial where they may be allocated to a placebo tablet instead of an active agent. Nevertheless, treatment research trials aim to evaluate a new therapy which is *potentially* more effective than standard management. They may offer a chance of greater benefit but they also carry a greater risk of damage because the treatment has not been evaluated in a large number of people over a period of many years. This explains why the participants in a trial undergo special investigations and supervision.

The doctor who enters his patient into a trial does *not* subordinate his patient's interests to the interests of scientific research for the benefit of future generations. Many doctors feel that such a trial offers their patients the opportunity for state-of-the-art care, while at the same time, helping in the need to advance medical science. Informed consent for research generally involves a more rigorous consent form than does informed consent for standard treatment, mainly to protect the doctor in case of complications. The difference between the two types of consent is however, blurred [38]. Informed consent for any procedure should not be an attempt to minimize a doctor's liability for any adverse effects which may arise; it should always represent decision making which is shared between doctor and patient out of respect for every individual's autonomy.

The publicly expressed misgivings about the USA Breast Cancer Prevention Trial [3] are based mainly on its uncertain benefits and uncertain hazards when given to healthy women. Even if five years Tamoxifen treatment is proved to reduce the incidence of breast cancer by one-third in such women, two-thirds of them have been treated unnecessarily. It may be useful to look at these misgivings in the light of the less than 20% of patients showing benefit after five years of Tamoxifen adjuvant treatment for breast cancer. The treatment is now practically routine in postmenopausal patients, *mainly because of patient demand*. Every woman makes her own assessment of the threat to her life and her own decision of what is a worthwhile treatment.

The possible adverse effects of long-term Tamoxifen administration may be offset by its possible advantage in reducing the risk of coronary heart disease and osteoporosis in postmenopausal women. Based on the experience in the adjuvant Tamoxifen trials, the potential benefit from the reduction of heart disease is likely to be significant only among women aged over 60. It will be the end of the century before results emerge both on this point and on its ability to reduce the risk of breast cancer.

It has been emphasized that the setting up of a trial to evaluate Tamoxifen protection against breast cancer in women at increased risk is not an endorsement of its use in all women irrespective of risk [29]. If however, the current studies show worthwhile protection without significant adverse effects, any woman who has had breast cancer in the past may request such treatment. Although not eligible for current trials, they are all potentially at risk to cancer in the second breast.

Its estrogenic activity may limit Tamoxifen's effectiveness in suppressing the development of breast cancer. This limitation might be avoided if we used a pure antiestrogen which could deprive developing breast cancer of all estrogenic stimulation. A new pure antiestrogen has recently undergone initial trials in women with primary breast cancer although so far, only the toxicity and biologic effects of short-term administration have been reported [39]. It appears to be well-tolerated and shows purely antiestrogenic effects. It must however be taken into account that the beneficial effects of Tamoxifen in reducing blood cholesterol levels and maintaining bone density in postmenopausal women may well be manifestations of its partial estrogenic potential. They would presumably be lost in the treatment of breast cancer by a pure antiestrogen.

An alternative approach which still awaits clinical investigation is the combination of Tamoxifen with Vitamin A analogues (retinoids). The latter are currently undergoing trials in protecting women against second breast cancers. A combination of Tamoxifen with retinoids has been shown to suppress the growth of breast cancer cells in the laboratory, more than does either agent by itself [40].

Conclusion

Women receiving adjuvant Tamoxifen therapy after primary surgery for breast cancer show a reduced risk of developing cancer in the second breast in subsequent years. Tamoxifen offers a preventive option for women considered to be at increased risk to breast cancer based on biopsy, family history, on childbearing/menstrual history. Currently, the potential adverse effects of long-term Tamoxifen administration limit its use to randomized clinical trials in women at increased risk to breast cancer. Women entering these trials accept that they may receive placebo therapy.

References

1. Howell, A. (1989). Clinical evidence for the involvement of oestrogen in the development and progression of breast cancer. *Proc. Roy. Soc. Edin.*, **95B**, 49–57.
2. Gray, R. (1993). Tamoxifen; how boldly to go where no women have gone before. *J. Natl Cancer Inst.*, **85**, 1358–1360.
3. Fugh-Berman, A., Epstein, S. (1992) Tamoxifen; disease prevention or disease substitution. *Lancet*, **340**, 1143–1145.
4. Stoll, B.A. (1983). Intermittent anti-estrogen therapy in advanced breast cancer. *Cancer Treat. Rep.*, **67**, 98–99.
5. Sunderland, M.C., Osborne, C.K. (1991). Tamoxifen in premenopausal patients with metastatic breast cancer; a review. *J. Clin Oncol.*, **9**, 1283–1297.
6. Early Breast Cancer Trialists Collaborative Group (1988). Effects of adjuvant tamoxifen and of cytotoxic therapy on mortality in early breast cancer. An overview of 61 randomized trials among 28, 896 women. *N. Engl. J. Med.*, **319**, 1681–1692.

7. Scottish Cancer Trials Office, MRC Edinburgh (1987). Adjuvant tamoxifen in the management of operable breast cancer; the Scottish trial. *Lancet*, **2**, 171–175.
8. Palshof, T., Mouridsen H.T., Daehnfeldt, J.L. (1985). Adjuvant endocrine therapy in pre and postmenopausal women with operable breast cancer. *Rev. Endoc. Rel. Cancer*, **17**, (Suppl.), 43–50.
9. Cummings, F.J., Gray, R., Davis, T.E. (1986). Tamoxifen versus placebo. Double blind adjuvant trial in elderly women with Stage 2 breast cancer. In *Proceedings of the NJH Consensus Development Conference on Adjuvant Chemotherapy and Endocrine Therapy for Breast Cancer*, Bethesda, Maryland, 119–123.
10. Rutqvist, L.E., Cedermark, B., Glas, U. (1987). The Stockholm trial on adjuvant tamoxifen in early breast cancer. *Breast Cancer Res. Treat*, **10**, 255–266.
11. Pritchard, K.J., Meakin, J.W., Boyd, N.F. (1987). Adjuvant tamoxifen in postmenopausal women with axillary node positive breast cancer; an update. In Salmon, S.E. (ed.), *Adjuvant Therapy of Cancer*, Grune & Stratton, New York, 391–400.
12. CRC Adjuvant Breast Trial Working Party (1988). Cyclophosphamide and tamoxifen as adjuvant therapies in the management of breast cancer. *Br. J. Cancer*, **57**, 604–607.
13. Nolvadex Adjuvant Trial Organisation (1988). Controlled trial of tamoxifen as a single adjuvant agent in the management of early breast cancer. *Br. J. Cancer*, **57**, 608–611.
14. Fisher, B., Costantino, J., Redmond, C. *et al*. (1989). A randomized clinical trial evaluating tamoxifen in the treatment of patients with node-negative breast cancer who have estrogen receptor positive tumors. *N. Engl. J. Med.*, **320**, 479–484.
15. Nayfield, S.G., Karp, J.E., Ford, L.G., Dorr, F.A., Kramer, B.S. (1991). Potential role of tamoxifen in prevention of breast cancer. *J. Natl. Cancer Inst.*, **83**, 1450–1459.
16. Wattenberg, L.W. (1993). Prevention therapy; basic science and the resolution of the cancer problem. *Cancer Res.*, **53**, 5890–5896.
17. Jordan, V.C., Gottandis, M.M., Robinson, S.P. (1989). Immune-deficient animals to study hormone dependent breast and endometrial cancer. *J. Steroid Biochem.*, **34**, 169–176.
18. Gottardis, M.M., Jordan, V.C. (1987). The antitumor actions of keoxifene and tamoxifen in the N–nitrosomethylurea–induced ratmammary carcinoma model. *Cancer Res.*, **47**, 4020–4024.
19. Chlebowski, R.T., Butler, J., Nelson, A., Lillington, L. (1993). Breast cancer chemoprevention. *Cancer*, **72**, 1032–1037.
20. Jones, A.L., Powles, T.J., Treleaven, J.G. *et al*. (1992). Haemostatic changes and thromboembolic risk during tamoxifen therapy in normal women. *Br. J. Cancer*, **66**, 744–747.
21. Rutqvist, L.E., Mattson, A. (1993). Cardiac and thromboembolic morbidity among postmenopausal women with early stage breast cancer in a randomized trial of adjuvant tamoxifen. *J. Natl. Cancer Inst.*, **85**, 1398–1406.
22. Hard, G.C., Williams, G.M., Iatropoulos, M.J. (1993). Tamoxifen and liver cancer. *Lancet*, **342**, 444–445.
23. Pavlidis, N.A., Petris, C., Briassoulis, E. *et al*. (1992). Clear evidence that long term, low dose tamoxifen treatment can induce ocular toxicity. *Cancer*, **69**, 2961–2964.
24. Magriples, U., Naftalin, F., Schwartz, P.E., Carcangiu, M.L. (1993). High grade endometrial cancer in tamoxifen-treated breast cancer patients. *J. Clin. Oncol.*, **11**, 485–490.
25. Van Leeuwen, F.E., Benraadt, J., Coebergh, J.W.W. *et al*. (1994) Risk of endometrial cancer after tamoxifen treatment of breast cancer. *Lancet*, **343**, 448–452.
26. Neven, P. (1993). Tamoxifen and endometrial lesions. *Lancet*, **342**, 452.
27. Powles, T.J., Tillyer, C.R., Jones, A.L. *et al*. (1990). Prevention of breast cancer with tamoxifen; an update on the Royal Marsden Hospital Pilot Programme. *Eur. J. Cancer*, **26**, 680–684.
28. Cuzick, J., Allen, D., Baum, M. *et al*. (1993). Long term effects of tamoxifen; biological effects of Tamoxifen Working Party. *Eur. J. Cancer*, **29A**, 15–21.
29. Fisher, B., Redmond, C. (1991). New perspective on cancer of the contralateral breast; a marker for assessing tamoxifen as a preventive agent. *J. Natl. Cancer Inst.*, **83**, 1278–1280.

30. Redmond, C.K., Wickerham, D.L., Cronin, W. (1993). The NSABP Breast Cancer Prevention Trial; a progress report. *Proc. ASCO*, **12**, 69.

31. Gail, M.H., Brinton, L.A., Byar, D.P. *et al.* (1989). Projecting individualized probabilities of developing breast cancer for white females who are being examined annually. *J. Natl. Cancer Inst.*, **81**, 1879–1886.

32. News (1993). Breast cancer chemoprevention trials launched in Europe. *Ann. Oncol.*, **4**, 2.

33. News (1993). Breast cancer prevention study initiated in Italy. *J. Natl. Cancer Inst.*, **84**, 1555–1556.

34. News (1993). UK prevention trial gets go-ahead and expands to other countries. *Ann. Oncol.*, **4**, 707–708.

35. News (1993). European tamoxifen studies moving ahead. *J. Natl. Cancer Inst.*, **85**, 145–1451.

36. Jordan, V.C. (1993). How safe is tamoxifen? *Br. Med. J.*, **307**, 1371–1372.

37. Paterson, H.G., Geggie, P.H.S. (1993). Can tamoxifen prevent breast cancer? *Can. Med. Assoc. J.*, **148**, 142–143.

38. Lantos, J. (1993). Informed consent; the whole truth for patients. *Cancer*, **72**, 2811–2815.

39. DeFriend, D.J., Howell, A., Nicholson, R.I. *et al.* (1994). Investigation of a new pure antiestrogen (ICI 182780) in women with primary breast cancer. *Cancer Res.*, **54**, 408–414.

40. McCormick, D., Moon, R. (1986). Retinoid-tamoxifen interaction in mammary cancer chemoprevention. *Cancinogenesis*, **7**, 193–196.

Chapter 11

Trial of Vitamin A Analogues for Protection

ALBERTO COSTA, FRANCA FORMELLI, ROSALBA TORRISI and
ANDREA DECENSI

A precursor or latent stage of cancer is well known [1]. Chemoprevention aims either to block the initiation of cancer or else to arrest or reverse further progression during the precursor phase. Thus, Vitamin A analogues (retinoids) have been shown to arrest or reverse the progression of leukoplakia in the mouth [2, 3], to reduce the occurrence of second primary cancers of the aero-digestive tract [4, 5] and to reduce, in association with vitamin E and selenium, mortality from gastric cancer in the Chinese population [6]. Similar too, is the ability of Tamoxifen to reduce the occurrence of second primary breast cancers in women at high risk [7].

Role of Retinoids in Differentiation and Proliferation

Seventy years ago, it was reported [8] that retinoid deficiency led to a failure of stem cells to mature into differentiated cells. This was accompanied by enhanced cell proliferation, with formation of lesions resembling those seen in malignant or premalignant tissues. Subsequently, it was shown that retinoids are required to maintain normal differentiation and proliferation of almost all cells in mammals during both embryonic and adult life [9].

Because retinoids exert this hormone-like control of cell differentiation and cell proliferation, it was logical to investigate whether they might also be useful for chemoprevention of cancer. The development of cancer is characterized by loss or arrest of cellular differentiation and growth control, and retinoids both suppress growth and induce or enhance cellular differentiation.

Retinoic acid receptors (RARs) in cell nuclei may mediate the growth control induced by both natural and synthetic retinoids. The potential chemopreventive effect of retinoids in breast cancers thus raises the question of whether these tumors express RARs [10]. In addition, a reciprocal effect of retinoids and antiestrogens

Basil A. Stoll (ed.), Reducing Breast Cancer Risk in Women, 103–108.
© 1995 *Kluwer Academic Publishers. Printed in the Netherlands.*

on their respective receptors has been observed [10] and may be the molecular basis for the increased inhibition of breast cancer cell growth seen when the two agents are given in combination [11].

The Synthetic Retinoid Fenretinide (4–HPR)

Retinoids play a crucial role in cellular and tissue differentiation but their poor clinical tolerability has prevented use of these agents as anticarcinogens. Toxic symptoms which may be acceptable in treating established cancer are not necessarily considered acceptable for reducing cancer risk. One of the less toxic vitamin A analogues studied for breast cancer chemoprevention is the synthetic retinoid fenretinide or N-(4-hydroxyphenyl)retinamide (4–HPR) [12]. The inhibition of chemically–induced mammary carcinoma in rats by 4–HPR was described by Moon *et al.* [13]. This compound has since been studied extensively and proved to be less toxic than many other retinoids [14]. On this basis, 4–HPR was proposed for chemopreventive trials in human breast cancer.

It was decided to study the ability of this retinoid, when given to patients with early stage breast cancer, to prevent the appearance of new primary cancers in the opposite breast [15]. The concept was that patients treated for an early breast cancer have a good prognosis, but also a known risk of developing a second primary tumor, totally independent in its origin. One advantage of studying these tumors in the opposite breast is that their incidence (about 0.8% per year) remains stable for the first ten years after surgery in patients with early breast cancer. Second, these patients are already under periodical follow-up and it is relatively easy to have them participate in the study for the prolonged period necessary. Third, compliance by these patients in taking the agent is likely to be higher than in the general population or in women at increased breast cancer risk.

Our first protocol for a randomized clinical trial to evaluate the efficacy of 4–HPR in preventing contralateral (second) breast cancers, was postponed after considering toxicity data from clinical studies using 600 mg and 800 mg daily doses [16]. The reported side effects (night blindness and erythema) were dose–related and a subsequent drug study led us to identify the best tolerated dose as 200 mg/day with a three-day interruption of treatment at the end of each month [17, 18].

The effects of 4–HPR on plasma retinol levels have been studied in breast cancer patients who participated in the study and continued to be treated and followed for 5 years [19, 20]. We have demonstrated that 4–HPR blood levels remain constant during administration for as long as five years, that the drug accumulates in the human breast, and that a significant decline of plasma retinol levels is responsible for the night blindness.

It was shown that 4–HPR causes early reduction of plasma retinol concentrations [19] and that the plasma level of N-(4-methoxyphenyl)retinamide (the principal metabolite of 4–HPR) is the major determinant of the retinol decrease. It is associated with diminished dark adaptation, a dose-dependent side effect reported in

4–HPR-treated patients [16, 17, 21, 22]. In order to minimise this side effect, it was decided to periodically and temporarily interrupt drug treatment to increase plasma retinol concentrations, thus allowing storage of retinol in the retina.

Randomized Trial of 4–HPR

On the basis of experimental data showing accumulation of 4–HPR in the rodent mammary gland [13] and good tolerability in humans [17, 18], a large randomized chemoprevention trial was started in 1987. The assumption was that, if 4–HPR succeeds in preventing second primaries in breast cancer patients, it would possibly be useful for a wider group of high risk subjects, such as families showing a high incidence of the disease [23].

Study participants are breast cancer patients between the age of 33 and 68. In order to be eligible, patients must have had an operated breast cancer (T1–2), without axillary lymph node involvement and without evidence of local recurrence and/or distant metastases. They must have normal metabolic, liver and renal function tests besides a normal blood count. Due to the teratogenic effect of 4–HPR, they must avoid pregnancy during the study and for 6 months after the end of treatment. Clinical examination and baseline mammography of the second breast are performed on all patients, and all the characteristics of the mammary gland are carefully recorded. Patients are randomized to receive 200 mg 4–HPR daily for five years (with a 3-day drug holiday at the end of each month) versus no treatment.

Before joining the study, each patient is counselled by the investigating physician on the aims of the study, the expected drug effects and side effects. After the informed consent form has been signed by the patient, a behavioural agreement is discussed in order to enhance long-term maintenance of drug administration, and it is explained that it is important to take the drug daily after dinner to increase the bioavailability of 4–HPR [24].

Follow-up continues for at least 2 years after stopping administration in order to evaluate the efficacy of the drug and also in terms of a possible 'rebound effect'. The main measurements of efficacy will be physical examination and mammography. Accrual was closed on July 31, 1993. Overall, 2,972 patients were randomised, 1,496 in the 4–HPR group and 1,476 in the control group. Protocol and treatment compliance is high with over 90% drug compliance in 81% of the women and over 80% in another 10% of women. Tolerability of the drug is good and only 51 of 1,397 women (3.6%) interrupted drug intake due to toxicity.

In August 1994, a first interim analysis of the study was performed showing no difference between the two groups in terms of incidence of new primaries in the contralateral breast. This data cannot be interpreted as conclusive since more than one-third of the patients are still on treatment. However an interesting preliminary finding is the protective effect apparently exerted by 4-HPR in younger patients (below 45 years of age): in this subgroup, and during the exposure to the retinoid, the incidence of new contralateral primaries is significantly lower than in the control group.

Toxicity of 4–HPR

One of the main reasons for selecting 4–HPR is its tolerability compared to other retinoids. In a study of different doses of 4–HPR, no acute or severe toxicity was observed [17] and the same applied to long-term daily oral administration of 200 mg 4–HPR in 53 patients treated for 42 months [18]. Dermatological and metabolic alterations were relatively uncommon (less than 5% of cases) and no liver function abnormalities were observed [25].

Diminished dark adaptation is relatively frequent. Goldmann–Weekers dark-adaptometry (a psychophysical test to detect subclinical vitamin A deficiency) has shown a 23% incidence of mild, and a 26% incidence of moderate, alteration of dark-adaptation. This is associated with the reduction of plasma retinol below the threshold levels of 160 and 100 ng/ml, respectively, in women treated with 200 mg 4–HPR daily [21]. Nearly 50% of the treated patients with altered dark-adaptation are asymptomatic and the implications of the finding are uncertain.

Future Developments

As regards further investigations, the combined administration of 4–HPR with Tamoxifen (TAM) appears to be of major interest. The combined administration of TAM and 4–HPR has proved to be additive or synergistic in both the growth inhibition of MCF–7 cells [26] and the prevention of N-methyl-N-nitrosourea (MNU)-induced mammary carcinoma in the rat [27]. The concept of different agents separately inhibiting the growth of hormone-dependent and-independent breast cancers is intriguing. Hypothetically, TAM would prevent ER^+ tumours, and retinoids ER^- tumours. At present this is purely theoretical, but on this premise, a pilot study preliminary to a larger clinical trial has been designed to evaluate the chemopreventive activity of the combination of TAM and 4–HPR in breast cancer.

Conclusion

Fenretinide (4–HPR), a synthetic derivative of retinoic acid, has proved effective in inhibiting breast cancer cell growth and preventing the progression of chemically-induced mammary carcinoma in rodents. A randomized clinical study was closed on July 31, 1993, having accrued 2,972 Stage I breast cancer patients. The aim is to evaluate the ability of a five-year administration of 4–HPR to prevent second primary breast cancers.

Compliance to protocol and treatment is high and the tolerability of the drug is good with only 51 women out of 1,397 (3.6%) having to interrupt drug intake due to toxicity. The only adverse effect of 4–HPR administration is diminished dark adaptation, which occurs in about one-fourth of the patients and is dependent on the decline of plasma retinol below the threshold level of 100 ng/ml. However, about 50% of the patients with altered dark-adaptometry are asymptomatic, thus leaving the implication of the finding unsettled. In addition, alterations of dark adaptation are promptly reversible upon drug discontinuation.

Since the combination of 4–HPR with the antiestrogen Tamoxifen has shown synergistic activity in the prevention of breast cancer in experimental models, it is an important avenue for future clinical investigation. If it permits dose reduction in one or both agents, thereby minimising toxicity while maintaining activity, it could represent a major improvement in breast cancer chemoprevention.

References

1. Boone, C.W., Kelloff, G.J., Freedman, L.S. (1993). Intraepithelial neoplasia as a stochastic continuum of clonal evolution, and its relationship to mechanisms of chemopreventive drug action. *J. Cell Biochem.*, **17G**, 14–25.
2. Hong, W.K., Endicott, J., Itri L.M., *et al.* (1986). 13–cis–retinoic acid in the treatment of oral leukoplakia. *N. Engl. J. Med.*, **315**, 1501–1505.
3. Chiesa, F., Tradati, N., Marazza, M. *et al.* (1992). Prevention of local relapses and new localisations of oral leukoplakias with the synthetic retinoid fenretinide (4–HPR). Preliminary results. *Oral. Oncol. Eur. J. Cancer*, **28B**, 97–102.
4. Hong, W.K., Lippmann, S.M., Itri, L.M. *et al.* (1990). Prevention of secondary primary tumors in squamous cell carcinoma of the head and neck with 13–cis–retinoic acid. *N. Engl. J. Med.*, **323**, 795–801.
5. Pastorino, U., Infante, M., Maioli, M. *et al.* (1993). Adjuvant treatment of Stage I lung cancer with high–dose vitamin A. *J. Clin. Oncol.*, **11**, 1216–1222.
6. Blot, W.J., Li, J.-Y., Taylor, P.R. *et al.* (1993). Nutrition intervention trials in Linxian, China: multiple vitamin/mineral supplementation, cancer incidence and disease specific mortality in the general population. *J. Natl. Cancer Inst.*, **85**, 1492–1498.
7. Early Breast Cancer Trialists' Collaborative Group (1992). Systemic treatment of early breast cancer by hormonal, cytotoxic, or immunotherapy. *Lancet*, **339**, 1–15, 71–85.
8. Wolbach, S.B., Howe, P.R. (1925). Tissue changes following deprivation of fat soluble A vitamin. *J. Exp. Med.*, **42**, 753–777.
9. Sporn, M.B., Dunlop, N.M., Newton, D.L. *et al.* (1976). Prevention of chemical carcinogenesis by vitamin A and its synthetic analogs (retinoids). *Fed. Proc.*, **35**, 1332–1338.
10. Roman, S.D., Clarke, C.L., Hall, R.E. (1992). Expression and regulation of retinoic acid receptors in human breast cancer cells. *Cancer Res.*, **52**, 2236–2242.
11. Moon, R.C., Mehta, R.G. (1989). Chemoprevention of experimental carcinogenesis in animals. *Prev. Med.*, **18**, 576–591.
12. Costa, A. (1992). Biological approaches to breast cancer prevention. *The Breast*, **1**, 119–123.
13. Moon, R.C., Thompson, H.J., Becci, P.L. *et al.* (1979). N–(4–hydroxyphenyl) retinamide, a new retinoid for prevention of breast cancer. *Cancer Res.*, **39**, 1339–1346.
14. Paulson, J.D., Oldham, J.W., Preston, R.F. *et al.* (1992). Lack of genotoxicity of the cancer chemopreventive agent N–(4–hydroxyphenyl) retinamide. *Fundam. Appl. Toxicol.*, **5**, 144–150.
15. Veronesi, U., De Palo, G., Costa, A. *et al.* (1992). Chemoprevention of breast cancer with retinoids. *NCI Monographs*, **12**, 93–97.
16. Kaiser-Kupfer, M.I., Peck, G.L., Caruso, R.C. *et al.* (1986). Abnormal retinal function associated with Fenretinide, a synthetic retinoid. *Arch. Ophtalmol.*, **104**, 69–70.

17. Costa, A., Malone, W., Perloff, M. *et al.* (1989). Tolerability of the synthetic retinoid fenretinide (HPR). *Eur. J. Cancer Clin. Oncol.*, **25**, 805–809.
18. Rotmensz, N., De Palo, G., Formelli, F. *et al.* (1991). Long term tolerability of fenretinide (4–HPR) in breast cancer patients. *Eur. J. Cancer*, **2**, 1127–1131.
19. Formelli, F., Carsana, R., Costa, A. *et al.* (1989). Plasma retinol level reduction by the synthetic retinoid fenretinide: A one year follow–up study of breast cancer patients. *Cancer Res.*, **49**, 6149–6152.
20. Formelli, F., Clerici, M., Campa, T. *et al.* (1993). Five-year administration of fenretinide: Pharmacokinetics and effects on plasma retinol concentrations. *J. Clin. Oncol.*, **11**, 2036–2042.
21. Decensi, A., Torrisi, R., Polizzi, A. *et al.* (1994). Effect of the synthetic retinoid fenretinide on dark-adaptation and the ocular surface. *J. Natl. Cancer Inst.*, **86**, 105–110.
22. Kingstone, T.P., Lowe, N.J., Winston, J. *et al.* (1986). Visual and cutaneous toxicity which occurs during N–(4–hydroxyphenyl)retinamide therapy for psoriasis. *Clin. Exp. Dermatol.*, **II**, 624–627.
23. Vasen, H.F.A., Beex, L.V.A.M., Cleton, F.J. *et al.* (1993). Clinical heterogeneity of hereditary breast cancer and its impact on screening protocols: the Dutch experience on 24 families under surveillance. *Eur. J. Cancer*, **29A**, 1111–1114.
24. Doose, D.R., Minn, F.L., Stellar, S. *et al.* (1992). Effects of meals and meal composition on the bioavailability of fenretinide. *J. Clin. Pharmacol.*, **32**, 1089–1095.
25. Pizzichetta, M., Rossi, R., Costa, A. *et al.* (1992). Lipoproteins in Fenretinide (4–HPR)–treated patients. *Diabetes Nutr. Metab.*, **5**, 71–72.
26. Fontana, J.A. (1987). Interaction of retinoids and tamoxifen on the inhibition of mammary carcinoma cell proliferation. *Exp. Cell Biol.*, **55**, 136–144.
27. Ratko, T.A., Detrisac, C.J., Dinger, M.N. *et al.* (1989). Chemopreventive efficacy of combined retinoid and tamoxifen treatment following surgical excision of a primary mammary cancer in female rats. *Cancer Res.*, **497**, 4472–4476.

Chapter 12

Trial of Low Fat Diet for Protection

ROWAN T. CHLEBOWSKI

A woman's intake of fat has been proposed as a factor which may influence her risk of developing breast cancer [1–3]. Excessive fat intake has also been claimed to affect the growth and spread of existing breast cancer [4–6]. Evidence which supports these two hypotheses has led to the setting up of large-scale clinical trials to clarify the issues [1, 4, 7]. Because a woman's fat intake is directly under her control, the basis of these trials is reviewed with a view towards its application to an individual woman.

Dietary Fat Intake and Breast Cancer Prognosis

Potential benefit may follow the reduction of fat intake by women who have had early breast cancer treated by surgery, possibly in conjunction with other therapy such as adjuvant chemotherapy or Tamoxifen administration [8].

A potential role for dietary fat reduction in improving prognosis for women with resected breast cancer is based on the following observations:

(i) Evidence of substantial differences in survival rates for patients with localized breast cancer, comparing countries with a low-fat diet (such as Japan) to those eating a high-fat diet (United States and Western Europe) [9–13].

(ii) Observations that weight gain occurring after primary surgery may worsen a woman's breast cancer prognosis [14–17].

(iii) Evidence of a correlation between a high dietary fat intake at the time of breast cancer diagnosis with a worse prognosis [18–21].

Basil A. Stoll (ed.), Reducing Breast Cancer Risk in Women, 109–118.
© 1995 *Kluwer Academic Publishers. Printed in the Netherlands.*

(iv) Animal studies showing an adverse influence by increased dietary fat intake (especially the polyunsaturated linoleic acid) on both growth and metastatic spread of breast cancer [6, 22].

 (v) Evidence of stimulation by linoleic acid of human breast cancer cell growth both in tissue culture and in tumor implanted in immune-deficient mice [23–25].

(vi) Plausible mechanisms of action have been suggested which could mediate the influence of dietary fat intake on breast cancer growth and metastatic spread [4–6].

(vii) Evidence that a major reduction in fat intake can be achieved by women who have been treated by primary surgery for breast cancer [26, 27].

A higher survival rate, especially in postmenopausal patients with breast cancer, has been reported in countries with low dietary fat intakes. For example, the survival rate of early breast cancer patients in Japan (low dietary fat) is 21% higher (73% versus 52%) than that in the United Kingdom [13]. It is unlikely that such differences in survival rates between Western and Japanese women with breast cancer are related to differences in either histopathology, treatment factors or treatment response [28]. Dietary intake is a plausible explanation for such differences.

Not all clinical observations however, support the relationship between dietary fat intake and breast cancer prognosis. Difficulties which are commonly associated with prospective studies on diet include small sample sizes, collection of dietary data mostly in one period, and the relatively limited variation in dietary fat intake which is found in the population of a given specific geographic area. These problems have precluded conclusive studies [1]. While some studies have reported that higher dietary fat intake is related to a poorer prognosis [18–21, 29] other have not confirmed such a relationship [30–32]. The narrow range of fat intake observed in such studies reflects the major problem limiting such studies.

Dietary Fat Intake Reduction Programs

Studies in the United States and Europe have tried to determine whether a decrease in dietary fat intake can be achieved in women with resected breast cancer [26, 27, 33].

The Women's Intervention Nutrition Study set up a feasibility study, enrolling 290 postmenopausal women after cancer resection [34]. Dietary fat intake decreased from 32% of calories at baseline to 20% of calories in the Intervention Group, while the Control Group (counseled for nutrition adequacy only) did not significantly change intake. Significant differences in fat intake were maintained for the 24 month observation period [26]. All categories of fat (saturated, polyunsaturated, and monounsaturated) were significantly reduced by approximately 50%, and a 16% reduction in caloric intake was observed.

Table 1. Current study of dietary fat intake reduction as adjuvant management after breast cancer surgery [39]

Title:	Women's Intervention Nutrition Study
Study Design:	Randomized, multicenter, five-year trial
Sample Size:	2,000 women with resected breast cancer
Eligibility:	Age $\geq$ 48 < 78 years; $\geq$ 25% of total kcal as fat
Objective:	To test whether dietary fat intake reduction will reduce breast cancer recurrence and increase patient survival
Dietary goals:	15% of total kcal as fat
Endpoints:	Breast cancer recurrence; patient survival

Physiological changes following dietary fat reduction included reduction in body weight [26], reduction in serum estradiol levels [35], and differences in free fatty acid profiles [36]. Similar results have been reported by other studies [27, 37, 38] involving changes in dietary fat, nutrient intake and patient weight in women with resected breast cancer subjected to fat intake reduction. Together, these data confirm that fat intake reduction can be achieved in women after breast cancer surgery.

Based on these results, a study of dietary fat intake restriction for women with resected breast cancer is now accruing patients, (Table 1). This study will assess the role of fat intake reduction as a form of adjuvant management after primary surgery for breast cancer. Such a trial has considerable practical advantages when compared with trials of dietary change for the purpose of breast cancer prevention [39]. Advantages include high patient motivation resulting in greater adherence to the regimen, easier follow-up of patients and easily-measured endpoints involving recurrence or death.

Would a dietary approach be effective if used at the same time as the anti-estrogen Tamoxifen? There is evidence suggesting that Tamoxifen and dietary fat intake reduction do not influence breast cancer growth by the same mechanism in patients with resected breast cancer. The ACETBC Japan Trial [8] evaluated two years of adjuvant tamoxifen therapy in Japanese women taking their normally low dietary fat intake [40]. Surprisingly, the magnitude of benefit associated with Tamoxifen in this setting was twice that seen in all other randomized trials comparing Tamoxifen to no intervention [8]. These results suggest that Tamoxifen benefit is not mediated exclusively through the same mechanism as a low-fat diet since if that were the case, little or no benefit would be expected from Tamoxifen in a population already consuming a low-fat diet.

Weight Gain and Breast Cancer Prognosis

Recent reports have confirmed a relationship between the presence of obesity at the time of breast cancer diagnosis and a subsequent poor prognosis [41–43]. Sub-

Table 2. Randomized trials of dietary intervention in patients with resected breast cancer: influence on body weight

			Result	
			(intervention vs. control)	
			On daily	On body
Trial	No.	Intervention target	fat intake	weight
North Central Oncology Group (46)	109	Weight maintenance [dietician referral]	Not reported	Weight increase: 3 kg in both groups
Women's Intervention Nutrition Study (26)	290	Fat reduction [centralized program]	50% reduced	Weight difference: 3.5 kg (P < 0.01) through 24 months
Karolinska Institute (27, 37)	257	Fat reduction [centralized program]	43% reduced	Weight difference: 2.4 kg (P < 0.05) through 24 months

stantial weight gain is commonly associated with systemic adjuvant therapy after primary breast surgery, especially after combination chemotherapy regimens [14–17, 44, 45]. Weight gain is also reported in postmenopausal breast cancer patients not given systemic adjuvant therapy [16]. The weight increase usually develops in the six months after breast cancer resection, ranging from 2–6 kilograms, and is largely retained subsequently. For patients receiving adjuvant chemotherapy, the weight gain is greater in premenopausal than in postmenopausal patients [17].

Observations suggest that weight increase in the post-resection period adversely influences breast cancer survival rates [15, 16]. After nearly 7 years of follow up in 646 breast cancer patients who were entered on adjuvant chemotherapy trials [16], those premenopausal women gaining more than the median weight at one year were found to be 1.5 times more likely to have relapsed, and 1.7 time more likely to have died, than women gaining less than the median weight. Similar trends were seen in postmenopausal populations. The mechanisms underlying such weight increase have not been identified but could include increased caloric intake, change of physical activity, and change in host metabolic status [17].

Trials of strategies to prevent systemic therapy-associated weight gain are summarized in Table 2. The North Central Cancer Treatment Group recently reported their experience with dietician-referral to prevent weight gain in such cases [46]. A total of 109 premenopausal women were randomized to receive either standard care or monthly referral to a dietician for counseling on weight maintenance during chemotherapy. Overall median weight gain was one and three kilograms at three and six months, respectively, but the dietician-counseling group did not achieve a significantly lower weight or reduction in caloric intake when compared to the no-counseling group.

In contrast, programs targeted specifically to dietary fat intake reduction have been successful in abrogating the weight increase in such cases [26, 27, 33]. In the Women's Intervention Nutrition Study referred to above [26], the program involved four bi-weekly visits to a nutritionist (Registered Dietician) trained to implement a defined 'Low Fat Eating Plan' [34]. Associated with the 50% reduction in daily fat intake, weight change was greater in the Intervention than in the Control Dietary Group, and an approximately 3.5 kilogram difference was maintained throughout the 24 months of observation [26]. A similar magnitude of weight reduction was also seen in a Scandinavian study evaluating a low-fat diet in a comparable study design [27].

Dietary Fat Intake and Breast Cancer Prevention

The potential role of dietary fat in breast cancer prevention is controversial [3, 47, 48]. To test a hypothesis relating dietary fat to primary breast cancer prevention, an extremely large population size is required, and adherence over a long period of time would have to be maintained. Motivation of women to a major dietary change in the absence of established disease would be difficult. However, some of these problems may be obviated when populations at extremely high risk of breast cancer development can be genetically identified [49].

There is evidence of consistent country-by-country associations between dietary fat intake and rates of breast cancer [2, 50] and combined analysis of 12 case control studies has demonstrated a significant association between dietary fat intake and breast cancer risk [50]. However, major prospective cohort studies show a less consistent picture. The Nurse's Health Study prospectively followed over 89,000 nurses in the United States and showed no relationship between intake of dietary fat and breast cancer risk. However, a cohort study with 56,000 Canadian women did show an effect of fat intake on breast cancer risk [51] and a cohort study with over 34,000 postmenopausal women showed a result comparable to the Canadian report [52]. Such studies have been criticized for their relatively narrow range of dietary fat intakes. For example, the lowest quintile dietary fat intake in the Nurse's Health Study exceeds the average intake found in the control population of some dietary intervention studies [26].

In spite of these uncertainties, the National Institutes of Health in the United States [7], is supporting a major prospective clinical trial to address the issue, (Table 3). The dietary component of the Women's Health Initiative will evaluate a reduced dietary fat strategy, designed to prevent breast and colon cancer as well as reduce cardiovascular disease in postmenopausal women. The dietary goals of the Women's Health Initiative include reduction of total dietary intake to 20% of calories; reduction of saturated fat intake to 7% of calories; and increased intake of fruits, vegetables and grain products. This study will enter 48,000 women over an approximately two to three year accrual period. Accrual is beginning in 1994 for this trial and results will require perhaps a decade to mature.

Rowan T. Chlebowski

Table 3. Prospective clinical trial of dietary fat intake reduction in relation to cancer prevention

Title:	Dietary component; Women's Health Initiative
Study Design:	Randomized, multicenter, 11 year trial
Sample Size:	48,000 women
Eligibility:	Postmenopausal; no prior breast or colon cancer; $\geq 34\%$ of total kcal as fat at baseline
Objective:	To determine whether a low-fat dietary program will reduce incidence of breast and colorectal cancer and coronary heart disease
Dietary goals:	20% of total kcal as fat; 7% of total kcal as saturated fat; increased fruits, vegetables and grains (5 or more daily servings)
Endpoints:	Breast cancer, colon cancer; cardiac events

The feasibility of implementing the proposed dietary change in postmenopausal women without disease is supported by an antecedent pilot study, the Women's Health Trial [53,54,55]. This randomized study, in postmenopausal women used a group intervention approach with centralized training of the nutritionists. In the intervention group, reductions in dietary fat intake from baseline values of 39% of calories from fat, to 23% of calories from fat, were rapidly achieved and maintained for 24 months [53,54]. In 524 of the original participants who were traced one year after the study period, only a 1.4 percent increase in percent calories from fat was reported, despite the absence of any contact during the post study period [55].

These self-reported dietary intake differences were associated with body weight reductions (3.4 kilograms), and reductions in estradiol (17%), remarkably similar to those seen in intervention studies in populations with resected breast cancer [26, 57]. In addition, cholesterol reduction consistent with those predicted by the Keys Equation [58] have been observed in women in the intervention arm of the Women' Health Trial [53]. Thus, in a multi-center trial, postmenopausal women have been successful in altering their dietary fat intake for a considerable period. Whether such a reduction in fat intake can be maintained over the longer period required to test the primary breast cancer prevention hypothesis remains to be determined.

At present, definitive recommendations on the optimal dietary fat intake needed to minimize breast cancer risk cannot be provided. Theoretical recommendations [3,59] largely involve more modest fat intake reductions than those currently being tested in clinical trials (i.e. dietary fat intake targets of approximately 25% of total energy intake). One must consider competing risks [60] and a women's individual medical and genetic [61] circumstances. One must also exercise caution in combining dietary and drug approaches, given the limited information on potential interactions between dietary change and pharmaceutical agents. For example, we have reported that dietary fat reduction, in combination with Tamoxifen may disproportionately *increase* HDL cholesterol with implications for cardiovascular risk [62].

Conclusion

Programs directed specifically at the reduction of dietary fat intake have proved successful in preventing weight increase in women with breast cancer following primary surgery. While clinical trials are under way evaluating these programs for their effect on breast cancer prognosis, such diets also offer the possibility of cardiovascular risk reduction. For women at increased risk of breast cancer, one could consider entry into a prospective trial or else the adoption of a somewhat less stringent dietary fat reduction target.

Acknowledgements

Some of the results presented have been supported by grant number CA 45502 from the National Cancer Institute, Bethesda, Maryland, USA.

References

1. Henderson, M.M. (1992). Role of intervention trials in research on nutrition and cancer. *Cancer Res.*, **52**, 2030s–2034s.
2. Howe, G.R. (1993). High–fat diets and breast cancer risk. The epidemiologic evidence. *J. Am. Med. Assoc.*, **268**, 2080–2081.
3. Miller, A.B., Berrino, F., Hill, M. *et al.* (1994). Diet in the aetiology of cancer: a review. *European J. Cancer*, **30A**, 207–220.
4. Chlebowski, R.T., Rose, D., Buzzard, I.M. *et al.* (1991). Adjuvant dietary fat intake reduction in postmenopausal breast cancer management. *Breast Cancer Res. Treat.*, **20**, 73–84.
5. Cohen, L.A., Rose, D.P., Wynder, E.L. (1993). A rationale for dietary intervention in the treatment of postmenopausal breast cancer patients; An update. *Nutr. Cancer*, **19**, 1–10.
6. Rose, D.P., Hatala, M.A. (1994). Dietary fatty acids and breast cancer invasion and metastasis. *Nutr. Cancer*, **21**, 103–111.
7. Greenwald, P. (1993). NCI cancer prevention and control research. *Prev. Med.*, **22**, 642–660.
8. Early Breast Cancer Trialists' Collaborative Group (1992). Systemic treatment of early breast cancer by hormonal cytotoxic or immune therapy. *Lancet*, **339**, 1–15.
9. Wynder, E.L., Kajitani, T., Kuno, J. *et al.* (1963). A comparison of survival rates between American and Japanese patients with breast cancer. *Gynecol. Obstet.*, **111**, 196–200.
10. Sakamoto, G., Sugano, H., Hartman, W.H. (1979). Stage-by-stage survival from breast cancer in the U.S. and Japan. *Jpn. J. Cancer*, **25**, 161–170.
11. Markita, M., Sakamoto G. (1990). Natural history of breast cancer among Japanese and Caucasian females. *Gan. to Kagaku Ryoho*, **17**, 1239–1243.
12. Morrison, A.S., Lowe, C.R., MacMahon, B. *et al.* (1976). Some international differences in treatment and survival in breast cancer. *Int. J. Cancer*, **18**, 269–273.
13. Allen, D.S., Bulbrook, R.D., Chauhdary, M.A. *et al.* (1991). Recurrence and survival rates in British and Japanese women with breast cancer. *Breast Cancer Res. Treat.*, **18**, S131–S134.
14. Dixon, J., Moritz, D.A., Baker, F.L. (1978). Breast cancer and weight gain: An unexpected finding. *Oncol. Nurs. Forum*, **5**, 5–7.
15. Chlebowski, R.T., Weiner, J.M., Reynolds, R. *et al.* (1986). Long term survival following relapse after 5–FU but not CMF adjuvant breast cancer therapy. *Breast Cancer Res. Treat.*, **7**, 23, 30.

16. Camoriano, J.K., Loprinzi, C.L., Ingle, J.N. *et al.* (1990). Weight change in women treated with adjuvant therapy or observed following mastectomy for node-positive breast cancer. *J. Clin. Oncol.*, **8**, 1327–1334.
17. Denmark-Wahnefried, W., Winer, E.P., Rimer, B.K. (1993). Why women gain weight with adjuvant chemotherapy for breast cancer. *J. Clin. Oncol.*, **11**, 1418–1429.
18. Normura, A., Le Marchand, L., Kolonel, L., Hankin, J. (1991). The effect of dietary fat on breast cancer survival among Caucasian and Japanese women in Hawaii. *Breast Cancer Res. Treat.*, **18**, 135–141.
19. Gregorio, D., Emrich, L., Graham, S., Marshall, J., Nemoto, T. (1985). Dietary fat consumption and survival among women with breast cancer. *J. Natl. Cancer Inst.*, **75**, 37–41.
20. Holm, L.E., Callmer, E., Hjalmar, M.L. *et al.* (1989). Dietary habits and prognostic factors in breast cancer. *J. Natl. Cancer Inst.*, **81**, 1218–1223.
21. Holm, L.E., Nordevang, E., Jhalmar, M.L. *et al.* (1993). Treatment failure and dietary habits in women with breast cancer. *J. Natl. Cancer Inst.*, **85**, P32–6.
22. Erickson, K.L., Hubbard, N.E. (1990). Dietary fat and tumor metastasis. *Nutr. Rev.*, **48**, 6–12.
23. Rose, D.P., Connolly, J.M., Meschter, C.L. (1991). Effect of dietary fat on human breast cancer growth and lung metastasis in nude mice. *J. Natl. Cancer Inst.*, **83**, 1491–1495.
24. Rose, D.P., Connolly, J.M. (1992). Influence of dietary fat intake on local recurrence and progression of metastases arising from MDA-MB–435 human breast cancer cells in nude mice after excision of the primary tumor. *Nutr. Cancer*, **18**, 113–122.
25. Rose, D.P., Hatala, M.A., Connolly, J.M. Rayburn, J. (1993). Effect of diets containing different levels of linoleic acid on human breast cancer growth and lung metastasis in nude mice. *Cancer Res.*, **53**, 4686–4690.
26. Chlebowski, R.T., Blackburn, G.L., Buzzard, I.M. *et al.* (1993). For the Women's Intervention Nutrition Study. Adherence to a dietary fat intake reduction program in postmenopausal women receiving therapy for early breast cancer. *J. Clin. Oncol.*, **11**, 2072–2080.
27. Holm, L.E., Nordevang, E., Ikkala, E. *et al.* (1990). Dietary intervention as adjuvant therapy in breast cancer patients: A feasibility study. *Breast Cancer Res. Treat.*, **16**, 103–109.
28. Henderson, I.C. (1991). Rapporteur's report – treatment and response. *Breast Cancer Res. Treat.*, **18**, S157–S158.
29. Jain, M., Miller, A.B., Teresa, T. (1994). Premorbid diet and the prognosis of women with breast cancer. *J. Natl. Cancer Inst.*, **86**, 1390–1397.
30. Rohan, T., Hiller, J., McMichael, A. (1993). Dietary factors and survival from breast cancer. *Nutrition and Cancer*, **20**, 167–177.
31. Newman, S.C., Miller, A.B., Howe, G.R. (1986). A study of the effect of weight and dietary fat on breast cancer survival time. *Amer. J. Epidemiology*, **123**, 767–74.
32. Kyogoku, S., Hirohata, T., Nomura, Y. (1992). Diet and prognosis of breast cancer. *Nutrition and Cancer*, **17**, 271–7.
33. Chlebowski, R.T., Nixon, D.W., Blackburn, G.L. *et al.* (1987). A breast cancer nutrition adjuvant study (NAS): protocol design and initial patient adherence. *Breast Cancer Res. Treat.*, **10**, 21–29.
34. Buzzard, I.M., Asp, E.H., Chlebowski, R.T., *et al.* (1990). Diet intervention methods to reduce fat intake: Nutrient and food group composition of self-selected low-fat diets. *J. Am. Diet. Assoc.*, **90**, 42–49.
35. Rose D.P., Chlebowski R.T., Connolly J.M. *et al.* (1992). The effects of tamoxifen adjuvant therapy and a low-fat diet on serum binding proteins and estradiol bioavailability in postmenopausal breast cancer patients. *Cancer Res.*, **52**, 5386–5390.
36. Chlebowski, R.T., Rose, D., Blackburn, G. *et al.* (1991). Feasbility of using dietary fat intake reduction in adjuvant breast cancer management. *Proc. Amer. Soc. Clin. Onc.*, **10**, 217.
37. Nordevang, E., Ikkala, E., Callmer, E. *et al.* (1990). Dietary intervention in breast cancer patients: Effects on dietary habits and nutrient intake. *Eur. J. Clin. Nutr.*, **44**, 681–687.
38. Nordevang, E., Callmes, E., Marmur, A., Holm, E.L. (1992). Dietary intervention in breast cancer patients: effects on food choice. *European J. Clin. Nutr.*, **46**, 387–396.

39. Willet, W.C. (1993). Dietary fat reduction among women with early breast cancer. *J. Clin. Oncol.*, **11**, 2061–2062.
40. Lands, W.E.M., Hamazaki, T., Yamazaki, K. *et al.* (1990): Changing dietary patterns in Japan and the U.S. *Am. J. Clin. Nutr.*, **51**, 991–993.
41. Senie, R.T., Rosen, P.P., Rhodes, P. *et al.* (1992). Obesity at diagnosis of breast carcinoma influences duration of disease–free survival. *Ann. Intern. Med.*, **116**, 26–32.
42. Tretli, S., Haldorsen, T., Ottestad, L. (1990). The effect of pre-morbid height and weight on the survival of breast cancer patients. *Brit. J. Cancer*, **62**, 299–304.
43. Bastarruchea, J., Hortobagyi, G.N., Smith, T.L., Kai, S.C., Buzdar, A.U. (1993). Obesity as an adverse prognostic factor for patients receiving adjuvant chemotherapy for breast cancer. *Ann. Intern. Med.*, **119**, 18–25.
44. Hoskin, P.J., Ashley, S., Yarnold, J.R. (1990). Changes in body weight after treatment for breast cancer and the effect of tamoxifen. *Br. J. Cancer*, **62**, (Suppl. XI), 26.
45. Heasman, K.Z., Sutherland, J.H., Campbell, J.A., Elhakim, T., Boyd, N.F. (1986). Weight gain during adjuvant chemotherapy for breast cancer. *Breast Cancer Res. Treat.*, **5**, 195–200.
46. Athmann, L., Loprinzi, C.L., Kardinal, C., O'Fallon, J.R. *et al.* (1994). Randomized evaluation of dietician counseling to prevent weight gain associated with breast cancer adjuvant chemotherapy. *Proc. Amer. Soc. Clin. Onc.*, **13**, 47.
47. Whittemore, A.S., Henderson, B.E. (1993). Dietary fat and breast cancer: Where are we? *J. Natl. Cancer Inst.*, **85**, 762–763.
48. Freedman, L.S., Prentice, R.L., Clifford, C., Harlan, W., Henderson, M. *et al.* (1993). Dietary fat and breast cancer: Where are we? *J. Natl. Cancer Inst.*, **85**, 764–765.
49. Eeler, R.A., Stratton, M.R., Goldgar, D.E., Easton, D.F. (1994). The genetics of familial breast cancer and their practical implications. *Europ. J. Cancer*, **9**, 1383–1390.
50. Howe, G.R., Hirohata, T., Hislop, T.G. *et al.* (1990). Dietary factors and risk of breast cancer: combined analysis of 12 case–control studies. *J. Natl. Cancer Inst.*, **82**, 561–569.
51. Howe, G.R., Freidenreich, C.M., Jain, M., Miller, A.B. (1991). A cohort study of fat intake and risk of breast cancer. *J. Natl. Cancer Inst.*, **83**, 336–340.
52. Kushi, L.H., Sellers, T.A., Potter, J.D. *et al.* (1992). Dietary fat and postmenopausal breast cancer. *J. Natl. Cancer Inst.*, **84**, 1092–1099.
53. Henderson, M.M., Kushi, L.H., Thompson, D.J. *et al.* (1990). Feasibility of a randomized trial of a low-fat diet for the prevention of breast cancer. *Prev. Med.*, **19**, 115–133.
54. Gorbach, S., Morrill-LaBrode, A., Woods, M.N. *et al.* (1990). Changes in food patterns during a low-fat dietary intervention in women. *J. Amer. Diet. Assoc.*, **90**, 802–809.
55. Kristal, A.R., White, E., Shattuck, A.C. *et al.* (1992). Long-term maintenance of a low-fat diet: durability of fat-related dietary habits in the Women's Health Trial. *J. Am. Diet. Assoc.*, **92**, 553–559.
56. Prentice, R., Thompson, D., Clifford, C. *et al.* (1990). Dietary fat reduction and plasma estradiol concentration in healthy postmenopausal women. *J. Natl. Cancer Inst.*, **82**, 129–134.
57. Rose, D.P., Connolly, J.M., Chlebowski, R.T., Buzzard, I.M., Wynder, E.L. (1993). The effects of a low-fat dietary intervention and tamoxifen adjuvant therapy on the serum estrogen and sex hormone-binding globulin concentrations of postmenopausal breast cancer patients. *Breast Cancer Res. and Treat.*, **27**, 253–262.
58. Keys, A. (1984). Serum cholesterol response to dietary cholesterol. *Am. J. Clin. Nutr.*, **40**, 351–359.
59. Wynder, E.L., Taioli, E., Rose, D.P. (1992). Breast cancer, the optimal diet. *Adv. Experiment. Med. Biol.*, **322**, 143–153.
60. Committee on Diet and Health (1989). *Diet and Health. Implication for Reducing Chronic Disease Risk*. National Academy Press, Washington, D.C.
61. Ford, D., Easton, D.F., Bishop, D.T. *et al.* (1994). Risks of cancer in BRCA 1–mutation carriers. *Lancet*, **343**, 692–695.

62. Chlebowski, R.T., Blackburn, G., Richie, J.P., Wynder, E. (1994). Unanticipated effect of dietary
     fat intake reduction on HDL cholesterol in postmenopausal women receiving tamoxifen. *Proc.
     Amer. Soc. Clin. Onc.*, **13**, 214.

Chapter 13

Trial of Ovarian Suppression for Protection

DARCY V. SPICER, ELIZABETH A. KRECKER and
MALCOLM C. PIKE

There is irrefutable evidence that ovarian hormones are intimately involved in the genesis of breast cancer and the protective effect of early menopause has been well documented. Natural menopause occurring before age 45 is associated with one-half the breast cancer risk of menopause occurring after age 55 [1]. Early artificial menopause has a similar effect.

Effect of Artificial Menopause

Women who had undergone an artificial menopause by either surgical oophorectomy or radiation ablation prior to age 35 were found to have a 64% reduction in breast cancer risk compared to women with menopause at age 45–54 [1]. Feinleib [2] noted a 75% reduction in breast cancer incidence among women with artificial menopause before age 40, while in the epidemiologic study of Hirayama and Wynder [3] the relative risk of breast cancer showed a 59% reduction in women who were oophorectomized before age 37.

A key observation was the long-term, probably life-long, persistence of the risk reduction and this has been confirmed [4]. Even 30 or more years later, breast cancer risk was reduced by two-thirds in women with menopause induced before age 35 [1].

The protective effect of early oophorectomy on breast cancer risk confirms that ovarian hormones are key factors in breast cancer etiology. It would be imprudent however, to consider oophorectomy for the prevention of breast cancer under most, if not all circumstances. Although oophorectomy at a young age is associated with a 60–70% reduction in breast cancer risk, it must be accompanied by some replacement of estrogen.

Basil A. Stoll (ed.), Reducing Breast Cancer Risk in Women, 119–123.
© 1995 *Kluwer Academic Publishers. Printed in the Netherlands.*

Prophylactic bilateral oophorectomy and hysterectomy has been advocated for the prevention of ovarian cancer in individuals from families with a well-documented familial (genetic) predisposition to ovarian cancer [5, 6]. In such cases, oophorectomy would also be expected to substantially decrease the risk of breast cancer.

Trial of GnRH Agonist

We have previously argued that it is possible to develop a GnRHA (gonadotropin releasing hormone agonist)-based contraceptive, combining it with an ultra-low dose of estrogen and progestogen. This should protect against breast cancer by reducing breast mitogen exposure during the period of contraceptive use [7, 8].

GnRH agonists (GnRHA) are small peptides that cannot be administered orally. However, the development of depot formulations of GnRHA permits sustained suppression of ovarian steroid production, and serum estradiol and progesterone levels are suppressed to postmenopausal levels [9, 10].

The use of GnRHA as an improved method of contraception was initially explored based on potentially greater convenience, effectiveness, or fewer side effects than combination-type oral contraceptives (COCs) [8]. Following a decade of research, the contraceptive use of GnRHAs was abandoned as it appeared to offer no advantage. However, by combining a GnRHA with the steroids in COCs, the dose of sex steroids can be substantially reduced. This reduction in sex steroids should provide protection against the development of breast cancer [8].

The design aim is to give sufficient add-back estrogen to counter the hypoestrogenic state induced by GnRHA, but no more estrogen than is absolutely necessary since estrogen will counteract the benefits of GnRHA in protecting against breast and endometrial cancer. Available evidence suggests that a dose similar to that used as estrogen replacement therapy (ERT) for postmenopausal women is adequate, such as 0.625 mg/day of conjugated estrogens (CE). The dose of estrogen in current COCs (such as 30 μg of ethinyl estradiol) is unnecessarily high when administered with a GnRHA. The replacement of estrogen at a dose similar to that used for postmenopausal replacement therapy is expected to slighly increase breast cancer risk over the use of a GnRHA alone, but still be associated with a substantial reduction in breast cancer risk [7, 8].

The prescribing of a progestogen every fourth 28-day cycle is our calculated attempt to ensure that no endometrial problems arise, while retaining the breast cancer and cardiovascular benefit of GnRHA plus estrogen replacement therapy. Progestogens appear to be important breast mitogens [11], and although the available epidemiological data are sparse [12], we believe that the addition of a progestogen will increase the risk of breast cancer above that of ERT alone. As medroxyprogesterone acetate (MPA) is the progestogen most commonly administered with CE, it was chosen as the replacement progestogen in our pilot study [8].

There is evidence to suggest that progestogen is not required every cycle [13]. The minimum duration of progestogen administration necessary to control endometrial hyperplasia completely, appears to be 12–13 days, [14, 15]. It was therefore decided to administer the progestogen for 13 days only every fourth 28-day cycle to minimize exposure of the breast epithelium to progestogen, while preserving the maximum beneficial effects of the estrogen on cardiovascular disease risk, and still prevent endometrial hyperplasia.

Preliminary Results of Pilot Trial

Criteria for eligibility were: premenopausal women aged 25 to 40 with a 5-fold greater than normal risk of breast cancer; no prior malignancy; bone mineral density not less than 2 standard deviations below normal for age; normal cholesterol levels; and a normal physical and pelvic examination. The women were randomized in a 2 to 1 ratio to the contraceptive group or a control group.

The contraceptive group received: the GnRHA leuprolide acetate depot (Lupron Depot®, TAP Pharmaceuticals, Abbott Laboratories, North Chicago, IL) 7.5 mg by intramuscular injection (IM) every 28 days; CE (Premarin®, Wyeth–Ayerst, Philadelphia, PA) 0.625 mg by mouth (PO) for 6 days out of 7 every week; and MPA (Provera®, Upjohn, Kalamazoo, MI) 10 mg PO for 13 days every fourth 28-day cycle, i.e. every 112 days. If the subject reported adverse effects such as hot flushes or vaginal symptoms, the dose of CE was increased to 0.9 mg. Contraceptive subjects are scheduled to receive the regimen for 24 cycles.

Bone mineral density (BMD) falls after a natural or surgical menopause, and effects of GnRHA on bone metabolism are thus to be expected. In our pilot trial, despite the use of a CE dose thought to be adequate, an annualized decline of 2–3% in the lumbar spine BMD was seen in the contraceptive subjects [16]. We have thus added a small dose of androgen to replace the ovarian androgens suppressed by the GnRHA, and preliminary results show no further change in BMD.

Estrogen has significant effects on cardiovascular disease and ERT given to postmenopausal women will reduce risk of cardiovascular disease [17]. In our pilot trial, favorable increases in high-density lipoprotein cholesterol (HDLC) were seen, greatest (a 14% increase) in the cycles in which MPA was not administered [16]. Unscheduled bleeding or spotting occurred infrequently, and declined with time on the prototype contraceptive [16]. Scheduled bleeding occurred following each period of MPA use, i.e. every four months.

The effects of the contraceptive regimen on mammograms were assessed by comparing the baseline to follow-up images with controls. When the individual subjects' average change scores of mammographic densities were combined, the women on the contraceptive regimen had statistically significantly less mammographic densities at one year than at baseline [18]; while the mammographic densities of the control women remained essentially unchanged. Because increased mammographic densities are associated with an increased risk of breast cancer [19,

20] we believe that such a reduction in densities will be associated with a reduced risk of breast cancer.

Suppression of ovulation by GnRHA should protect against ovarian cancer to the same extent as do COCs, and the addition of CE and MPA to the GnRHA should have no effect on this reduced risk. Early menopause will substantially reduce endometrial cancer risk [21], and use of a GnRHA alone would similarly achieve a substantial reduction in a woman's risk of endometrial cancer. The addition of CE to the GnRHA will, however, increase the endometrial cancer risk when compared to use of GnRHA alone; while the addition of a progestogen, even if given only every fourth cycle, will reduce this risk.

Conclusion

It is presently possible to develop approaches which will reduce exposure of the premenopausal breast to estrogen and progestogens. In a pilot trial with a prototype using a GnRHA plus add-back CE and MPA, a substantial reduction in mammographic densities is evident. Development of more simplified regimens could prove an important advance in the prevention of breast cancer.

References

1. Trichopoulos, D., MacMahon, B., Cole, P. (1972). Menopause and breast cancer risk. *J. Natl. Cancer Inst.*, **48**, 605–613.
2. Feinleib, M. (1968). Breast cancer and artificial menopause: a cohort study. *J. Natl. Cancer Inst.*, 41, 315–329.
3. Hirayama, T., Wynder, E.L. (1962). A study of the epidemiology of cancer of the breast II. The influence of hysterectomy. *Cancer*, **15**, 28–38.
4. Brinton, L.A., Schairer, C., Hoover, R.N. (1988). Menstrual factors and risk of breast cancer. *Cancer Invest.*, **6**, 245–254.
5. Tobacman, J., Tucker, M., Kase, R. *et al.* (1982). Intra-abdominal carcinomatosis after prophylactic oophorectomy in ovarian-cancer-prone families. *Lancet*, **ii**, 795–797.
6. Cruickshank, D., Haites, N. *et al.* (1992) The multidisciplinary management of a family with epithelial ovarian cancer. *Br. J. Obstet. Gynaecol.*, **99**, 226–231.
7. Pike, M.C., Ross, R.K., Lobo, R.A. *et al.* (1989). LHRH agonists and the prevention of breast and ovarian cancer. *Br. J. Cancer*, **60**, 142–148.
8. Spicer, D.V., Shoupe, D., Pike, M. (1991). GnRH agonists as contraceptive agents: Predicted significantly reduced risk of breast cancer. *Contraception*, **44**, 289–310.
9. Friedman, A., Rein, M., Harrison-Atlas, D., Garfield, J., Doubilet, P. (1989). A randomized, placebo-controlled, double-blind study evaluating leuprolide acetate depot treatment before myomectomy. *Fertil. Steril.*, **52**, 728–733.
10. Schlaff, W., Zerhouni, E., Huth, J. *et al.* (1989). A placebo-controlled trial of a depot gonadotropin-releasing hormone analogue (Leuprolide) in the treatment of uterine leiomyomata. *Obstet. Gynecol.*, **74**, 856–862.
11. Pike, M.C., Spicer, D.V., Dahmoush, L., Press, M.F. (1993). Estrogens, progestogens, normal breast cell proliferation and breast cancer risk. *Epidemiol. Rev.*, **15**, 17–35.
12. Stanford, J., Thomas, D. (1993). Exogenous progestins and breast cancer. *Epidemiol. Rev.*, **15**, 98–107.

13. Schiff, I., Sela, H., Cramer, D., Tulchinsky, D., Ryan, K. (1982). Endometrial hyperplasia in women on cyclic or continuous estrogen regimens. *Fertil. Steril.*, **37**, 79–82.
14. Studd, J., Thom, M., Paterson, M. (1980). The prevention and treatment of endometrial pathology in postmenopausal women receiving exogenous oestrogens. In Pasetto, W., Pavletti, R., Lambrus, J. (eds.), *The Menopause and Postmenopause*, MTP Press, Lancaster, England, 127–138.
15. Whitehead, M., Lane, G., Siddle, N., Townsend, P., King, R. (1983). Avoidance of endometrial hyperstimulation in estrogen-treated postmenopausal women. *Semin. Reprod. Endocrin.*, **1**, 41–54.
16. Spicer, D.V., Pike, M.C., Pike, A. *et al.* (1993). Pilot trial of a gonadotropin hormone agonist with replacement hormones as a prototype contraceptive to prevent breast cancer. *Contraception*, **47**, 427–444.
17. Henderson, B., Ross, R., Lobo, R., Pike, M., Mack, T. (1988). Re-evaluating the role of progestogen therapy after the menopause. *Fertil. Steril.*, **49**, (Suppl.), 9–15.
18. Spicer, D., Ursin, G., Parisky, Y. *et al.* (1994). Changes in mammographic densities induced by a hormonal contraceptive designed to reduce breast cancer risk. *J. Natl. Cancer Inst.*, **86**, 431–436.
19. Saftlas, A.F., Szklo, M. (1987). Mammographic parenchymal patterns and breast cancer risk. *Epidemiol. Rev.*, **9**, 146–74.
20. Warner, E., Lockwood, G. (1992). The risk of breast cancer associated with mammographic parenchymal patterns: a meta – analysis of the published literature to examine the effect of method of classification. *Cancer Detect. Prev.*, **16**, 67–72.
21. Key, T.J.A., Pike, M.C. (1988). The dose-effect relationship between 'unopposed' oestrogens and endometrial mitotic rate: its central role in explaining and predicting endometrial cancer risk. *Br. J. Cancer*, **57**, 205–212.

Chapter 14

Compliance by High-Risk Women

HENRY T. LYNCH, JANE F. LYNCH and THERESA CONWAY

Inherited susceptibility to breast cancer includes several distinct syndromes [1–3], each involving heritable genetic mutations [4–6]. Compliance by families in the control of hereditary breast cancer (HBC) is increased if its members are educated about the genetics and natural history of the disease. We initiate education in the mid-to-late teens but breast self-examination and semi-annual physician breast examination should begin at age 20. We begin mammography at age 25 and perform this annually.

In families where there is strong evidence of the BRCA1 gene indicating high susceptibility to breast and ovarian cancers, we advise women identified as BRCA1 carriers to consider having their families early and undergo prophylactic oophorectomy by about age 35. In spite of oophorectomy however, evidence of peritoneal spread of cancer appears later in about 5% of cases, even though the ovaries may have appeared normal at the time of the operation.

Should hereditary breast cancer be managed differently from the so-called sporadic type of breast cancer? The answer to this question is uncertain but we prefer mastectomy to lumpectomy on the basis of what is known about the natural history of HBC. Because of the early onset of breast cancer in HBC, the patient remains at risk for a number of years after the initial cancer treatment, and because of the known danger of multiple foci of cancer in the breast, new lesions may appear. We are also concerned about the danger of lesions arising in the opposite breast, and we recommend prophylactic mastectomy for the opposite breast when the original lesion has been adequately controlled.

One must also consider that radiation therapy is associated with lumpectomy and there are possible dangers from its long-term effects, apart from potential danger from scattered radiation to the opposite breast or other organs. Thus, an excess incidence of lung cancer has been reported on the same side as that given radiation [7]. There is also the possibility of genetic sensitivity to radiation in some

Basil A. Stoll (ed.), Reducing Breast Cancer Risk in Women, 125–131.
© 1995 *Kluwer Academic Publishers. Printed in the Netherlands.*

HBC syndromes, for example, in patients homozygous for the gene for ataxia telangiectasia.

Psychological Management for HBC

What proportion of people would like to be informed about their genetic susceptibility to cancer? In a sample of the public, 83% of respondents expressed interest in a genetic test for colon cancer susceptibility [8]. In a study of first-degree relatives of ovarian cancer patiennts [9] 75% said they would definitely want to obtain a genetic test for BRCA1. It appears that persons with a strong interest in genetic testing were more likely to exhibit psychological distress and to anticipate serious consequences of receiving adverse test results.

While a heavy emotional burden is placed on an individual testing positive for a cancer-prone gene [9,10], emotional stress may also be observed among persons told that they are *not* carriers of a deleterious gene, the so-called survival guilt [11–14]. It is also reported that individuals who withdraw from testing or receive uninformative results may be at the greatest risk for adverse psychological consequences [15].

An adverse emotional reaction to testing positive for BRCA1 could interfere with adherence to cancer prevention practices [10]. In previous studies, anxiety was shown to be associated with a reduced likelihood of adherence to mammography [16, 17], as well as to clinical breast examination and breast self-examination [18]. Lerman *et al.* [17, 19] and Li and Fraumeni [20], who researched the psychological impact of cancer risk notification, demonstrated that it can cause anxiety, traumatic stress symptoms and impaired daily functioning [17, 19, 20] and that such distress can impair adherence to breast cancer screening [16, 17]. Recent studies have focused on psychological issues in relation to genetic testing for cancer susceptibility [8, 9, 17, 21].

Counselors must be aware of the patient's need to understand the natural history of the disease in order to make informed decisions about surveillance and to ensure compliance. Merely dispensing accurate genetic information may be ineffective or even harmful. Education of patients from HBC families can be provided individually or in groups of up to fifteen or twenty family members. Both approaches enable the clinician to present detailed information about the natural history of HBC and its genetic basis to family members. Questions are encouraged both to evaluate the level of understanding and also to reinforce the impact of the educational message.

Advantages of the group approach are the relaxed atmosphere, the discussion of issues among members of the group and the reduced inhibitions about asking pertinent questions. It also enables multiple family members to hear questions asked by their relatives which are representative of their own concerns. We also believe that group education enhances the ability of individual family members to use the resources for emotional support within the family. It also may be a less expensive method of providing education.

On the other hand, individual sessions may facilitate attention to concerns of particular family members, and may reduce the effect of intrafamily pressure to see things and do things in a particular way. Group precounseling education may lead some persons to request genetic testing who otherwise would not do so.

In both group and individual approaches, education can be enhanced by providing written descriptive material about HBC in advance. We have developed material written at the level of understanding of the average patient. It contains descriptive material relevant to the age of onset, organs involved, and the rationale for our specific surveillance and management recommendations. We also provide a pedigree of their family, depicting their position in the pedigree and its risk significance. With the patients' consent, a detailed letter is sent to primary physicians explaining their patients' cancer genetic risk, as well as the information provided to them about the natural history of cancer in the family and our surveillance and management recommendations.

Psychosocial Problems in Selected HBC Families

In Family A (Figure 1) the 39 year old proband (IV–1), at 50% risk for breast cancer due to her position in an HBC kindred, contacted our Hereditary Cancer Institute for personal cancer risk assessment. Her mother (III–1) had recently been diagnosed with recurrent, Stage IV breast cancer. The proband was being monitored by her physician for a palpable and painful breast mass occurring during the middle of her menstrual cycle. Mammograms had been performed annually since she was 35 years of age and were negative. Her physician did not recommend a biopsy, believing that the mass was related to her cycle and probably benign. Although the patient wanted a breast biopsy, she felt she had no 'authority' to request this from her physician. Her fear of breast cancer increased to the extent that she elected to undergo prophylactic bilateral mastectomy with immediate reconstruction. Could a biopsy have reduced the fear? In a follow-up telephone call five months after her surgery, the patient reported that she was psychologically less fearful of breast cancer and very pleased with reconstruction results.

Patient II–6 (Figure 2) identified as an obligate gene carrier in Family B was counseled and given the options of intensive breast cancer surveillance or prophylactic bilateral mastectomy. She selected prophylactic surgery with immediate reconstruction. Pathological review of the breast tissue revealed bilateral ductal hyperplasia with no atypia noted. Following her surgery, she expressed to us the gratitude she felt for the knowledge about HBC that she had gained from participating in the family study. She wished this information could have been available to her sister (II–5), who had been diagnosed with *bilateral* breast cancer and died fifteen years earlier of metastatic disease.

Family C (Figure 3) is a hereditary breast-ovarian cancer (HBOC) kindred that was found to be linked to the BRCA1 locus at chromosome 17q and given individual risk assessment. The significance of linkage findings, as well as the

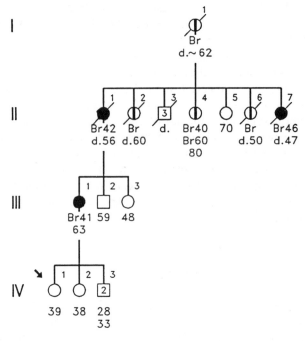

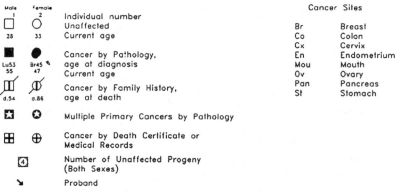

Figure 1. Pedigree of hereditary breast cancer family A whose psychosocial aspects are discussed in the text.

benefits and limitations of receiving personal risk assessment based on the linkage data were discussed with family members first by letter, and then by a family group information session. Individual sessions to reveal carrier status were then provided if requested by family members. The proband (II–I) attended the family information session with her husband. However, she elected *not* to be told her risk status because of her fear of insurance discrimination. Because of an anticipated change of insurance providers, the patient felt that she would be obligated to report

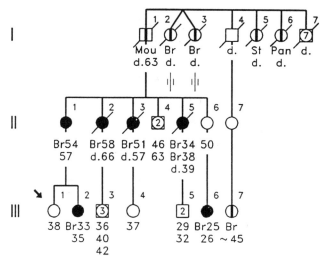

Figure 2. Pedigree of hereditary breast cancer family B whose sociopsychological dynamics are discussed in the text. (For key see Figure 1.)

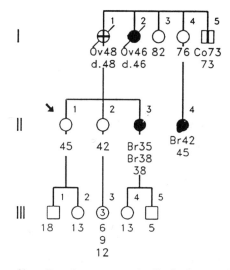

Figure 3. Pedigree of hereditary breast cancer family C whose sociopsychological dynamics are discussed in the text. (For key see Figure 1.)

the results of genetic counseling. She feared that if she was found to be a BRCA1 gene carrier, then she, her family, and the family's small business might be denied coverage or be required to pay increased insurance rates.

Family D (Figure 4) depicts extremely early age onset breast cancer in the proband (IV–4) of this HBC kindred. The proband presented to her primary care physician at the age of 18 with a pea-size breast mass. The clinical evaluation was

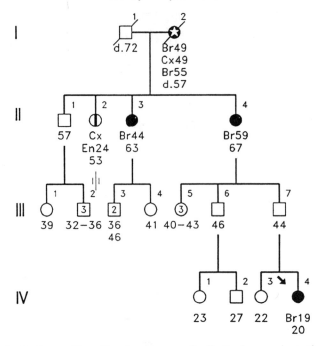

Figure 4. Pedigree of hereditary breast cancer family D whose sociopsychological dynamics are discussed in the text. (For key see Figure 1.)

a possible fibroadenoma and she was told to return in six months. Nine months later the patient returned, at which time the mass was found to have grown to the size of a grape. A mammogram was positive. Biopsy revealed mucinous carcinoma and ductal carcinoma *in situ*, comedo type. A modified radical mastectomy was performed with no tumor found in thirteen lymph nodes. The patient elected to have contralateral prophylactic total mastectomy with immediate bilateral reconstruction. Adjuvant chemotherapy was initiated. Five months following her diagnosis, however, the proband's father reported that his daughter was having difficulty expressing her fears and concerns. She had discontinued chemotherapy after completing only two cycles. She had attended local breast cancer support groups, but felt alone in that there were no other women in attendance who had her similar circumstances – single, young with cancer, and lacking all breast tissue.

Conclusion

There are undoubtedly many similarities between the emotional responses and behavior of breast cancer patients belonging to hereditary breast cancer families and those without such family histories. A major difference is, however, that most patients from breast cancer syndrome families have witnessed early-onset cancer in one or more close relatives. As reflected in our examples, these cancer experiences usually lead to a sense of high personal cancer risk. They can accentuate psychological problems such as depression, anger, denial or bewilderment, but they can also inform patients about cancer and motivate them to seek further information and treatment.

References

1. Easton, D.F., Bishop, D.T., Ford, D. *et al.* (1993). Genetic linkage analysis in familial breast and ovarian cancer: results from 214 families. *Am. J. Hum. Genet.*, **52**, 678–701.
2. Lynch, H.T., Lynch, J.F. (1986). Breast cancer genetics in an oncology clinic: 328 consecutive patients. *Cancer Genet. Cytogenet.*, **22**, 369–371.
3. Lynch, H.T., Albano, W.A., Danes, B.S., *et al.* (1984). Genetic predisposition to breast cancer. *Cancer*, **53**, 612–622.
4. Malkin, D., Li, F.P., Stron, L.C. *et al.* (1990). Germ line p53 mutations in a familial syndrome of breast cancer, sarcomas and other neoplasms. *Science*, **250**, 1233–1238.
5. Hall, J.M., Lee, M.K., Newman, B. *et al.* (1990). Linkage of early-onset breast cancer to chromosome 17q21. *Science*, **250**, 1684–1689.
6. Narod, S.A., Feunteun, J., Lynch, H.T. *et al.* (1991). Familial breast-ovarian cancer locus on chromosome 17q12–q23. *Lancet*, **338**, 82.
7. Neugut, A.I., Murray, T., Santos, J. *et al.* (1994). Increased risk of lung cancer after breast cancer radiation therapy in cigarette smokers. *Cancer*, **73**, 1615–1620.
8. Croyle, R.T., Lerman, C. (1993). Interest in genetic testing for colon cancer susceptibility: cognitive and emotional correlates. *Prev. Med.*, **22**, 284–292.
9. Lerman, C., Croyle R. (1994). Psychological issues in genetic testing for breast cancer suscep- tibility. *Arch. Intern. Med.* (In press).
10. Lerman, C., Rimer, B., Engstrom, P. (1991). Cancer risk notification: Psychological and ethical implications. *J. Clin. Oncol.*, **9**, 1275–1282.
11. Lynch, H.T., Watson, P., Conway, T.A., *et al.* (1993). DNA screening for breast/ovarian cancer susceptibility based on linked markers. *Arch. Intern. Med.*, **153**, 1979–1987.
12. Hayden, M.R. (1991). Predictive testing for Huntington's disease: are we ready for widespread community implementation? *Am. J. Med. Genet.*, **40**, 515–517.
13. Meissen, G.J., Mastromauro, C.A., Kiely, D.K. *et al.* (1991). Understanding the decision to take the predictive test for Huntington's disease. *Am. J. Med. Genet.*, **39**, 404–410.
14. Perry, T.L. (1981). Some ethical problems in Huntington's chorea. *Can. Med. Assoc. J.*, **125**, 1098–1100.
15. Wiggins, S., Whyte, P., Huggins, M. *et al.* (1993). The psychological consequences of predictive testing for Huntington's disease. *N. Engl. J. Med.*, **327**, 1401–1405.
16. Lerman, C., Rimer, B.K., Trock, B. *et al.* (1990). Factors associated with repeat adherence to breast cancer screening. *Prev. Med.*, 19, 279–290.
17. Lerman, C., Daly, M., Sands, C. *et al.* (1993). Mammography adherence and psychological distress among women at risk for breast cancer. *J. Natl. Cancer Inst.*, **85**, 1074–1080.
18. Kash, K.M., Holland, J.C., Halper, M.S., Miller, D.G. (1992). Psychological distress and surveil- lance behaviors of women with a family history of breast cancer. *J. Natl. Cancer Inst.*, **84**, 24–30.
19. Lerman, C., Rimer, B., Engstrom, P. (1991). Cancer risk notification: Psychological and ethical implications. *J. Clin. Oncol.*, **9**, 1275–1282.
20. Li, F.O., Fraumeni, J.F., Jr. (1992). Predictive tesing for inherited mutations in cancer- susceptibility genes. *J. Clin. Oncol.*, **10**, 1203–1204.
21. Daly, M., Lerman, C. (1993). Ovarian cancer risk counseling. *Semin. Oncol.*, **7**, 27–34.

PART THREE

AVOIDANCE OF POSSIBLE RISK FACTORS

Chapter 15

Dietary Guidelines

MICHELLE D. HOLMES, DAVID J. HUNTER and
WALTER C. WILLETT

There are five-fold differences in breast cancer incidence rates around the world
[1], and migrants moving from low- to high-incidence countries acquire rates close
to those of the new country after one generation [2]. Differences in diet, among
other lifestyle influences, may explain these observations but no dietary component
except alcohol can yet be confidently associated with increased risk of breast cancer.

The most prominent hypothesis has been that high fat intake increases risk.
Alcohol and caffeine have also been proposed as increasing risk while dietary
fiber, as well as the antioxidant micronutrients selenium and vitamins A, C and E
have been proposed as protective. The fat hypothesis will not be reviewed here as
it is discussed fully in another chapter.

Dietary Fiber

Fiber may reduce the intestinal reabsorption of estrogens excreted via the biliary
system. It has been hypothesized that diets high in fiber may be protective against
breast cancer [3], but few epidemiologic studies have reported on the association
of fiber with breast cancer risk. A meta-analysis of 10 case-control studies reported
a protective effect involving a relative risk (RR) of 0.85 for a 20 g/day increase in
dietary fiber [4]. In a case-control study of 519 cases, a high fiber intake was associated with a marginally significant decreased risk, but this association appeared to
be confounded by vitamin A intake [5].

An association has not been shown in cohort studies. In the largest of these, the
Nurses' Health Study with 1,439 cases, there was virtually no effect of total dietary
fiber intake on subsequent breast cancer incidence [6]. In another cohort with 344
cases there was no suggestion of a protective association [7]. This suggests that

135

Basil A. Stoll (ed.), Reducing Breast Cancer Risk in Women, 135–144.
© 1995 *Kluwer Academic Publishers. Printed in the Netherlands.*

any protective effect of dietary fiber is unlikely to be large but it is possible that some subfractions of fiber intake may be relevant in breast cancer etiology.

Vitamin A

Vitamin A consists of two forms: (i) preformed vitamin A (retinol, retinyl esters and related compounds) found in animal sources; (ii) carotenoids which are partially converted to retinol in the intestinal epithelium (carotenoid vitamin A) found primarily in fruits and vegetables. Many carotenoids are potent antioxidants.

Most studies of vitamin A intake and breast cancer risk have been case-control studies [8–22]. Four studies have reported data for total vitamin A intake (retinol plus carotenoids with vitamin A activity); all report a protective association. The largest case-control study reports a protective association (RR = 0.8) comparing the highest quartile of vitamin A consumption with the lowest [8]. A meta-analysis of nine other case-control studies also found a significant protective association between total vitamin A and the risk of breast cancer [4].

The results for preformed vitamin A are mixed: Of nine case-control studies comparing the highest and lowest categories of intake, four found either no association or an increased risk of breast cancer (RR over 1.0), and five found decreased risk (RR less than 0.9). Fourteen studies evaluated carotenoid vitamin A. Four studies found no effect or increased risk (RR $\geq$ 1.0), and ten found a protective effect (RR $\leq$ 0.8). In a meta-analysis of case-control studies, eight studies with data on β-carotene showed a significant protective effect, while no association was present among eight studies with data for preformed vitamin A [4]. Thus, the data from case-control studies more strongly support a protective association for carotenoid vitamin A than for preformed vitamin A.

Fewer data from cohort studies are available [5, 7, 23, 24]. The Nurses' Health Study, assessed these associations among the cohort of 89, 494 women described earlier. It observed a modest (RR = 0.8), but significant, protective association for total vitamin A. This association was somewhat stronger for preformed vitamin A than for carotenoid vitamin A [24]. In another cohort in a California retirement community with 123 cases of breast cancer, there was a protective effect for both total vitamin A and β-carotene (RR for each = 0.8) [23]. In a New York State cohort (344 cases) there was no association [7]. In a Canadian cohort (519 cases) a marginally significant protective association between total vitamin A intake and breast cancer risk was observed; both preformed vitamin A and β-carotene contributed to this inverse association [5]. Thus, the data from cohort studies support a modest protective effect of vitamin A.

An alternative to the dietary assessment of vitamin A intake, is the measurement of vitamin A compounds in blood. Unfortunately, most studies have assessed blood retinol which is unresponsive to retinol intake in well-nourished populations [25]. Blood levels of β-carotene do reflect β-carotene intake. However, there is little consistency among these studies. Case-control studies in Italy and Boston did not find a protective association [11,22]. Another case-control study in New York did observe a significant protective association [15]. Only one out of three cohort studies reported a protective effect; however, these studies were limited by the small number of cases (52 in the largest) [22–28]. A potential limitation in these studies is that blood β-carotene levels are unstable, and may degrade even at -70°C [29].

In summary, available data are suggestive, but not conclusive, of a protective association between vitamin A intake and breast cancer risk. A randomized trial of the synthetic retinoid fenretinide, to prevent second breast cancer development in women following surgery for a first breast cancer, is underway in Italy. In addition, the recently commenced Women's Health Study will test the effect of β-carotene among 44,000 post-menopausal women in the U.S.

Vitamin E

Vitamin E is also an antioxidant. Vitamin E has been proposed as a treatment for benign breast disease for almost 30 years [30]. Relatively few studies have reported on the association between dietary vitamin E intake and breast cancer risk. Five case-control studies have had mixed results; three reported a protective association (RR = 0.6 to 0.7) [17, 19, 22], while another two have reported either no association or increased risk (RR = 1.0 to 1.3) [13, 20]. None of the three published cohort studies has reported a significant protective effect [5, 7, 24]. The largest of these, the Nurses' Health Study, included almost as many cases as the five case-control studies combined. In this study, an initially weak protective association with vitamin E disappeared entirely when vitamin A was controlled for, and there was no evidence of a protective association with consumption of vitamin E supplements [24].

Blood levels of vitamin E reflect vitamin E intake, especially after controlling for blood lipid levels [31]. Two case-control studies have examined blood levels of vitamin E; one showed an association with increased risk and one showed a weak protective association [22, 32]. An initial report of a protective association with higher serum vitamin E from a cohort in Guernsey with 39 cases may have been due to differential degradation of vitamin E between cases and controls. Results were not confirmed in a further follow-up of this cohort [26, 33]. The two other prospective studies offer little support for the hypothesis that higher levels of serum vitamin E are protective [28, 34].

Vitamin C

The largest case-control study reported did not observe a protective association with breast cancer risk for vitamin C [8]. However, in a subsequent study by the same group a significant protective association was found for the highest compared to the lowest intake (RR = 0.6) [17]. A meta-analysis of nine other case-control studies found vitamin C to be protective (RR = 0.69 for each 300 mg/day increase in vitamin C) [4].

Three cohort studies have reported on the relation of vitamin C to breast cancer risk [5, 7, 24]. Only one observed a protective effect, and that was not statistically significant [7].

Thus, the existing data on intake of vitamin C and breast cancer risk are inconsistent. The available cohort data do not support a protective effect and more prospective data with longer periods of follow-up, are needed. As intake of the different antioxidant micronutrients is often positively correlated, careful attention should be given to controlling intake of each micronutrient for the others.

Selenium

Selenium is an important component of the antioxidant enzyme glutathione peroxidase. Studies have shown strong inverse associations between measures of selenium exposure and breast cancer rates [35–37] but should be interpreted with caution. In the US for instance, high-selenium areas tend to be sparsely populated rural areas which differ in many respects from low-selenium areas. Selenium intake cannot be measured accurately by dietary assessment because the selenium content of individual foods may vary up to 100-fold depending on the geographic area in which the foods were grown [38].

Fortunately, selenium levels in tissues such as blood and toenails do reflect selenium intake [39, 40]. Two case control studies of breast cancer risk and selenium give mixed results. A small study of 38 cases showed an elevated risk (RR = 2.0) with higher red blood cell selenium levels, but the results were not statistically significant [41]. The second study observed a protective association of high selenium as measured in plasma, while there was virtually no association when selenium was measured in red blood cells and toenails [42]. Since red blood cell and toenail selenium levels reflect longer term intake, these results are consistent with breast cancer itself decreasing plasma levels in the cases.

In contrast, a recent prospective study of postmenopausal Dutch women found that women with breast cancer had levels of toenail selenium which were (non-significantly) higher than controls [43]. The largest cohort study observed no association between toenail selenium levels and risk of breast cancer over four years of follow-up [44]. Of the four other cohort studies, three showed no significant effect [45–47].

One study from Finland showed evidence of increased risk among women in the lowest level category of selenium [48]. As Finland has the lowest dietary selenium levels of any of the countries studied, this observation is consistent with the possibility that a threshold exists below which low selenium intake does increase breast cancer risk. While this possibility deserves further exploration, it seems unlikely that selenium is significantly associated with breast cancer risk for most women in countries with moderate or high levels of selenium intake.

Alcohol

The association between alcohol and breast cancer has been controversial but in recent years, substantial evidence has accumulated to support an association of increased breast cancer risk with alcohol consumption. A meta-analysis of 30 epidemiologic studies estimated an 11% increased risk for one drink daily of alcohol [49].

Cohort studies of alcohol intake and breast cancer are summarized in Table 1 [50–58]. The meta-analysis mentioned above examined four cohort studies, and calculated a combined increased risk of 40% for women drinking 12 g/day (1 drink), and a 70% increased risk for 24 g/day of alcohol [49]. Five more cohort studies have been published subsequent to this meta-analysis. The two smallest studies showed no effect [51, 52]. However, the three largest studies (all of which controlled for major breast cancer risk factors) showed increased risks of 1.5 to 3 times higher for the highest category of alcohol consumption compared with no consumption [53–55].

Until recently, the association between alcohol intake and breast cancer seen in epidemiological studies suffered from the lack of a plausible mechanism for increased risk. A recent controlled metabolic study has demonstrated increases in total estrogen and bioavailable estrogen blood levels with daily intake of 30 g of alcohol (about 2 drinks) [59].

Thus, an increased risk among women consuming moderate amounts of alcohol is probably the best established dietary risk factor for breast cancer. However, if this knowledge is to be translated into public health recommendations, then it is important to establish whether quitting alcohol consumption in middle life is beneficial. Unfortunately, relatively few data are available to link age-specific drinking patterns with breast cancer risk.

The preliminary analyses of a large case-control study reported that recent consumption of 3+ drinks per day was associated with a relative breast cancer risk of 2.2, while the relative risk was only 0.9 for consumption of 3+ drinks per day from ages 16–29 [60]. This study suggests that drinking later in life may be more important than early adult drinking patterns. Conflicting results were found in another study however, where women who drank before age 30 and later stopped, experienced a similar elevation in risk to those who continued to drink [61].

Similarly, another study observed an increase in risk among past drinkers compared with women who never drank (RR = 2.2), although the age at quitting alcohol consumption was unspecified [56]. These findings are consistent with other data indicating that the breast is more susceptible to cancer risk factors during adolescence and early adult life, and suggest that in order to reduce their risk, women may have to reduce their alcohol consumption at an early age.

Table 1. Prospective studies of alcohol consumption in relation to risk of breast cancer

Study (Reference)	Population	Number of cases	Comparison	Relative risk (95% confidence interval) for high vs. low categories	Controlled for
Seidman et al., 1982* (58)	U.S.	3,130	Daily vs. < Daily Alcohol	1.2	–
Hiatt and Bawol, 1984 (53)	U.S.	1,169	≥ 3 drinks/day vs. 0	1.4 (p = 0.03)	Race, education, smoking, BMI, 1 or more reproductive risk factors.
Schatzkin et al., 1987 (57)	U.S.	88	≥ 5 g/day vs. 0	2.0 (1.1–3.7)	Age, education, race, BMI, dietary fat, 1 or more reproductive risk factors.
Willet et al., 1987 (50)	U.S.	601	≥ 15 g/day vs. 0	1.6 (1.3–2.0)	Age, menopausal status, maternal history of breast cancer, 1 or more reproductive risk factors.
Hiatt et al., 1988 (56)	U.S.	303	≥ 6 drinks/day vs. 0	3.3 (1.2–9.3)	Age, race, BMI, smoking.
Garfinkel et al., 1988+ (54)	U.S.	2,933	≥ 6 drinks/day vs. 0	1.6 (1.0–2.6)	Age, education, smoking, meat consumption, family history of breast cancer, 1 or more reproductive risk factors.
Schatzkin et al., 1989 (51)	U.S.	141	≥ 5 g/day vs. 0	0.8 (0.5–1.2)	Age, BMI, menopausal status, 1 or more reproductive risk factors.
Simon et al., 1991 (52)	U.S.	87	≥ 2 drinks/day vs. 0	1.1 (0.3–5.0)	Age, BMI, skinfold measurements, education, smoking, family history of breast cancer, 1 or more reproductive risk factors.
Gapstur (55)	??	493	??	1.5 (1.0–2.0)	??

*Rates for Seidman et al. study are interpolated from figure, among women with no other risk factors. +Mortality, not incidence, used as endpoint. BMI = Body Mass Index.

Caffeine

A report that women with benign breast disease experienced relief from symptoms after eliminating caffeine from their diet led to speculation that caffeine may be a risk factor for breast cancer [62]. The majority of case-control studies however, have not observed evidence of a positive association. A cohort study of Seventh Day Adventist women showed no increase in breast cancer risk among those who consumed coffee [63]. The Nurses Health Study actually observed a weak, but significant protective association between caffeine consumption and risk of breast cancer [64]. Thus, the epidemiologic evidence is not compatible with any substantial increase in breast cancer risk associated with caffeine intake.

Conclusion

Among environmental factors, it remains likely that diet is an important determinant of breast cancer. Dietary fat intake in middle life is probably not strongly related to breast cancer development, at least within the range of typical Western diets. However, the hypothesis that very low fat intakes (<20% of calories) may be protective has not been fully tested.

It is possible that vitamin A or other antioxidant or antiproliferative agent, may reduce breast cancer risk. Further investigations are however required.

Evidence for an association between moderate alcohol intake and increased breast cancer risk is substantial but it is unclear whether the risk is associated primarily with consumption during youth or throughout life. Making recommendations for an individual is complicated by the fact that moderate alcohol drinking may decrease the risk of cardiovascular disease [65].

Cost-benefit analysis for individual women depends on their relative cardiovascular or breast cancer risk factors. Women who do not smoke and are otherwise at low risk of coronary heart disease may, on balance, benefit by limiting alcohol consumption to not more than a few drinks per week.

While public health pronouncements are not yet possible on dietary changes which may prevent cancer, useful information can be given to women on ways which *potentially* lower heart cancer risk yet cause no harm; (i) Dietary reduction of saturated and hydrogenated fat is unlikely to cause harm and is likely to lower the risk of cardiovascular disease [66] and colon cancer [67], even if breast cancer risk is not influenced. (ii) Diets high in fresh fruits and vegetables are likely to reduce risk from other cancers [68] and may reduce breast cancer risk as well.

Motivated patients with breast cancer who wish to follow diets high in fruits and vegetables and low in fat, appear to have little to lose.

Acknowledgement

Our thanks to Tracey Corrigan, for manuscript preparation.

References

1. Muir, C.S., Waterhouse, J., Mack, L. *et al.* (1987). Cancer incidence on five continents. In *International Agency for Research on Cancer* IARC Scientific Publication, No. 88, Lyon, 882–883.
2. Kelsey, J.L., Horn-Ross, P.L. (1993). Breast cancer: Magnitude of the problem and descriptive epidemiology. *Epidemiol. Rev.*, **15**, 7–16.
3. Goldin, B.R., Aldercreutz, H., Gorbach, S.L., *et al.* (1982). Estrogen excertion patterns and plasma levels in vegetarian and omnivorous women. *N. Engl. J. Med.*, **307**, 1542–1547.
4. Howe, G.R., Hirohata, T., Hislop, T.G. *et al.* (1990). Dietary factors and risk of breast cancer: combined analysis of 12 case–control studies. *J. Natl. Cancer Inst.*, **82**, 561–569.
5. Rohan, T.E., Howe, G.R. Friedenreich, C.M. *et al.* (1993). Dietary fiber, vitamins A, C, and E, and risk of breast cancer: a cohort study. *Cancer Causes and Control*, **4**, 29–37.
6. Willett, W.C., Hunter, D.J., Stampfer, M.J. *et al.* (1992). Dietary fat and fiber in relation to risk of breast cancer. *J. Am. Med. Assoc.*, **268**, 2037–2044.
7. Graham, S., Zielezny, M., Marshall, J. *et al.* (1992). Diet in the epidemiology of postmenopausal breast cancer in the New York State cohort. *Am. J. Epidemiol.*, **136**, 1327–1337.
8. Graham, S., Marshall, J., Mettlin, C. *et al.* (1982). Diet in the epidemiology of breast cancer. *Am. J. Epidemiol.*, **116**, 68–75.
9. LaVecchia, C., Decarli, A., Franceschi, S. *et al.* (1987). Dietary factors and the risk of breast cancer. *Nutr. Cancer.*, **10**, 205–214.
10. Katsouyanni, K., Willett, W., Trichopoulos, D. *et al.* (1988). Risk of breast cancer among Greek women in relation to nutrien intake. *Cancer*, **61**, 181–185.
11. Marubini, E. Decarli, A., Costa, A. *et al.* (1988). The relationship of dietary intake and serum levels of retinol and β-carotene with breast cancer. *Cancer*, **61**, 173–180.
12. Rohan, T.E., McMichael, A.J., Baghurst, P.A. (1988). A population-based case-control study of diet and breast cancer in Australia. *Am. J. Epidemiol.*, **61**, 173–180.
13. Toniolo, P., Riboli, E., Protta, F. *et al.* (1989). Calorie–providing nutrients and risk of breast cancer. *J. Natl. Cancer Inst.*, **81**, 278–286.
14. Ewertz, M., Gill, C. (1990). Dietary factors and breast-cancer risk in Denmark. *Int. J. Cancer*, **46**, 779–784.
15. Potischman, N., McCullock, C.F., Byers, T. *et al.* (1990). Breast cancer and plasma concentrations of carotenoids and vitamin A. *Am. J. Clin. Nutr.*, **52**, 909–915.
16. Van 't Veer, P., Kalb, C.M., Verhoef, P. *et al.* (1990). Dietary fiber, β-carotene and breast cancer: results from a case-control study. *Int. J. Cancer*, **45**, 825–828.
17. Graham, S., Hellmann, R., Marshall, J., *et al.* (1991). Nutritional epidemiology of postmenopausal breast cancer in western New York. *Am. J. Epidemiol.*, **134**, 552–566.
18. Ingram, D.M., Nottage, E., Roberts, T. (1991). The role of diet in the development of breast cancer: a case-control study of patients with breast cancer, benign epithelial hyperplasia and fibrocystic disease of the breast. *Br. J. Cancer*, **64**, 187–191.
19. Lee, H.P., Gourley, L., Duffy, S.W. *et al.* (1991). Dietary effects on breast-cancer risk in Singapore. *Lancet*, **337**, 1197–1200.
20. Richardson, S., Gerber, M., Cenee, S. (1991). The role of fat, animal protein and some vitamin consumption in breast cancer: a case-control study in Southern France. *Int. J. Cancer*, **48**, 1–9.
21. Zaridze, D., Lifanova, Y., Maximovitch, D. *et al.* (1991). Diet, alcohol consumption and reproductive factors in a case-control study of breast cancer in Moscow. *Int. J. Cancer*, **48**, 493–501.
22. London, S.J., Stein, E.A., Henderson, I.C., *et al.* (1992). Carotenoids, retinol, and vitamin E and risk of proliferative benign breast disease and breast cancer. *Cancer Causes and Control*, **3**, 503–512.
23. Paganini-Hill, A., Chao, A., Ross, R.K., *et al.* (1987). Vitamin A, β-carotene and the risk of cancer: a prospective study. *J. Natl. Cancer Inst.*, **79**, 443–448.

24. Hunter, D.J., Manson, J.E., Colditz, G.A., *et al.* (1993). A prospective study of consumption of vitamins C, E and A and breast cancer risk. *N. Engl. J. Med.*, **329**, 234–240.
25. Willett, W.C., Stampfer, M.J., Underwood, B.A., *et al.* (1984). Vitamin A supplementation and plasma retinol levels: a randomized trial among women. *J. Natl. Cancer Inst.*, **73**, 1445–1448.
26. Wald, N.J., Boreham, J., Hayward, J.L., *et al.* (1984). Plasma retinol, beta-carotene and vitamin E levels in relation to the future risk of breast cancer. *Br. J. Cancer*, **49**, 321–324.
27. Knekt, P., Aromaa, A., Maatela, J., *et al.* (1990). Serum vitamin A and the subsequent risk of cancer: cancer incidence follow-up of the Finnish Mobile Clinic Health Examination Survey. *Am. J. Epidemiol.*, **132**, 857–870.
28. Comstock, G.W., Helzlsouer, K.J., Bush, T.L. (1991). Prediagnostic serum levels of carotenoids and vitamin E as related to subsequent cancer in Washington County, Maryland. *Am. J. Clin. Nutr.*, **53**, 260S–264S.
29. Ziegler, R.G. (1991). Vegetables, fruits, and carotenoids and the risk of cancer. *Am. J. Clin. Nutr.*, **53**, 251S–259S.
30. Abrams, A.A. (1965). Use of vitamin E in chronic cyctic mastitis (letter). *N. Engl. J. Med.*, **272**, 1080–1081.
31. Willett, W.C., Stampfer, M.J., Underwood, B.A. *et al.* (1983). Validation of a dietary questionnaire with plasma carotenoid and alpha–tocopherol levels. *Am. J. Clin. Nutr.*, **38**, 631–639.
32. Gerber, M., Cavallo, F., Marubini, E. *et al.* (1988). Liposoluable vitamins and lipid parameters in breast cancer. A joint study in northern Italy and southern France. *Int. J. Cancer*, **42**, 489–494.
33. Wald, N.J., Nicolaides–Bouman, A., Hudson, G.A. (1988). Plasma retinol, β-carotene and vitamin E levels in relation to future risk of breast cancer. *Br. J. Cancer*, **57**, 235.
34. Knekt, P. (1988). Serum vitamin E level and risk of female cancers. *Int. J. Epidemiol.*, **17**, 281–286.
35. Shamberger, R.J., Tytko, S.A., Willis, C.E. (1976). Antioxidants and cancer, VI: selenium and age–adjusted human cancer mortality. *Arch. Environ. Health*, **31**, 231–235.
36. Clark, L.C. (1985). The epidemiology of selenium and cancer. *Fed. Proc.*, **44**, 2584–2589.
37. Schrauzer, G.N., White, D.A., Schneider, C.J. (1977). Cancer mortality correlation studies, III: statistical associations with dietary selenium intakes. *Bioinorg. Chem.*, **7**, 23–35.
38. Levander, O.A. (1986). The need for a measure of selenium status. *J. Am. Coll. Toxicol.*, **5**, 37–44.
39. Hunter, D.J. (1990). Biochemical indicators of dietary intake. In Willett, W. (ed.), *Nutritional Epidemiology*, Oxford University Press New York, 143–216.
40. Hunter, D.J., Morris, J.S., Chute, C.G. *et al.* (1990). Predictors of selenium concentration in human toenails. *Am. J. Epidemiol.*, **132**, 114–122.
41. Meyer, F., Verreault, R. (1987). Erythrocyte selenium and breast cancer risk. *Am. J. Epidemiol.*, **125**, 917–919.
42. Van 't Veer, P., Van Der Wielen, R.P., Kok, F.J. *et al.* (1990). Selenium in diet, blood, and toenails in relation to breast cancer: a case–control study. *Am. J. Epidemiol.*, **131**, 987–994.
43. Van Noord, P.A.H., Maas, M.J., Van der Tweel, I., Collett, C. (1993). Selenium and the risk of postmenopausal breast cancer in the DOM cohort. *Breast Cancer Res. Treat.*, **25**, 11–19.
44. Hunter, D.J., Morris, J.S., Stampfer, M.J. *et al.* (1990). A prospective study of selenium status and breast cancer risk. *J. Am. Med. Assoc.*, **264**, 1128–1131.
45. Van Noord, P.A., Collette, H.J., Maas, M.J. *et al.* (1987). Selenium levels in nails of premenopausal breast cancer patients assessed prediagnostically in a cohort-nested case-referent study among women screened in the DOM project. *Int. J. Epidemiol.*, **16**, (Suppl.) 318–322.
46. Coates, R.J., Weiss, N.S., Daling, J.R. *et al.* (1988). Serum levels of selenium and retinol and the subsequent risk of cancer. *Am. J. Epidemiol.*, **128**, 515–523.
47. Overvad, K., Wang, D.Y., Olsen, J. *et al.* (1991). Selenium in human mammary carcinogenesis: a case-cohort study. *Eur. J. Cancer*, **27**, 900–902.
48. Knekt, P., Aromaa, A., Maatela, J. *et al.* (1990). Serum selenium and subsequent risk of cancer among Finnish men and women. *J. Natl. Cancer Inst.*, **82**, 864–868.

144   *Michelle D. Holmes et al.*

49. Longnecker, M., Berlin, J.A., Orza, M.J. *et al.* (1988). A meta–analysis of alcohol consumption in relation to breast cancer risk. *J. Am. Med. Assoc.*, **260**, 642–646.
50. Willett, W.C., Stampfer, M.J., Colditz, G.A. *et al.* (1987). Dietary fat and risk of breast cancer. *N. Engl. J. Med.*, **316**, 22–28.
51. Schatzkin, A., Carter, C.C., Green, S.B. *et al.* (1989). Is alcohol consumption related to breast cancer? Results from the Framingham Heart Study. *J. Natl. Cancer Inst.*, **81**, 31–35.
52. Simon, M.S., Carman, L.S., Wolfe, R. *et al.* (1991). Alcohol consumption and the risk of breast cancer: a report from the Tecumseh Community Health Study. *J. Clin. Epidemiol.*, **44**, 755–761.
53. Hiatt, R.A., Bawol, R.D. (1984). Alcoholic beverage consumption and breast cancer incidence. *Am. J. Epidemiol.*, **120**, 676–683.
54. Garfinkel, L., Bofetta, P., Stellman, S.D. (1988). Alcohol and breast cancer: a cohort study. *Prev. Med.*, **17**, 686–693.
55. Gapstur, S.M., Potter, J.D., Sellers, T.A., Folsom, A.R. (1992). Increased risk of breast cancer with alcohol consumption in postmenopausal women. *Am. J. Epidemiol.*, **136**, 1221–1231.
56. Hiatt, R.A., Klatsky, A.L., Armstrong, M.A. (1988). Alcohol consumption and the risk of breast cancer in a prepaid health plan. *Cancer Res.*, **48**, 2284–2287.
57. Schatzkin, A., Jones, D.Y., Hoover, R.N. *et al.* (1987). Alcohol consumption and breast cancer in the epidemiologic follow-up study of the first National Health and Nutrition Examination Survey. *N. Engl. J. Med.*, **316**, 1169–1173.
58. Seidman, H., Stellman, S.D., Muchinski, M.H. (1982). A different perspective on breast cancer risk factors: some implications of nonattributable risk. *CA*, **32**, 3–15.
59. Reichamn, M.E., Judd, J.T., Longcope, G. *et al.* (1993). Effects of alcohol consumption on plasma, and urinary hormone concentrations in premenopausal women. *J. Natl. Cancer Inst.*, **85**, 722–727.
60. Longnecker, M., Newcomb, P.A., Mittendorf, R. *et al.* (1992). Risk of breast cancer in relation to past and recent alcohol consumption. *Am. J. Epidemiol.* **136**, 1001, (Abstract).
61. Harvey, E.B., Schairer, C., Brinton, L.A. *et al.* (1987). Alcohol consumption and breast cancer. *J. Natl. Cancer Inst.*, **78**, 657–661.
62. Minton, J.P., Foecking, M.K., Webster, D.J. *et al.* (1979). Response of fibrocystic disease to caffeine withdrawal and correlation of cyclic nucleotides with breast disease. *Am. J. Obstet. Gynecol.*, **135**, 157–158.
63. Snowden, D.A., Phillips, R.L. (1984). Coffee consumption and risk of fatal cancers. *Am. J. Public Health*, **74**, 820–823.
64. Hunter, D.J., Manson, J.E., Stampfer, M.J. *et al.* (1992). A prospective study of caffeine, coffee, tea, and breast cancer. *Am. J. Epidemiol.*, **136**, 1000–1001, (Abstract).
65. Maclure, M. (1993). Demonstration of deductive meta–analysis: ethanol intake and risk of myocardial infarction. *Epidemiol. Rev.*, **15**, 1–24.
66. Shekelle, R.B., Shryock, A.M., Paul, O. *et al.* (1981). Diet, serum cholesterol, and death from coronary heart disease. The Western Electric Study. *N. Engl. J. Med.*, **304**, 65–70.
67. Willett, W.C., Stampfer, M.J., Colditz, G.A., Rosner, B.A., Speizer, F.E. (1990). Relation of meat, fat, and fiber intake to the risk of colon cancer in a prospective study among women. *N. Engl. J. Med.*, **323**, 1664–1672.
68. Steinmetz, K.A., Potter, J.D. (1991). Vegetables, fruit, and cancer. I. Epidemiology. *Cancer Causes Control*, **2**, 325–357.

Chapter 16

Risks Associated with Obesity

KATHY L RADIMER and CHRISTOPHER BAIN

In childhood, an energy-rich diet may lead to overweight which can promote earlier ovarian maturation and consequently early onset of menstruation and breast tissue proliferation [1]. Thus, childhood and adolescent overweight may be relevant to breast cancer risk. For adult women, overweight is generally considered to be a risk factor for breast cancer, perhaps primarily via the formation of estrogen in adipose tissue [2]. Obesity is probably most relevant to increased risk after the menopause, when ovarian production of estrogen no longer predominates. The effect of adult obesity on breast cancer risk, therefore, needs to be considered according to the ovarian status of a woman.

The role of body size (other than height) in relation to breast cancer has been examined using either absolute or relative weight, weight change or the distribution of fat tissue in the body. Absolute weight, the number of kilograms or pounds a person weighs, reflects a combination of adipose tissue and lean body mass [3]. A measure more directly indicating adiposity *per se* is relative weight. This 'corrects' weight for height, resulting in weight per unit of height, and the formula most commonly used is the Quetelet index [weight (kilograms)/height (metres)^2] also referred to as the Body Mass Index (BMI).

Adult weight gain has also been used as an indicator of adiposity, as it mostly reflects gain of adipose tissue [4]. Finally, fat distribution has been assessed either with the Waist-to-Hip Ratio (WHR), comparing the girth of the waist to that of the hip, or by measuring skinfold thickness, usually in the triceps and subscapular skin areas.

Basil A. Stoll (ed.), Reducing Breast Cancer Risk in Women, 145–153.

Body Mass and Breast Cancer Risk

Childhood Body Mass

A number of studies have investigated the association of body mass in pre-teen years with the risk of breast cancer [5–8]. The results suggest that higher adiposity in childhood (approximately 9–14 years) is probably not associated with increased risk of premenopausal breast cancer and may even be protective, although one study [8] suggests otherwise. Postmenopausally there is less evidence of a protective effect, however, the data are sparse, not entirely consistent, and rarely significant. Overall, the data do not support the notion that higher body mass in childhood affects the risk of breast cancer.

Teenage Body Mass

All six studies investigating the association of teenage (15–19 years) body mass with premenopausal breast cancer [6–11] found an inverse association (decreased risk with increased mass) which was significant in four studies. The reduction in risks generally ranged from 20 to 40%. For postmenopausal breast cancer, [5–7, 9–14] the relationship was again found to be inverse overall but less clearly so. The consistency and significance of these results suggest that relative adiposity in teenage years is associated with a 20 to 40% lowering of risk of developing premenopausal breast cancer. Postmenopausally the inverse association is neither so consistent nor so striking.

Early Adult Body Mass

A variety of investigations have examined the relationship of early adult body mass (generally between ages 20 and 30) to the risk of premenopausal or postmenopausal breast cancer [6, 7, 11, 15–22]. The associations with body mass in early adulthood are less uniform than those at younger ages, and do not support either direct or inverse associations of early adult mass with breast cancer before or after menopause.

Adult Body Mass and Premenopausal Breast Cancer

The bulk of the data on adult body mass measured at various ages prior to the diagnosis of cancer come from prospective studies which collected body size data before the onset of disease. Overall, these data point to a modestly decreased risk of premenopausal breast cancer in association with increased mass [5–10, 23–27]. The range of effect was fairly wide, however, varying from a 10% increase in risk to a 40% decrease associated with the greatest level of overweight.

Much of the data supporting this view come from three large Scandinavian studies [23–25], all using measured data, with excellent follow-up. None adjusted for possible confounders, however, and it is unclear what effect full adjustment might have, as there has been little effect on risk in some studies [16, 28], but a significant increase in risk in at least one other [4]. The other supporting data come from three US studies [5, 6, 9], two of which did adjust for relevant variables.

Assessment of the relationship between breast cancer risk and weight at or near the time of diagnosis, on the other hand, has been based mostly upon data recalled by the patient [7, 9, 11, 13–18, 27–35]. The support for an inverse association provided by these studies was much more modest. This may be due in part to weight loss associated with the onset of the disease and non-participation of some of the more obese cases, as obesity is associated with a poorer prognosis for breast cancer.

Overall, though, these data imply that an increased adult body mass decreases the risk of breast cancer occurring prior to the menopause. There is some evidence that this relationship applies most strongly to women in their forties [5, 9, 13, 23, 27] and differences in age distribution may account in part for different findings. The overall inverse relation is at best likely to be weak however; perhaps no more than a 20 to 30% lowering of risk across a wide range of body mass.

Does the finding of an overall inverse association mean that overweight is actually protective at these ages? It has been suggested that some of the observed association may be due to later detection of disease in more obese women. While a number of authors have calculated that not all the decreased risk can be attributed to delayed detection [6, 9, 23], many studies have found smaller tumours in leaner women, supporting the premise that this accounts for at least some of the effect. [9, 14, 15, 23, 27]. Further, it has been found that obese cases were less likely to have examined their breasts or had a mammogram [101]. These factors and the weakness of the overall association do not provide a good basis for assuming a causal protective effect of overweight, especially as no repeatable dose-response effect is evident. However, the general consistency in findings should not be ignored, and biologically there is the possibility of a protective role of reduced progesterone levels among obese premenopausal women [36].

Adult Body Mass and Postmenopausal Breast Cancer

Data relating body mass measured prior to diagnosis of breast cancer to the risk of postmenopausal breast cancer come mainly from 10 prospective studies. Almost all showed a correlation between increased mass and increased breast cancer risk. In general, the increased risk ratios (RR) were between 1.1 and 1.3 [6, 12, 23, 25, 26, 37]. Two papers reported larger RRs (3.0, 1.7) [5, 38], but these pertained only to women over 55 years of age, while two others reported slightly inverse associations, neither including older women [9, 24].

The relationship of body mass at or near diagnosis to the risk of postmenopausal breast cancer was investigated in 20 studies, nearly all of which were retrospective. Most of these studies found positive associations, although many were not significant, with increased risk of between 20 and 90%. However, a small number found no or inverse associations, particularly if BMI rather than absolute weight was used [7, 9, 11, 13–15, 17–20, 27–34, 39].

Overall, the data on adult body mass support the suggestion that heaviness or obesity is associated with an increased risk of postmenopausal breast cancer. The strength of the relationship tended to be moderate, frequently less than a 50% excess, although it was greater among older women.

A number of factors could have affected the risk estimates. Some of these are similar to those for premenopausal breast cancer, such as weight loss at the time of diagnosis, poorer detection of tumours in obese women, non-participation of those with a poorer prognosis (in which the obese may be over-represented), and lack of adjustment for potential confounders. Overall, the most likely result of these factors would be underestimation of the effect of obesity, i.e. the true relation is likely to be stronger than the reported risk estimate. It seems reasonable to conclude that overweight in adulthood is causally linked to breast cancer after menopause, given the fair strength and general consistency of the data, along with an accepted biological basis. In the absence of functioning ovaries, obesity produces a hormonal milieu potentially conducive to breast neoplasia via production of estrone in adipose tissue, and increased availability of estrogen due to lowered levels of sex hormone binding globulin [2]. However the lack of a consistent dose-response effect still casts some doubt on the causal association.

Weight Change

Eight population studies reported findings on the association of body mass change from 18–25 years of age to adulthood with premenopausal breast cancer [5, 6, 9, 10, 13, 15, 16, 18]. The data suggest a possibly lower risk of premenopausal breast cancer associated with weight gain from early to later adulthood, although one significantly increased risk was also found. The studies which found significant inverse associations tended to be larger and to have a broader distribution of weight and BMI for comparison, and used age 18 as the baseline age. The single significant positive result also came from a larger study and dated from age 18, but compared relative rather than an absolute increase in BMI, which may account for some of the difference.

The findings for postmenopausal women stand in marked contrast to the pattern seen above. Twelve studies [4–6, 9, 10, 12–15, 18–20] examined weight gain in relation to postmenopausal breast cancer, using various time frames. All but one found a positive association, and eight of these were significant, although in one instance only for women diagnosed after age 55 [5]. The data are thus quite consistent in finding an increase in risk associated with weight gain assessed in a variety of circumstances. This may be strongest in women with a longer duration of weight gain and for older women, with up to a four-fold increase in risk for older women who put on most weight.

Central Adiposity

Central adiposity is another measure of excess body mass. Because of the scarcity of studies measuring adiposity, six of the eight reviewed here did not meet the selection criteria (see Addendum). Three studies used skinfold measurements to estimate central adiposity [40–42]. All found increased measurements to be associated with increased risk. One study found this to be stronger for women over than under 50.

Six studies examined the waist-to-hip ratio (WHR) to estimate central adiposity, each using a slightly different protocol for measuring waist circumference. One prospective study, containing only postmenopausal women, found an overall increase in risk of borderline significance (RR = 1.4) with increased WHR [12]. This relationship strengthened with age, higher BMI and family history [43]. Three case-control studies found no risk associated with increased WHR, [44–46] while two others found a positive association between breast cancer risk and a higher mean WHR [42, 47].

The data suggest that central adiposity may be associated with increased risk of breast cancer, particularly for older women, however this relationship may be due in part to the association between central and overall adiposity. Further and more precise research in this area will allow better exploration of this relationship.

The Effect of Age on Risk from Obesity

Twelve studies, including five which did not meet the selection criteria [6–10, 23, 38, 48–52], examined differences in the association of risk of postmenopausal breast cancer and obesity by age at diagnosis or years since menopause. All but two [38, 52] found a greater increase in risk for women older or further past the menopause. This effect was seen for a variety of measures: weight, BMI, weight change, and WHR. It appears that the increase in risk has begun by about 55–60 years of age, and is especially strong after 70 [11, 52]. This appears to be part of a gradual change in the effect of body mass over much of a woman's life. The risk of breast cancer prior to age 50 or so may be reduced by up to 40% among women who are heavier in their late teens, and perhaps by 20% in those who are heavier in their twenties and thirties. There is a less consistent effect for women in their fifties, but by their sixties, the risk associated with increased body mass is clearly increased.

A number of studies have found that age is more closely associated with risk than menopausal status [4, 6, 9, 27], and a very large cohort study [23] presents data demonstrating the effect of age. There is a nearly linear increase in risk with increasing age, beginning with a decreased risk at age 30 and gradually evolving to an increased risk by age 55 which continues increasing through to age 69, the oldest age in this study.

In summary, higher childhood and teenage body mass appear to be associated with a modestly decreased risk of breast cancer presenting at any age. For breast cancer, before the age of 50, which is generally premenopausal, the relationship with increased adult body mass remains slightly inverse, particularly for early stage tumors, indicating that the relationship may result in part from impaired detection of small tumors in the obese. There may also be, however, some protective effect.

For older-onset breast cancer, the relationship with body mass is generally positive, with increases of 10 to 40% in risk for heavier or more obese women. This relationship may be weak or non-existent in women in their fifties, with some evidence that age, rather than menopausal status, is a better predictor of risk. The clearest evidence is that there is a higher breast cancer risk associated with obesity or heaviness in older women, and that this risk continues to increase with increasing age.

Conclusion

Maintenance of a moderate body weight throughout adulthood is advisable in view of the evidence that weight, body mass, maximum weight, weight at menopause, and weight gain (especially over a prolonged period) were all associated with an increased risk of breast cancer in postmenopausal women. This is especially important for women over 60, who appear to be at greatest risk from an increased body mass.

The data hint that obesity in teenage years may be slightly protective against breast cancer. It is, however, not desirable to advise children or teenagers to become obese, given other adverse health effects associated with obesity and the correlation of childhood obesity with adult obesity [53].

There is also some evidence suggesting an even more modest decrease in early onset breast cancer risk with increasing adult body mass, although again, over-weight should not be advised. Because there is some evidence of lower tumor detection in more obese premenopausal women, however, it may be wise to monitor obese premenopausal women who have other risk factors, particularly those with a family history of breast cancer.

Monitoring of women with greater central adiposity also may be warranted, especially those who are older or who have a family history of breast cancer. The data on central adiposity are as yet too sparse to determine whether it assesses breast cancer risk better than does body mass.

Acknowledgments

The assistance of Amanda Hudson in preparing the manuscript is gratefully acknowledged. Funding for Dr. Radimer was provided by the Public Health Research and Development Committee of the Australian National Health and Medical Research Council.

Addendum

Study Identification and Selection Criteria

We used the MEDLINE database for 1980 to 1993 to find articles in English which assessed the relationship of anthropometry and breast cancer and drew additional papers from the reference lists of these articles. To be included, papers needed to include at least 50 cases of breast cancer and present results by menopausal status or age. The comparison group had to be appropriate – i.e. from the same population as the cases. Hospital-based studies were accepted only where the authors excluded controls with other malignancies and conditions linked to obesity. 37 papers (of 74 identified) describing 32 studies (of 62 identified) were included. For some specific topics where data from the studies were limited, results from otherwise included studies are used.

References

1. DeWaard, F., Trichopoulos, D. (1988). A unifying concept of the aetiology of breast cancer. *Int. J. Cancer*, **41**, 666–669.
2. Morabia, A., Wynder, E.L. (1990). Epidemiology and natural history of breast cancer. Implications for the body weight–breast cancer controversy. *Surg. Clin. North Am.*, **70**, 739–52.
3. Willett, W. (1990). *Nutritional Epidemiology*. Oxford University Press, New York.
4. Ballard-Barbash, R., Schatzkin, A., Taylor, P.R. *et al.* (1990). Association of change in body mass with breast cancer. *Cancer Res.*, **50**, 2152–2155.
5. LeMarchand, L., Kolonel, L.N., Earle, M.E. *et al.* (1988). Body size at different periods of life and breast cancer risk. *Am. J. Epidemiol.*, **128**, 137–152.
6. Brinton, L., Swanson, C. (1992). Height and weight at various ages and risk of breast cancer. *Ann. Epidemiol.*, **2**, 597–609.
7. Hislop, T.G., Coldman, A.J., Elwood, J.M. *et al.* (1986). Childhood and recent eating patterns and risk of breast cancer. *Cancer Detect. Prev.*, **9**, 47–58.
8. Pryor, M., Slattery, M.L., Rovison, L.M. *et al.* (1989). Adolescent diet and breast cancer in Utah. *Cancer Res.* **49**, 2161–2167.
9. London, S.J., Colditz, G.A., Stampfer, M.J. et al. (1989). Prospective study of relative weight, height, and risk of breast cancer. *J. Am. Med. Assoc.*, **262**, 2853–2858.
10. Chu, S.Y., Lee, N.C., Wingo, P.A. *et al.* (1991). The relationship between body mass and breast cancer among women enrolled in the cancer and steroid hormone study. *J. Clin. Epidemiol.*, **44**, 1197–1206.
11. Choi, N., Miller, A., Matthews, V. *et al.* (1978). An epidemiologic study of breast cancer. *Am. J. Epidemiol.*, **107**, 510–521.

12. Folsom, A.R., Kaye, S.A., Prineas, R.J. *et al.* (1990). Increased incidence of carcinoma of the breast associated with abdominal adiposity in postmenopausal women. *Am. J. Epidemiol.*, **131**, 794–803.

13. Lubin, F., Ruder, A.M., Wax, Y. *et al.* (1985). Overweight and changes in weight throughout adult life in breast cancer etiology. *Am. J. Epidemiol.*, **122**, 579–588.

14. Harris, R.E., Namboodiri, K.K., Wynder, E.L. (1992). Breast cancer risk: effects of estrogen replacement therapy and body mass. *J. Natl. Cancer Inst.*, **20**, 1575–1582.

15. Radimer, K., Siskind, V., Bain, C., Schofield, F. (1993). Relation between anthropometric indicators and risk of breast cancer among Australian women. *Am. J. Epidemiol.*, **138**, 77–89.

16. Lund, E., Adami, H.-O., Bergstrm, R., Meirik, O. (1990). Anthropometric measures and breast cancer in young women. *Cancer Causes and Control*, **1**, 169–172.

17. Ewertz, M. (1988). Influence on non-contraceptive exogenours and endogenous sex hormones on breast cancer risk in Denmark. *Int. J. Cancer*, **42**, 832–838.

18. Paffenbarger, R.S., Jr., Kampert, J.B., Chang, H.–G. (1980). Characteristics that predict risk of breast cancer before and after the menopause. *Am. J. Epidemiol.*, **112**, 258–268.

19. Kyogokui, S., Hirogata, T., Takeshita, S. *et al.* (1990). Anthropometric indicators of breast cancer risk in Japanese women in Fukuoka. *Jpn. J. Cancer Res.*, **81**, 731–737.

20. Kolonel, L.N., Nomura, A., Lee, J. *et al.* (1986). Anthropometric indicators of breast cancer risk in postmenopausal women in Hawaii. *Nutr. Cancer*, **8**, 247–256.

21. Whittemore, R.S., Paffenberger, J., Anderson, K., Lee, J.E. (1985). Early precursors of site-specific cancers in college men and women. *J. Natl. Cancer Inst.*, **74**, 43–51.

22. Iscovich, J.M., Iscovich, R.B., Howe, G., Shiboski, S., Kaldor, J.M. (1989). A case-control study of diet and breast cancer in Argentina. *Int. J. Cancer*, **44**, 770–776.

23. Tretli, S. (1989). Height and weight in relation to breast cancer morbidity and mortality. A prospective study of 570,000 women in Norway. *Int. J. Cancer*, **44**, 23–30.

24. Tornberg, S.A., Holm, L.-E., Carstensen, J.M. (1988). Breast cancer risk in relation to serum cholesterol, serum beta-lipoprotein, height, weight, and blood pressure. *Acta Oncol.*, **27**, 31–37.

25. Vatten L.J., Kvinnsland, S. (1992). Prospective study of height, body mass index and risk of breast cancer. *Acta Oncol.*, **31**, 195–200.

26. DeStavola, B.L., Wang, D., Allen, D.S. *et al.* (1993). The association of height, weight, menstrual and reproductive events with breast cancer: result from two prospective studies on the island of Guernsey (United Kingdom). *Cancer Causes and Control*, **4**, 331–340.

27. Swanson, C.A., Brinton, L.A., Taylor, P.R. *et al.* (1989). Body size and breast cancer risk assessed in women participating in the breast cancer detection demonstration project. *Am. J. Epidemiol.*, **130**, 1133–1141.

28. LaVecchia, C., Decarli, A., Parazzini, F. *et al.* (1987). General epidemiology of breast cancer in northern Italy. *Int. J. Epidemiol.* **16**, 347–355.

29. Rosenberg, L., Palmer, J.R., Miller, D.R. *et al.* (1990). A case-control study of alcoholic beverage consumption and breast cancer. *Am. J. Epidemiol.*, **131**, 6–14.

30. Adami, H., Rimsten, A., Stenkvist, B. *et al.* (1977). Influence of height, weight and obesity on risk of breast cancer in an unselected Swedish population. *Br. J. Cancer*, **36**, 787–792.

31. Helmrich, S.P., Shapiro, S., Rosenberg, L. *et al.* (1983). Risk factors for breast cancer. *Am. J. Epidemiol.*, **117**, 35–44.

32. Parazzini, F., LaVecchia, C., Negri, E., *et al.* (1990). Anthropometric variables and risk of breast cancer. *Int. J. Cancer*, **45**, 397–402.

33. Schatzkin, A., Palmer, J.R., Rosenberg, L. *et al.* (1987). Risk factors for breast cancer in black women. *J. Natl. Cancer Inst.*, **78**, 213–217.

34. Tao, S.-C., Yu, M.C., Ross, R.K., Ziu, K.-W. (1988). Risk factors for breast cancer in Chinese women of Beijing. *Int. J. Cancer*, **42**, 495–498.

35. Toti, A., Aguaiaro, S., Amadori, D. *et al.* (1986). Breast cancer risk factor in Italian women: a multicentric case-control study. *Tumori*, **72**, 241–249.

36. Key, T.J.A., Pike, M.C. (1988). The role of oestrogens and progestagens in the epidemiology and prevention of breast cancer. *Eur. J. Cancer Clin. Oncol.*, **24**, 29–43.
37. Swanson, C.A., Jones, D.Y., Schatzkin, A. *et al.* (1988). Breast cancer risk assessed by anthropometry in the NHANES I epidemiological follow-up study. *Cancer Res.*, **48**, 5363–5367.
38. De Waard, F., Baanders-van Halewijn, E.A. (1974). A prospective study in general practice on breast-cancer risk in postmenopausal women. *Int. J. Cancer*, **14**, 153–160.
39. Graham, S., Hellmann, R., Marshall, J. *et al.* (1991). Nutritional epidemiology of postmenopausal breast cancer in western New York. *Am. J. Epidemiol.* **134**, 552–566.
40. Ballard-Barbash, R., Schatzkin, A., Carter, C.L. *et al.* (1990). Body fat distribution and breast cancer in the Framingham Study. *J. Natl. Cancer Inst.*, **82**, 286–290.
41. Den Tonkelaar, I., Seidell, J.C., Collette, H.J.A., de Waard, F. (1991). Obesity and subcutaneous fat patterning in relation to breast cancer in postmenopausal women participating in the diagnostic investigation of mammary cancer project. *Cancer*, **69**, 2663–2667.
42. Schapira, D.V., Kumar, N.B., Lyman, G.H., Cox, C.E. (1990). Abdominal obesity and breast cancer risk. *Am. Coll. Physicians*, **112**, 182–186.
43. Sellers, T.A., Kushi, L.H., Potter, J.D. *et al.* (1992). Effect of family history, body-fat distribution, and reproductive factors on the risk of postmenopausal breast cancer. *N. Engl. J. Med.*, **326**, 1323–1329.
44. Lapidus, L., Helgesson, O. Merck, C. Bjorntorp, P. (1988). Adipose tissue distribution and female carcinomas. A 12-year-follow-up of participants in the population study of women in Gothenburg, Sweden. *Int. J. Obesity*, **12**, 361–368.
45. Petrek, J.A., Peters, M., Cirrincione, C., Rhodes, D., Bajorunas, D. (1993). Is body fat topography a risk factor for breast cancer? *Ann. Int. Med.*, **118**, 356–362.
46. Sonnichsen, A.C., Richter, W.O., Schwandt, P. (1990). Body fat distribution and risk for breast cancer. *Ann. Int. Med.*, **112**, 882.
47. Kodama, M., Kodama, T., Miura, S. Yoshida, M. (1991). Nutrition and breast cancer risk. *Anticancer Res.* **11**, 745–754.
48. de Waard, F. (1975). Breast cancer incidence and nutritional status with particular reference to body weight and height. *Cancer Research*, **35**, 3351–3356.
49. Dubin, N., Pasternack, B.S., Strax, P. (1984). Epidemiology of Breast Cancer in a Screened Population. *Cancer Detection and Prevention*, **7**, 87–102.
50. Kelsey, J.L., Fisher, D.B., Holford, T.R. *et al.* (1981). Exogenous estrogens and other factors in the epidemiology of breast cancer. *JNCI*, **67**, 327–333.
51. Hirayama, T. (1978). Epidemiology of breast cancer with special reference to the role of diet. *Prev Med*, **7**, 173–195.
52. Bouchardy, C., Le, M.G., Hill, C. (1990). Risk factors for breast cancer according to age at diagnosis in a French case-control study. *J. Clin Epidemiol*, **43**, 267–275.
53. National Research Council. Diet and Health: Implications for reducing chronic disease risk. (1989). Washington D.C. National Academy Press.

Chapter 17

Choosing Hormonal Contraception

KATHRYN F. McGONIGLE and GEORGE R. HUGGINS

In the US, oral contraceptives (OCs) have had changes in formulation and usage patterns since their introduction about 35 years ago and these changes complicate the evaluation of their role in breast disease. Most OCs now contain only 20 to 35 μg of ethinyl estradiol and 0.3 to 1 mg of progestogen compared with up to 150 μg and 10 mg, respectively, in the earliest formulations. However, although OC content decreased dramatically between 1960 and 1975, actual use of lower-dose formulations lagged behind their introduction. As late as 1985, over 30% of OCs prescribed in the US contained more than 35 μg of ethinyl estradiol. Consequently, most published studies reflect the use of high-dose OCs.

With regard to their pattern of usage, women are now using OCs for a longer time and at a younger age. They are being used especially before a first pregnancy in order to delay childbearing rather than to space pregnancies. Fewer than 0.5% of women aged 45 to 50 have used OCs before age 20, compared with 25% of women younger than age 23 [1]. Moreover, the number of women using OCs perimenopausally is rising, and this population of women is likely to represent a high proportion of OC users in the future.

The incidence of breast cancer in women has been rising in the USA since the mid 1940s and most of the rise has been since 1980 [2]. Reasons often cited for the increased incidence, such as delayed child bearing, less breast feeding, and increased mammographic screening [3, 4], can only partially explain it. The increased incidence is more marked in postmenopausal women in their late 60's and 70's who were rarely exposed to oral contraceptives (OCs) [2] and this observation, like most other scientific data, fails to support a contribution of OCs to this rise.

Yet, aggregate data suggest an increased breast cancer risk for a small proportion of women who used high dose OCs for prolonged periods of time, although there remains some controversy. The noncontraceptive health benefits of OCs must be weighed against the small potential risks. The decreased risk of ovarian

Basil A. Stoll (ed.), Reducing Breast Cancer Risk in Women, 155–164.
© 1995 *Kluwer Academic Publishers. Printed in the Netherlands.*

and endometrial cancers associated with OC use is estimated to be responsible for averting 1,700 cases of ovarian [5] and 2,000 cases of endometrial cancer [6] in the United States each year. Oral contraceptives are also known to decrease the incidence of ectopic pregnancy, pelvic inflammatory disease, benign ovarian cysts, iron-deficiency anemia, rheumatoid arthritis, dysmenorrhea and premenstrual tension [7]. Despite the fact that such benefits were identified and included in OC labeling over one decade ago, women today are largely unaware of the noncontraceptive health benefits of OCs [7].

Furthermore, significant misconceptions about OC-related side effects are common. A poll in 1985 demonstrated that 33% of women believed OCs caused cancer. Such fear is a powerful deterrent to OC use. Studies show cumulative OC termination rates in the United Kingdom at nearly 16% after reports in the lay media suggesting an adverse effect of OCs [8]. This was followed by a rise in unwanted pregnancies and their associated risks. Clearly, more public education is needed and health care professionals must keep themselves informed of current risks and benefits of OCs.

Benign Breast Disease and OC Use

Some types of breast disease are associated with an increased risk of subsequent breast cancer [9]. The mean age of women with benign breast disease is 15 to 20 years younger than that of women with breast cancer [10, 11] suggesting benign breast lesions may be premalignant. Conversely, they may develop independently of malignant breast lesions but share some risk factors [12]. This hypothesis is difficult to evaluate because benign breast disease is not a single well-defined disease. The histologic diagnoses are sometimes confusing and inconsistent and fibrosis, fibrocystic disease, fibroadenoma, cystic mastitis, adenosis, hypermetaplastic disease, and intraductal papillomas are all terms used in the literature [13]. Because there is no standard terminology for benign proliferative breast disorders, direct comparisons between various studies are difficult.

In attempts to analyze the risk of breast cancer in women with benign breast disorders, studies have demonstrated that most types are not associated with an increased risk of breast cancer [9, 14, 15]. A 1985 consensus conference sponsored by the College of American Pathologists and the American Cancer Society to determine the risk relationship between benign breast lesions and cancer, concluded that only those patients with marked hyperplasia had an increased risk of breast cancer (1.5 to 5 times) [9]. The most common symptomatic benign breast conditions (lobular hyperplasia, cystic duct dilation, fibroadenoma, and sclerosing adenosis) were not associated with an increased risk.

Numerous studies have demonstrated that OC use is associated with a significantly decreased risk of benign breast disease [16–23]. However, a few have failed to support this link [24–26]. Relative risks were generally 0.3 to 0.7 that of non-OC users. Most studies do not include women with biopsy-proven benign breast disease, making the data less clear-cut. Overall, most studies suggest that the high progestogen dose OCs used in the 1970s were protective.

The protective effect against benign breast disease is related to both length and recency of OC use. Most studies indicate that it begins after only 2 to 5 years of OC use [18, 19, 23]. Some have found that the protective effect is lost within a few months to 1 year of stopping OCs [23]. However, others have reported that it persisted for 24 months or more after ceasing therapy [18–20].

The progestogen dose in OCs may be important for protection. Two studies found that the lowest risk of benign breast disease was in users of OCs containing the highest progestogen dose. Both groups investigated women taking OCs with 50 μg of ethinyl estradiol and varying dosages of norethisterone acetate. One of the groups, the RCGP Study group [16], reported the lowest risk for benign breast disease in the highest progestogen group (4.0 mg) (risk ratio of 0.27), intermediate risk for the 2.5 to 3.0 mg pills (risk ratio of 0.5), and virtually no decrease in risk for the lowest dose or 1.0 mg pills. Berkowitz *et al.* [25], in a recent analysis that primarily examined women using low progestogen dose OCs, found no decreased risk of benign breast disease. For women taking 20 to 50 μg ethinyl estradiol and 1 to 2.5 mg progestogen preparations, the risk ratios were close to 1 or greater.

Excellent data support the hypothesis that the high progestogen dose OCs used before the mid 1970s protected against most forms of benign breast disease. But it is not clear whether current low progestogen dose OCs will confer comparable protection. Ory *et al.* [27] calculated from pre-1979 study estimates that the protective effect of OCs on benign breast disease resulted in 23,490 fewer breast biopsies per year among the eight million US women taking OCs at that time. Based on more recent studies, beneficial effects of current OCs may be much less than these estimates.

Breast Cancer and OC Use

Those studies showing protection against benign breast disease have failed to show the same protection against breast cancer. The aggregate data fail to demonstrate an effect on the aggregate life-time risk of breast cancer up to about age 60 [28–40].

Although a few studies have suggested otherwise [41–42], most studies suggest that long-term use does not confer elevated risk for women up to the time of the menopause. However, when the cohort is limited to women developing breast cancer at a young age, a positive association emerges in many studies [32, 34, 43–50]. In assessing nine case-control studies on breast cancer development before age 45, looking at years of OC use overall and prior to a first full term pregnancy [29], for each group of women there is a subtle increase in risk with duration of OC use. These studies suggested there may be increased risk of *early*-occurring breast cancer associated with long-term use of high-dose combination OCs used in the 1960s and 1970s. These types of reports have prompted investigators to analyze data on OC use for development of breast cancer at a young age.

Some groups noted an increased risk for young women [32, 42, 43, 46] while in some studies the association was found only in certain subgroups of this cohort of young women [44, 45, 47–49]. Each of the studies demonstrated an increased risk for development of breast cancer at a young age. Although the increased risk sometimes occurred in somewhat different subgroups of women, the data suggest that long-term high dose use of OCs confers an increased risk for the development of breast cancer in a small proportion of women at a young age.

Full development of the human breast occurs only after a first term birth and there is concern that exposure of the breast to OCs before this time may increase risk of breast cancer. Most studies have found no association with OC use before a first term pregnancy for women under age 60 at diagnosis of breast cancer [35–40]. Data from some studies suggests otherwise [37, 51, 52]. When the evaluation is limited to those women developing breast cancer at a younger age, more data are available, and several studies have identified an increased risk of breast cancer for this group with increasing OC use before a first term pregnancy. [43, 44, 47–49, 53].

In a meta-analysis summarizing data from studies on OC use and breast cancer, an increased risk for women less than age 45 was found. The risk was significantly elevated (risk ratio of 1.72) among those using OCs for at least four years before a first term pregnancy [34]. Overall, data suggest a slightly increased risk of breast cancer in young women with increasing length of high-dose OC use before a first term pregnancy. However, the inconsistencies make definitive conclusions difficult.

Currently, many women are using OCs for a prolonged time at young ages and near menarche, when the breast is still maturing. Before complete differentiation of breast epithelial ductal cells, they may be highly susceptible to the action of a carcinogen. The question of whether early onset of OC use and/or prolonged use at a young age is an important determinant of risk has been addressed by many studies [30, 34, 37, 42, 46, 54–57]. Preliminary data do not suggest that the young breast is more susceptible to adverse effects of OCs.

A recent case-control analysis from New Zealand (where a high proportion of young women aged 15 to 24 use OCs) failed to find an increased risk with use starting at very young ages, even before age 17 [37]. This and most other studies failed to find an increased risk of breast cancer with duration of OC use at a young age or with early onset of OC use. Overall, the largest and best conducted studies failed to identify an association, suggesting that these are not significant risk factors. However, since a few studies suggest some association, more data are required.

Several studies have evaluated the risk of breast cancer with OC use in women with a history of benign breast disease. Unfortunately, many of these studies have failed to confirm the diagnosis of benign breast disease by a history of previous biopsy. Some have found an increased risk of breast cancer in women with a history of benign breast disease [30, 36, 48], but other studies have found no increased risk [38, 42, 56, 58]. An analysis of the Cancer and Steroid Hormone study data [59] actually demonstrated a significantly decreased risk of breast cancer (risk ratio of

0.7) for women with a history of OC use and surgery for benign breast disease compared with that for non-users with the same history.

In assessing overall risk for women with *existing* benign breast disease and OC use, investigators have pointed out that many studies fail to exclude clearly the possibility that some of the study patients developed benign breast disease subsequent to the initiation of OCs. They suggest there is insufficient evidence to show that OC use increases the risk of breast cancer in women with a pre-existing history of benign breast disease.

Breast cancer risk is elevated in women with a family history of breast cancer. Although findings have varied considerably regarding the risk of breast cancer in an OC user with a family history of breast cancer, overall, OC use does not appear to affect this risk. Some have suggested that women with a family history of breast cancer had a slightly greater risk associated with OC use than those without [56, 60], but other studies have failed to find a positive association [61, 62]. Although some data are conflicting, the largest and best conducted studies suggest that women with a family history of breast cancer are not at increased risk because of OC use.

Several studies showed no significant difference in histopathology of breast cancer tissue, extent of disease at presentation or prognosis, in OC users compared to non-OC users [63–65]. Other studies have found that a history of OC use results in a more favorable prognosis with either more favorable clinical and histologic features than controls, prolonged survival or both [46, 66, 67]. While some have identified a history of OC use to be associated with poor prognostic factors [43, 58, 68]. In view of the inconsistent data, it is unclear whether a history of OC use changes the stage at presentation or the prognosis of breast cancer.

OC formulations have changed dramatically since their introduction about 35 years ago and most women have used more than one type. Because the majority of studies evaluating the effects of hormone content are retrospective and depend on patient recall, the quality of these analyses is questionable. Although a few studies suggest one formulation or another may be associated with an increased risk, there is no consensus. Overall, there is no particular formulation or hormone type associated with an increased risk of breast cancer [44, 46, 49]. The Cancer and Steroid Hormone study with large numbers of women, [69] failed to demonstrate an increased risk of breast cancer with any particular type of OC for a duration of over five years. Similarly, other studies have been unable to identify a change in breast cancer risk associated with a particular OC formulation.

It has been suggested that a long-term latent effect may be present in which women are at an increased risk of breast cancer many years after the onset of OC use and therefore OCs may play a role in cancer initiation. Most of the data fail to support a long-term latent effect of OCs on the development of breast cancer [30, 55, 70], although a few studies suggest it may be important [34, 37, 43]. Most studies have failed to identify an increased risk with a latency period, suggesting there is not an elevated risk of breast cancer within 10 to 20 years of stopping OCs, even with long-term use.

Clinical Implications

The one most consistent finding is an increase in risk for breast cancer at a young age. It has been suggested that this occurrence may represent a promotional effect with long-term use of the discontinued, high-dose OC formulations so that an increased incidence of breast cancer in young women may be associated with a concurrent decreased incidence in older women. In such a case, the lifetime risk of breast cancer would not be increased, but the disease would occur at younger ages. Given the marked over-all inconsistency of the data, it is likely that the increasing risk is small and affects a small proportion of women who used high-dose OCs.

Furthermore, if we accept the hypothesis that long-term use of high-dose OCs is associated with a slight increase risk of breast cancer in young women, it is important to understand what this increased risk means to a given population of women. In the CASH analysis [44] where an increased risk of breast cancer before age 45 was found only for nulliparous women who had menarche before age 13 and had used OCs for more than 8 years, only 1.3% of the cases of breast cancer occurred in the 'at risk group' (39 women). Moreover, for the RCGP study [43] where a 40 to 70% increased risk was found, the authors calculate that the absolute excess risk was about one in 7,000 ever-users per year less than age 35. In considering potential risk to current OC users, it is important to remember that these data are based on the use of high-dose formulations of the 1960 to 1970s. It is reasonable to expect that the current lower-dose formulations carry even less risk. Indeed, this is suggested by data from the UK National Case-Control Study Group where combination low-dose OCs conferred less risk [46].

Current data cannot fully evaluate the risk of breast cancer for OC exposure in women over age 60, who have the highest underlying risk. Because of the significantly higher baseline incidence of breast cancer in older women an increase or decrease in risk ratio conveys a more significant absolute change in risk than for younger women. Based on the differences in biological behavior, hormone receptor expression and risk factors, pre- and postmenopausal breast cancers appear to be quite different diseases. It is therefore reasonable to expect that the effects of OCs on breast cancer risk may differ for these two groups of women. The Centers for Disease Control's CASH data analysis found that women aged 45 to 54 who have used OCs have a 10% decreased risk of breast cancer [32]. If this decrease is real, we would expect that as women who have used OCs age, they will actually be protected from breast cancer.

The reason for the increasing incidence of breast cancer is largely unexplained. It is unlikely that OCs have contributed significantly for several reasons. First, the increase began in the mid-1940s, long before the introduction of OCs. Secondly, although increased incidence is noted for all age groups, it is greatest for older women who were rarely exposed to OCs [4]. Further, the aggregate data suggest that if OCs increased for breast cancer risk, it is primarily in younger women [4]. Thirdly, if an increased incidence has occurred as a result of OC exposure, it should be seen more in younger women than older women. Overall, the data suggest that a very small number of women may have developed breast cancer as a result of OC exposure.

Based on the combined evidence, authoritative bodies in the United States, Great Britain, and other countries independently came to similar conclusions in 1989. These included the United States Food and Drug Administration's Fertility and Maternal Health Drugs Advisory Committee, American College of Obstetricians and Gynecologists, the United Kingdom Committee on the Safety of Medicines, the Swedish national drug authorities, the World Health Organization, and the International Planned Parenthood Federation. Each recommended no change in OC labeling, prescribing, or use [71, 72]. However, in August 1990, the manufacturers of OCs in the United Kingdom, as a result of discussions with the United Kingdom Medicines Control Agency, inserted a statement in the OC leaflets about the possible association between the prolonged use of OCs and breast cancer in young women [73].

Conclusion

Epidemiologic data support the hypothesis that the types of OCs used before the mid-1970s protected against most forms of benign breast disease. It is unclear whether current low-dose progestogen OCs will confer the same protection. For breast cancer, the relationship is more complex. It is possible that prolonged use of high-dose OCs is associated with a small increased risk for breast cancer development in women at a young age and that prolonged use before a first term pregnancy may slightly increase risk for breast cancer in young women. Studies on the effect of current low-dose OCs are necessary to elucidate whether they exert any effect on breast cancer development.

As our population ages, studies will determine what effect prior OC use has on the breasts of older women. Moreover, as more and more women use OCs for prolonged periods near menarche, before a first term pregnancy, and perimenopausally, studies will need to examine whether use of OCs at these periods of a woman's reproductive life affect breast cancer risk.

References

1. Committee on the Relationship Between Oral Contraceptives and Breast Cancer, Institute of Medicine (1991). *Oral Contraceptives and Breast Cancer*. National Academy Press, Washington, D.C., 1.
2. National Cancer Institute (1989). *Animal Cancer Statistics Review, Including Cancer Trends: 1950–1985*. National Institutes of Health, Bethesda.
3. Baker, L.H. (1982). Breast cancer detection demonstration project: five-year summary report. *CA*, **32**, 194.
4. White, E. (1987). Projected changes in breast cancer incidence due to the trend toward delayed childbearing. *Am. J. Public Health*, **77**, 495.

5. Centers for Disease Control Cancer and Steroid Hormone Study (1983). Oral contraceptive use and the risk of ovarian cancer. *J. Am. Med. Assoc.*, **249**, 1596.

6. Centers for Disease Control Cancer and Steroid Hormone Study (1983). Oral contraceptive use and the risk of endometrial cancer. *J. Am. Med. Assoc.*, **249**, 1600.

7. Mishell, D.R. (1994). Noncontraceptive benefits of oral contraceptives. *J. Reprod. Med.*, **38**, 1021–1029.

8. Grimes, D.A. (1989). Breast cancer, the pill and the press. In Mann, R.D. (ed.), *Oral Contraceptives and Breast Cancer*, Parthenon Publishing Co., Park Ridge, New Jersey, 309.

9. Concensus Conference (1986). Is fibrocystic disease of the breast precancerous? *Arch. Pathol. Lab. Med.*, **110**, 171.

10. Frantz, V.K., Pickren, J.W., Melcher, G.W., Auchincloss, H. (1951). Incidence of chronic cystic disease in so-called 'normal breasts': a study based on 225 postmortem examinations. *Cancer*, **4**, 762.

11. Cook, M.G., Rohan, T.E. (1985). The patho-epidemiology of benign proliferative epithelial disorders of the female breast. *J. Pathol.*, **146**, 1.

12. Parazzini, F., LaVecchia, C., Franceschi, S. *et al.* (1984). Risk factors for pathologically confirmed benign breast disease. *Am. J. Epidemiol.*, **120**, 115.

13. Kodlin, D., Winger, E.E., Morgenstern, N.L., Chen, V. (1977). Chronic mastopathy and breast cancer. *Cancer*, **39**, 2603.

14. Hutchinson, W.B., Thomas, D.B., Hamlin, W.B. *et al.* (1980). Risk of breast cancer in women with benign breast disease. *J. Natl. Cancer Inst.*, **65**, 13.

15. Dupont, W.D., Page, D.L. (1985). Risk factors for breast cancer in women with proliferative breast disease. *N. Engl. J. Med.*, **312**, 146.

16. Royal College of General Practitioners (1974). *Oral Contraceptives and Health*. Pitman Publishing Co., New York, 1.

17. Vessey, M.P., Doll, R., Peto, R., Johnson, B., Wiggins, P. (1976). A longterm follow-up study of women using different methods of contraception: an interim report. *J. Biosoc. Sci.*, **8**, 375.

18. Ory, H., Cole, P., MacMahon, B., Hoover, R. (1976). Oral contraceptives and reduced risk of benign breast diseases. *N. Engl. J. Med.*, **294**, 419.

19. Hislop, T.G., Threlfall, W.J. (1984). Oral contraceptives and benign breast disease. *Am. J. Epidemiol.*, **120**, 273.

20. Pastides, H., Kelsey, J.L., LiVolsi, V.A. *et al.* (1983). Oral contraceptive use and fibrocystic breast disease with special reference to its histopathology. *J. Natl. Cancer Inst.*, **71**, 5.

21. Brinton, L.A., Vessey, M.P., Flavel, R., Yeates, D. (1981). Risk factors for benign breast disease. *Am. J. Epidemiol.*, **113**, 203.

22. Boston Collaborative Drug Surveillance Programme (1973). Oral contraceptives and venous thromboembolic disease, surgically confirmed gallbladder disease, and breast turnours. *Lancet*, **1**, 1399.

23. Franceschi, S., LaVecchia, C., Parazzini, *et al.* (1984). Oral contraceptives and benign breast disease: a case-control study. *Am. J. Obstet. Gynecol.*, **149**, 602.

24. Nomura, A., Comstock, G.W. (1976). Benign breast tumor and estrogenic hormones: a population-based retrospective study. *Am. J. Epidemiol.*, **103**, 439.

25. Berkowitz, G.S., Kelsey, J.L., LiVolsi, V. A., *et al.* (1984). Oral contraceptive use and fibrocystic breast disease among pre and postmenopausal women. *Am. J. Epidemiol.*, **120**, 87.

26. Sartwell, P.E., Arthes, F.G., Tonascia, J.A. (1973). Epidemiology of benign breast lesions: lack of association with oral contraceptive use. *N. Engl. J. Med.*, **288**, 551.

27. Ory, H.W., Forrest, J., Lincoln, R. (1983). *Making Choices: Evaluating the Health Risks and Benefits of Birth Control Methods*. Alan Guttrencher Institute, New York, 11.

28. Schlesselman, J.J. (1989). Cancer of the breast and reproductive tract in relation to use of oral contraceptives. *Contraception*, **40**, 1.

29. Schlesselman, J.J. (1990). Oral contraceptives and breast cancer. *Am. J. Obstet. Gynecol.*, **163**, 1379.

30. Rohan, T.E., McMichael, A.J. (1988). Oral contraceptive agents and breast cancer: a population-based case-control study. *Med. J. Aust.*, **149**, 520.
31. LaVecchia, C., Parazzini, F., Negri, E. *et al.* (1989). Breast cancer and combined oral contraceptives: an Italian case-control study. *Eur. J. Cancer Clinic. Oncol.*, **25**, 1613.
32. Wingo, P.A., Lee, N.C., Ory, H.W. *et al.* (1991). Age-specific differences in the relationship between oral contraceptive use and breast cancer. *Obstet. Gynecol.*, **78**, 161–170.
33. Mills, P.K., Beeson, W.L., Phillips, R.L., Fraser, G.E. (1989). Prospective study of exogenous hormone use and breast cancer in Seventh-day Adventists. *Cancer*, **64**, 591.
34. Romieu, I., Berlin, J.A., Colditz, G. (1990). Oral contraceptives and breast cancer: review and meta-analysis. *Cancer*, **66**, 2253.
35. Harris, R.E., Zang, E.A., Wynder, E.L. (1990). Oral contraceptives and breast cancer risk: a case-control study. *Int. J. Epidemiol.*, **19**, 240.
36. Schildkraut, J.M., Hulka, B.S., Wilkinson, W.E. (1990). Oral contraceptives and breast cancer: a case-control study with hospital and community controls. *Obstet. Gynecol.*, **76**, 395.
37. Paul, C., Skegg, D.C.G., Spears, G.F.S. (1990). Oral contraceptives and risk of breast cancer. *Int. J. Cancer.*, **46**, 366.
38. Rosenburg, L., Miller, D.R., Kaufman, D.W. *et al.* (1984). Breast cancer and oral contraceptive use. *Am. J. Epidemiol.*, **119**, 167.
39. Vessey, M.P., McPherson, K., Yeates, D., Doll, R. (1982). Oral contraceptive use and abortion before first term pregnancy in relation to breast cancer risk. *Br. J. Cancer*, **45**, 327.
40. Paul, C., Skegg, D.C.G., Spears, G.F.S., Kaldor, J.M. (1986). Oral contraceptives and breast cancer: a national study. *Br. Med. J.*, **293**, 723.
41. Ravnihar, B., Zakelj, P., Kosmelj, K., Stare, J. (1988). A case-control study of breast cancer in relation to oral contraceptive use in Slovenia. *Neoplasma*, **35**, 109.
42. WHO Collaborative Study of Neoplasia and Steroid Contraceptives (1990). Breast cancer and combined oral contraceptives: results from a multinational study. *Br. J. Cancer*, **61**, 110.
43. Kay, C.R., Hannaford, P.C. (1988). Breast cancer and the pill – a further report from the Royal College of General Practitioners' oral contraception study. *Br. J. Cancer*, **58**, 675.
44. Stadel, B.V., Lai, S. (1988). Oral contraceptives and premenopausal breast cancer in nulliparous women. *Contraception*, **38**, 287.
45. Miller, D.R., Rosenberg, L., Kaufman, D.W. *et al*, (1989). Breast cancer before age 45 and oral contraceptive use: new findings. *Am. J. Epidermiol.*, **129**, 269.
46. UK National Case-Control Study Group (1989). Oral contraceptive use and breast cancer risk in young women. *Lancet*, **1**, 973.
47. Meirik, O., Farley, T.M.M., Lund, E. *et al.* (1989). Breast cancer and oral contraceptives: patterns of risk among parous and nulliparous women – further analysis of the Swedish–Norwegian material. *Contraception*, **39**, 471.
48. Pike, M.C., Henderson, B.E., Casagrande, J.T., Rosario, I., Gray, G.E. (1981). Oral contraceptive use and early abortion as risk factors for breast cancer in young women. *Br. J. Cancer*, **43**, 72.
49. McPherson, K., Vessey, M.P., Neil, A. *et al.* (1987). Early oral contraceptive use and breast cancer: results of another case-control study. *Br. J. Cancer*, **56**, 653.
50. Lund, E., Meirik, O., Adami, H. *et al.* (1989). Oral contraceptive use and premenopausal breast cancer in Sweden and Norway: possible effects of different pattern of use. *Int. J. Epidemiol.*, **18**, 527.
51. Harris, N.V., Weiss, N.S., Francis, A.M., Polissar, L. (1982). Breast cancer in relation to patterns of oral contraceptive use. *Am. J. Epidemiol.*, **116**, 643.
52. Hawley, W., Nuovo, J., DeNeef, C.P., Carter, P. (1993). Do oral contraceptive agents affect the risk of breast cancer? A meta-analysis of the case-control reports. *J. Am. Board Fam. Pract.*, **6**, 123–135.
53. Ursin, G., Aragaki, C.C., Paganini-Hill, A. *et al.* (1992). Oral contraceptives and premenopausal bilateral breast cancer; a case-control study. *Epidemiol.*, **3**, 414–419.

54. Vessey, M.P., McPherson, L., Viilard-Mackintosh, L., Yeates, D. (1989). Oral contraceptives and breast cancer: latest findings in a large cohort study. *Br. J. Cancer*, **59**, 613.
55. Ellery, C., MacLennan, R., Berry, G., Shearman, R.P. (1986). A case-control study of breast cancer in relation to the use of steroid contraceptive agents. *Med. J. Aust.*, **144**, 173.
56. Ravnihar, B., Zakelj, P., Kosmelj, K., Stare, J. (1988). A case-control study of breast cancer in relation to oral contraceptive use in Slovenia. *Neoplasma*, **35**, 109.
57. Olsson, H., Muller, T.R., Ransram, J. (1988). Early oral contraceptive use and breast cancer. *Res.*, **8**, 29.
58. Romieu, I., Willett, W.C., Colditz, G.A. *et al.* (1989). Prospective study of oral contraceptive use and risk of breast cancer in women. *J. Natl. Cancer Inst.*, **81**, 1313.
59. The Cancer and Steroid Hormone Study of the Centers for Disease Control and the National Institute of Child Health and Human Development (1986). Oral-contraceptive use and the risk of breast cancer. *N. Engl. J. Med.*, **315**, 405.
60. Black, M.M., Barclay, T.H.C., Polednak, A. *et al.* (1983). Family history, oral contraceptive usage, and breast cancer. *Cancer*, **51**, 2147.
61. UK National Case-Control Study Group (1990). Oral contraceptive use and breast cancer risk in young women: subgroup analyses. *Lancet*, **335**, 1507.
62. Murray, P.P., Stadel, B.V., Schlesselman, J.J. (1989). Oral contraceptive use in women with a family history of breast cancer. *Obstet. Gynecol.*, **73**, 977.
63. Schlesselman, J.J., Stadel, B.V., Murray, P., Lai, S. (1987). Breast cancer risk in relation to type of estrogen contained in oral contraceptives. *Contraception*, **36**, 595.
64. Miller, N., McPherson, K., Jones, L., Vessey, M. (1989). Histopathology of breast cancer in young women in relation to use of oral contraceptives. *J. Clin. Pathol.*, **42**, 387.
65. Spencer, J.D., Millis, R.R., Hayward, J.L. (1978). Contraceptive steroida and breast cancer. *Br. Med. J.*, **1**, 1024.
66. Vessey, M., Baron, J., Doll, R., McPherson, K., Yeates, D. (1983). Oral contraceptives and breast cancer: final report of an epidemiological study. *Br. J. Cancer*, **47**, 455.
67. Matthews, P.N., Millis, R.R., Hayward, J.L. (1981). Breast cancer in women who have taken contraceptive steroids. *Br. Med. J.*, **282**, 774.
68. LaVecchia, C., Parazzini, F., Negri, E. *et al.* (1989). Breast cancer and combined oral contraceptives: an Italian case-control study. *Eur. J. Cancer Clinic. Oncol.*, **25**, 1613.
69. Centers for Disease Control (1984). Oral contraceptive use and the risk of breast cancer in young women. *MMWR*, **33**, 353.
70. Schlesselman, J.J., Stadel, B.V., Murray, P., Lai, S. (1988). Breast cancer in relation to early use of oral contraceptives: no evidence of a latent effect. *J. Am. Med. Assoc.*, **259**, 1828.
71. OCs and breast cancer: a round table discussion. (1989). *Dialogues in Contraception*, **2**, 1.
72. Alan Guttmacher Institute (1989). FDA panel examines link between breast cancer, pill, says more research needed. *Washington Memo.*, W–3, 3.
73. Information on oral contraceptives. (1990). *Lancet*, **336**, 498.

Chapter 18

Choosing Hormone Replacement Therapy

RICHARD L. THERIAULT, LAURA L. BOEHNKE and
RENA V. SELLIN

The menopause may have serious health consequences but maintaining the semblance of the premenopausal state by means of hormone replacement therapy also involves problems. The decision to use hormone replacement therapy is not simple and the best agent or agents to be used are not defined. The studies which have examined risks and benefits have not made clear which is greater – risk or benefit. Clinical application of such therapy involves careful assessment in each individual.

Consequences of Estrogen Deficiency

Hormone replacement therapy aims mainly to relieve estrogen deprivation occurring as a consequence of ovarian failure (Table 1). Lack of estrogen leads to genitourinary atrophy. This can result in atrophic vaginitis, urinary bladder dysfunction, and sexual dysfunction. Vasomotor instability and hot flushes are a frequent accompaniment of menopause and are severe enough in some women to interfere with sleep and cause emotional dysfunction.

Osteoporosis can lead to loss of bone of 3–5% per year immediately after menopause [1–3]. The loss of trabecular bone may lead to osteoporotic fracture of vertebral bodies and the development of femoral fractures. Skeletal-related disability and mortality have been estimated to result in health expenditures of 10 billion dollars per year in the USA. Estimates of 1.3 million osteoporotic fractures per year include approximately 250,000 hip fractures in US women [4, 5]. Hip fractures lead to death in 12–20% of women affected and 25% require extended nursing home or rehabilitation care [6]. Greater than 50,000 deaths per year are assessed to be the consequence of osteoporotic fractures.

Basil A. Stoll (ed.), Reducing Breast Cancer Risk in Women, 165–175.
© 1995 *Kluwer Academic Publishers. Printed in the Netherlands.*

Table 1. Physiologic consequences of estrogen deprivation and non-hormonal treatment alternatives

Estrogen Deficiency	Treatment Alternatives
Vasomotor instability (hot flushes)	Bellergal, clonidine, progesterone, herbal
Genital atrophy	Topical estrogen creams
Dyspareunia	Vaginal lubricants
Osteoporosis prevention	Calcium, biphosphonates, calcitonin, ?fluoride
Cardiovascular disease	Bile acid binding resins
Dyslipidemia-related	Fibric acid derivatives
	HMC–CoA reductase inhibibors
	Nicotinic acid, antioxidants

Cardiovascular disease remains the leading cause of death for women [7]. The risk of cardiovascular disease may increase as much as 18 fold after the menopause, a risk which is directly linked to estrogen deprivation [8].

Risks of Hormone Replacement Therapy

Unopposed estrogen used as replacement therapy has been associated with an increased risk of endometrial cancer. The risk has been shown to increase with longer duration of use and higher dosage [9]. A decline in risk is seen after the cessation of therapy. The increased incidence of endometrial cancer has been seen with the use of both conjugated estrogens, ethinyl estradiol and diethylstilbestrol. The risk of endometrial cancer with estrogen alone increases from 2–3 fold up to 15 fold for those with prolonged unopposed estrogen exposure [10, 11]. The use of cyclic progestins with estrogen for seven to ten days per month has been shown to decrease the risk of endometrial cancer in women using estrogen replacement therapy.

Gall bladder disease is increased in women taking estrogen therapy. This may require surgical intervention, but with modern techniques is unlikely to result in death [12–14].

Estrogen replacement therapy (ERT) may interact with other risk factors towards the development of breast cancer. Most analyses on the epidemiology of breast cancer concur that age is the most significant risk factor for the disease. The incidence increases during the sixth decade of life and continues to rise gradually but steadily [15–18]. Since ERT is also prescribed at this juncture for most women, it is difficult to clearly distinguish the potential contribution of ERT from the impact of age as a separate risk factor. Additional risk factors for breast cancer include positive family history, prior benign breast disease and age at onset of

Table 2. Postmenopausal estrogen replacement and increased risk for development of breast cancer: summary from six meta-analyses

Ref. No., Year	ERT Use	Overall Effect	Dose/Duration ERT	Family History of Cancer	Benign Disease
24, (1988)	N.S.	N.S.[a]	N.S.[a]	Incr.	N.S.
25, (1991)	N.S.	N.S.	Incr.[b]	Incr.	N.S.
23, (1991)	N.S.	N.S.	N.S.	–	N.S.
26, (1992)	Incr.	N.S.	Incr.[c]	–	–
27, (1992)	N.S.	N.S.	Incr.[c]	–	–
28, (1993)	N.S.	N.S.	N.S.[d]	N.S.	N.S.

N.S. = not significant .
[a] Total dose calculated to incorporate both dose/day and duration; summary RR = 1.28 with 95% confidence interval of 1.06–1.54 and a P value for heterogeneity of 0.09
[b] Trend for increased risk suggested after > 10 years
[c] Increased risk only in women with natural menopause
[d] Increased risk only among European studies

menstruation and childbearing [19–22]. In addition, prior diagnosis of breast cancer creates special concerns both in terms of developing second primary lesions and metastases.

The potential of ERT to increase breast cancer risk has been extensively studied during recent decades and overall, postmenopausal ERT has not been associated with significant increase of cancer risk. There are six recent meta-analyses on the subject [23–28] confirming that estrogen use *in general* has no significant impact on breast cancer risk (relative risk of 1.01–1.07). Attention has therefore focused on identifying ERT users who may be at increased risk by virtue of their personal or family medical history (Table 2), but in over 50 different analyses there is no consensus regarding special risk individuals. Although subsets of women at heightened risk emerge in some studies, these subsets vary between reports.

For example, no consistent trend suggests that an increasing estrogen dose alters the cancer risk. Reports also conflict regarding the potential effect of ERT duration on breast cancer risk. Reviewing individual studies, Dupont and Page [23] and Armstrong [24] reported no significant effect. Sillero-Arenas *et al* [26] suggested a dose – response relationship only in women with natural menopause. Steinberg *et al* [25] observed a duration-related increase only among European studies, while Grady *et al.* calculated a significant increase in risk in women treated with long-term ERT. Colditz *et al.* [28] calculated a significant increase in risk for ERT use longer than 10 years, although there was no relationship between the number of years of ERT and risk of breast cancer across 17 individual studies. Prior benign breast disease has been analyzed as another potential variable but available studies show either no effect [20, 21], or a small increase in risk [25, 28]. Similarly, family history of breast cancer does not appear to have a significant impact on ERT-related risk.

A small number of studies have considered the question of prognosis in women who develop breast cancer while on ERT. Some suggest that such women may have an improved prognosis compared to non-users [29–31] and this may reflect some unknown effect of estrogen replacement therapy or else the possibility that women have improved cancer surveillance while on ERT. This latter interpretation is supported by the observation that women on ERT have earlier stage disease at the time of diagnosis [32].

While two case-control studies suggest increased breast cancer risk in women treated with estrogen and progestin, a recent review concludes that there are inadequate data to assess risk of breast cancer in those who have received long-term estrogen plus progestin [27]. The effect of the type of estrogen formulation has also been studied. Conjugated estrogens are more often used in North American practice while synthetic preparations are more common in Europe. The observation that higher risk estimates are reported from European studies has, therefore, been interpreted by some investigators to suggest, indirectly, that the type of estrogen may have an independent effect on cancer risk.

Benefits of Hormone Replacement Therapy

Estrogen replacement is the only effective therapy for vasomotor symptoms (hot-flushes) and the genitourinary atrophy which accompanies the menopause [32, 34]. The benefits of estrogen on osteoporosis manifest as reduction in fracture risk by maintaining bone integrity. Estrogen has been shown to reduce menopausal bone loss at all sites thus resulting in reductions in hip and vertebral fractures with their attendant disability and mortality [4–6, 27, 35, 36].

All types of studies have shown a cardiovascular disease benefit [30,34] in postmenopausal women treated with estrogen. Reductions of approximately 50% in cardiac disease, heart attacks and sudden death, are attributable to estrogen therapy. Whether these favorable effects are mediated by the known reductions in low density lipoprotein, increase in high-density lipoprotein or a favorable effect on changes in blood vessels is unknown [37–39, 41, 42].

Reduced mortality from all causes has been reported for estrogen users. The decrease in mortality was due not only to reductions in death due to cardio-vascular disease, but also in all deaths due to cancer [43].

Hormone Replacement Therapy Agents

Hormone replacement therapy has consisted of numerous agents, combinations of hormones and combinations of hormones with other drugs. The major estrogen preparation used in the US has been oral conjugated estrogens and in the 1960's, the dose most frequently prescribed was 1.25 to 2.5 mg/day [44]. With the recognition of endometrial cancer risk and the demonstration that progestins could reduce this risk, prescribing practices changed dramatically in the 1970's. The dose of oral estrogens decreased to an average of 0.625 mg/day and the duration of use was shortened to encompass only the time necessary for the menopausal symptoms to subside (generally up to two years after cessation of menses). The most common agent used was still oral conjugated estrogens, but cyclic administration of progestins became the general practice [9, 39, 43, 45]. The use of estrogens combined with androgens fell out of favor.

A variety of administration routes have been shown to be effective for estrogen replacement therapy. Skeletal benefit has been shown for oral and transdermal estrogen [46, 47]. Clinical studies have not resolved whether the addition of progestins to estrogen affects the cardiovascular benefits of estrogen alone, but, it appears that progestins do not adversely affect bone integrity [27].

The decision to request or recommend ERT remains a controversial and often emotional argument both within the medical community and among the lay public [48–54]. While most physicians and many women recognize the cardiovascular and skeletal medical benefits of estrogen replacement, the motivating factors often revolve around the correction of subjective climacteric symptoms. It is important to point out that short-term ERT is frequently sufficient for alleviation of the climacteric symptoms, but longterm ERT is required to provide continued protection against cardiovascular disease and osteoporosis [27]. Failure to clarify this crucial point may account, in part, for widespread non-compliance with the use of prolonged ERT [55–57].

Women with a prior history of hormone-sensitive cancers which have been successfully treated raise special concerns in considering hormone therapy. If there are occult metastases, changes in hormonal milieu theoretically may promote their growth or dissemination. While many are beginning to question the proscription against hormone therapy in cancer patients, the definitions of risk and benefit remain unknown [58–62]. Limited clinical data suggests ERT may be prescribed for limited periods of time [63–65]. We have developed a structure for a prospective trial of estrogen replacement in breast cancer patients and a clinical trial has been initiated [66, 67].

The variety of agents available for hormone replacement therapy includes oral estrogen, oral estrogen and cyclic progestin, oral estrogen with continuous progestin, and transdermal estrogen with or without cyclic or continuous progestin (Tables 3 and 4). Commonly used regimens include daily oral conjugated estrogen, 0.625 mg which is satisfactory for women without concern for the endometrial affects of estrogen.

Alternatives for women with an intact uterus include conjugated estrogen 0.625 mg orally daily with cyclic medroxyprogesterone acetate five to ten mg orally for 10–14 days per month or conjugated estrogen plus continuous progestin-medroxy progesterone acetate 2.5 mg orally daily. The use of unopposed estrogen in women with an intact uterus requires careful gynecologic monitoring and surveillance for

Table 3. Progestational agents studied for hormone replacement therapy

Ref.	Agent	Dose*	Steroid Deriv.	AWP ($) per month**	Notes
70	Medroxyprogesterone Provera®, generic #	2.5–1.0 mg/day	17-HPG	2.38 (7 days) 9.52 (28 days)	Duration of action is prolonged and variable.
	Megestrol Megace®, generic	2.5–7.5 mg/day	17-HPG	–	Only dosage forms in U.S. are 20 mg or 40 mg tabs or 40 mg/ml suspension.
71	Norgestrel Ovrette®, Cyclabil® (UK)	0.15–2.5 mg/day	19-NT	5.48 (7 days) 43.80 (28 days)	Tablets available as 0.075 mg in the U.S. Price based on 2 tabs per day.
72	Norethindrone Micronor®, Nor-Q.D.®, Norlutin®	0.25–1 mg/day	19-NT	6.96 (7 days) 27.84 (28 days)	Tablets available as 0.35 mg in the U.S. Price based on 1 tablet per day.
73	Norethindrone Acetate Aygestin®, Norlutate®	0.25–1 mg/day	19-NT	6.44 (7 days) 25.76 (28 days)	Only available in 5 mg tablets in the U.S. Price based on 1 tablet per day.
	Cyproterone Androcur®	1 mg/day	17-HPT	–	Not available in the U.S.
	Desogestrel	0.15 mg/day	19-NT	–	Not available in the U.S. as single-agent tablet.
74	Combination products Norethindrone/Estradiol Estragest-TTS®	0.25 mg/day & 0.05 mg/day	–	–	Not available in the U.S.
75	Calendar packs Estradiol/Norgestrel Cyclo-Progynova® (11 tabs est. val. alone & 10 tabs est. val. + norgestrel)	1–2 mg estradiol valerate 0.15 mg norgestrel	–	–	Not available in the U.S.

* In combination with estrogens, cyclical (7 days/month) or daily progestins are recommended.

** Average wholesale price of the lowest recommended dose. Generic agents are less expensive.

Bioequivalency has been established between Provera® and generic products, allowing for substitution.

^ 17-HPG = 17-hydroxyprogesterone derivative; 19-NT = 19-nortestosterone derivative. All of these agents possess more potent progestational activity than androgenic activity. However, the 19-NT derivatives may have more androgenic side effects than the 17-HPG derivatives.

Table 4. Estrogenic agents studied for hormone replacement therapy

Agents	Admin. Schedule*	Route of Doses	Equipotent per month**	AWP ($)	Comments
Estradiol Estrace®	0.5–2 mg/day	PO	50 mcg	9.24 (21 days) 12.32 (28 days)	Use in U.S. is limited, but use in Europe is more common.
Estraderm®	0.05–0.1 mg/24 h twice weekly	TD	2.5 mcg	12.12 (21 days) 16.16 (28 days)	Skin metabolizes estradiol to a small extent, requiring smaller doses.
Estradiol Valerate	1–2 mg/day	PO	62.5 mcg	–	Not availabe in the U.S. in oral dosage form.
Conjugated Estrogens Premarin®, generic #	0.625–1.25 mg/day	PO	5 mg	7.77 (21 days) 10.36 (28 days)	Most common estrogen in U.S. 50–65% sodium estrone sulfate & 20–35% sodium equilin sulfate.
Esterified Estrogens Estratab®, Menest®	0.3–1.25 mg/day	PO	5 mg	4.20 (21 days) 5.60 (28 days)	75–85% sodium estrone sulfate & 6–15% sodium equilin sulfate.
Estropipate Ogen®, Ortho-Est®, generic	0.625–5 mg/day	PO	5 mg	10.29 (21 days) 13.72 (28 days)	Crystalline estrone solubilized as the sulfate and stabilized with piperazine 0.625 mg equivalent to 0.75 mg estropipate.
Ethinyl Estradiol Estinyl®	0.02–1.5 mg/day	PO	50 mcg	5.67 (21 days) 7.56 (28 days)	

PO = oral, TD = transdermal.

*Lowest possible dose is recommended when treating vasomotor symptoms of menopause. Cyclical administration (3 weeks on & 1 week off) is recommended. However, many other cyclic schedules are used. Concomitant progestin therapy daily or for 7 days/month is also recommended. However, many other cyclic schedules are used.

** Average wholesale price of the lowest dose recommended of the brand name agents. Generic products are less expensive.

Bioequivalency between Premarin® and generic conjugated estrogens has not been established and should not be assumed.

endometrial hyperplasia or malignancy. The oral route is preferred for cardiovascular benefits since there are inadequate data regarding cardiovascular disease risk reduction with transdermal preparations [68].

Tailoring the prescription to the clinical circumstances requires a definition of the goals of therapy and an assessment of benefits and risks in relation to bone disease, cardiovascular disease and cancer risk. Detailed discussion and patient education must define the measurement of treatment benefit and the surveillance necessary for maintenance therapy [69].

Conclusion

Non-hormonal alternatives exist for the management of the diverse consequences of estrogen deprivation, (Table 1). Their efficacy, patient acceptability and costs are variable. In contrast, ERT may be viewed as a comprehensive, inexpensive and effective therapy which may be required for a prolonged period of time. It becomes very important, therefore, to weigh carefully the known advantages of this approach against potential risks. Given the extended life expectancy of our population it is, perhaps, even more important to emphasize that many postmenopausal women remain healthy and may not require any specific intervention.

The severity of climacteric symptoms and the relative risk of developing other diseases of older women, including breast cancer, vary greatly from person to person. The decision to provide any medical therapy for postmenopausal women should be carefully individualized. Moderate doses of conjugated estrogens appear to optimize the risk-benefit ratio. Because ERT continues to protect the cardiovascular, genitourinary and skeletal systems in proportion to its duration, and because postmenopausal estrogen deficiency persists for several decades in healthy women, it is important to recognize that chronic estrogen administration may be appropriate for some individuals.

References

1. Cann, C., Genant, H., Ettinger, B., Gordon, G. (1980). Spinal mineral bone loss in oophorectomized women. *J. Am. Med. Assoc.*, **244**, 2056–2059.
2. Mazess, R. (1982). On aging bone loss. *Clin. Orthop.*, **165**, 239–252.
3. Riggs, B., Melton, L. (1986). Involutional osteoporosis. *N. Engl. J. Med.*, **314**, 1676–1685.
4. Riggs, B., Melton, L. (1992). The prevention and treatment of osteoporosis. *N. Engl. J. Med.* **327**, 620–627.
5. Proceedings of the National Conference on Women's Health Series (1987). Special Topic conference on Osteoporosis. *J.U.S. Public Health Service*, **48**, (Suppl.), 50–51.
6. Consensus Development Conference (1991). Prophylaxis and treatment of osteoporosis. *Am. J. Med.*, **90**, 107–110.
7. Gordon, T., Kannel, W.B., Hjortland, M.C. *et al.* (1978). Menopause and coronary heart disease. *Ann. Intern. Med.*, **85**, 157–161.
8. Rosenberg, L., Hennekens, C.H.E., Rosner, B. *et al.* (1981). Early menopause and the risk of myocardial infarction. *Am. J. Obstet. Gynecol.*, **139**, 47–51.

9. Thomas, D.B. (1988). Steroid hormones and medications that alter cancer risks. *Cancer*, **62**, 1755–1767.
10. Persson, I., Adami, H., Bergkvist, L. *et al.* (1989). Risk of endometrial cancer after treatment with estrogens alone or in conjunction with progestogens: Results of a prospective study. *Br. Med. J.*, **298**, 147–151.
11. Antunes, C.M.F., Stolley, P.D., Rosenshein, N.B. *et al.* (1979). Endometrial cancer and estrogen use. Report of a large case-control study. *N. Engl. J. Med.*, **300**, 9–13.
12. A Report from the Boston Collaborative Drug Surveillance Program, Boston University Medical Center (1974). Surgically confirmed gallbladder disease, venous thromboembolism and breast tumors in relation to postmenopausal estrogen therapy. *N. Engl. J. Med.*, 290, 9–15.
13. Petitti, D.B., Sydney, S., Perlman, J.A. (1988). Increased risk of cholecystectomy in users of supplemental estrogen. *Gastroenterology*, **94**, 91–95.
14. Van Erpecum, K.J., Van Berge-Henegouwen, G.P., Verschoor, L., Stoelwinder, B., Willikens, F.L. (1991). Different hepatobiliary effect of oral and transdermal estradiol in postmenopausal women. *Gastroenterology*, **100**, 482–488.
15. Dupont, W.B., Page, D.L. (1987). Breast cancer risk associated with proliferative disease, age at first birth and family history of breast cancer. *Am. J. Epidemiol.*, **125**, 769–779.
16. Henderson, I.C. (1993). Risk factors for breast cancer development. *Cancer*, **71**, 2127–2140.
17. Colditz, G.A., Willett, W.C., Hunter, D.J. *et al.* (1993). Family history, age and risk of breast cancer. Prospective data from the nurse's health study. *J. Am. Med. Assoc.*, **270**, 338–343.
18. Kelsey, K.J., Gammon, M.D. (1990). Epidemiology of breast cancer. *Epidemiol. Rev.*, **12**, 228–240.
19. Sellers, T.A., Kushi, L.H., Potter, J.D. *et al.* (1992). Effect of family history, body-fat distribution and reproductive factors on the risk of postmenopausal breast cancer. *N. Engl. J. Med.*, **326**, 1323–1329.
20. Nab, H.W., Googd, A.C., Coommelin, M.A. *et al.* (1993). Breast cancer incidence in the Southeastern Netherlands, 1960–1989: Trends in incidence and mortality. *Eur. J. Cancer*, **29A**, 1557–1559.
21. Calle, E.E., Martin, L.M., Thun, M.J., Miracle, H.L., Heath, C.W. (1993). Family history, age, and risk of fatal breast cancer. *Am. J. Epidemiol.*, **138**, 675–681.
22. Radimer, K., Siskind, V., Bain, C., Schofield, F. (1993). Relation between anthropometric indicators and risk of breast cancer among Australian women. *Am. J. Epidemiol.*, **138**, 77–89.
23. Dupont, W.D., Page, D.L. (1991). Menopausal estrogen replacement therapy and breast cancer. *Arch. Int. Med.*, **151**, 67–72.
24. Armstrong, B.K. (1988). Oestrogen therapy after the menopause – boon or bane? *Med. J. Austral.*, **148**, 213–214.
25. Steinberg, K.K., Thacker, S.B., Smith, S.J. *et al.* (1991). A meta-analysis of the effect of estrogen replacement therapy on the risk of breast cancer. *J. Am. Med. Assoc.*, **265**, 1985–1990.
26. Silero-Arenas, M., Delgado-Rodriquez, M., Rodiques-Canteras, R., Bueno-Cavanillas, A., Galvey-Vargas, R. (1992). Menopausal hormone-replacement therapy and breast cancer: a meta-analysis. *Obstet. Gynecol.*, **79**, 286–294.
27. Grady, D., Rubin, S.M., Petitte, D.B. *et al.* (1992). Hormone therapy to prevent disease and prolong life in postmenopausal women. *Ann. Intern. Med.*, **117**, 1016–1037.
28. Colditz, G.A., Egan, K.M., Stampfer, M.J. (1993). Hormone replacement therapy and risk of breast cancer: Results from epidemiologic studies. *Am. J. Obstet. Gynecol.*, **168**, 1473–1480.
29. Byrd, B.F., Burch, J.C., Vaughn, W.K. (1927). The impact of long-term estrogen support after hysterectomy: a report of 1016 cases. *Ann. Surg.*, **185**, 574–580.
30. Hunt, K., Vessey, M., McPherson, K. (1990). Mortality in a cohort of long-term users of hormone-replacement therapy: our updated analysis. *Br. J. Obstet. Gynecol.*, **97**, 1080–1086.
31. Bergkvist, L., Adami, H., Persson, I. *et al.* (1989). Prognosis after breast cancer diagnosis in women exposed to estrogen and estrogen-progestogen-replacement therapy. *Am. J. Epidemiol.*, **130**, 221–228.

32. Brinton, L.A., Hoover, R., Fraumeni, J.F. (1986). Menopausal oestrogens and breast cancer risk: an expanded case-control study. *Br. J. Cancer*, **54**, 825–832.
33. Lufkin, E., Carpenter, P., Ory, S., Malkasion, G., Edmanson, J. (1988). Estrogen replacement therapy: current recommendations. *Mayo Clin. Proc.*, **63**, 453–456.
34. Stuerkel, C. (1989). Menopause and estrogen replacement therapy. *Psychiatr. Clin. North. Am.*, **12**, 133–152.
35. Hillmer, B., Hollenberg, J., Parker, S. (1986). Post-menopausal estrogens in prevention of osteoporosis benefit virtually without risk if cardiovascular effects are considered. *Am. J. Med.*, **80**, 1115–1127.
36. Harris, S., Genant, H., Baylink, D. *et al.* (1991). The effects of estrone (ogen) on spinal bone density of postmenopausal women. *Arch. Intern. Med.*, **157**, 1980–1984.
37. Haarbo, J., Hassager, C., Jensen, S., Riis, B., Christianson, C. (1991). Serum lipids, liproproteins and apolipoproteins during postmenopausal estrogen replacement therapy combined with either 19- nor testosterone derivatives or 17-hydroxy progesterone derivatives. *Ann. J. Med.*, **90**, 584–589.
38. Hazzard, W. (1989). Estrogen replacement and cardiovascular disease: serum lipids and blood pressure effects. *Am. J. Obstet. Gynecol.*, **161**, 1847–1853.
39. Barrett-Connor, E. (1992). Risks and benefits of replacement estrogen. *Ann. Rev. Med.*, **43**, 239–251.
40. McGill, H. (1989). Sex steroid hormone-receptors in the cardiovascular system. *Post Grad. Med.*, **17**, 64–68.
41. Williams, J.K., Adams, M.R., Kopfenstein, H.S. (1990). Estrogen modulates responses of atherosclerotic coronary arteries. *Circulation*, **81**, 1680–1687.
42. Pines, A., Fishman, E.Z., Levo, Y. *et al.* (1991). The effects of hormone replacement therapy in normal postmenopausal women: measurements of Doppler-derived parameters of aortic flow. *Am. J. Obstet. Gynecol.*, **164**, 806–812.
43. Henderson, B.E., Paganini-Hill, A., Ross, R.K. (1991). Decreased mortality in users of estrogen replacement therapy. *Arch. Intern. Med.*, **151**, 75–78.
44. Kennedy, D.L., Baum, C., Forbes, M.B. (1985). Non-contraceptive estrogens and progestins: use pattern over-time. *Obstet. Gynecol.*, **65**, 441–446.
45. Hemminski, E., Kennedy, D.L., Baum, C. *et al.* (1988). Prescribing of noncontraceptive estrogen and progestins in the United States, 1974–86. *Am. J. Public. Health* **78**, 1478–1481.
46. Reginster, J.Y., Christiansen, C., Dequinze, B. *et al.* (1993). Effect of transdermal 17 beta-estradiol and oral conjugated equine estrogens on biochemical parameters of bone resorption in natural menopause. *Calcif.-Tissue-Int.*, **53**, 13–16.
47. Lindsay, R. (1993). Hormone replacement therapy for prevention and treatment of osteoporosis. *Am. J. Med.*, **95**, 375–395.
48. Ferguson, K.J., Hoegh, C., Johnson, S. (1989). Estrogen replacement therapy: survey of women's knowledge and attitudes. *Arch. Intern. Med.*, **149**, 133–136.
49. Schmitt, N., Gogate, J., Rothert, M. *et al.* (1991) Capturing and clustering women's judgement policies. The case of hormonal therapy for menopause. *J. Geronto.*, **46**, 92–101.
50. Kadri, A.Z. (1991). Hormone replacement therapy – a survey of perimenopausal women in a community setting. *Brit. J. General Practice*, **41**, 109–112.
51. Vassilopoulou-Sellin, R., Zolinski, C. (1992). Estrogen replacement therapy in women with breast cancer: A survey of patient attitudes. *Am. J. Med. Sci.*, **304**, 145–149.
52. Groeneveld, F.P.M.J., Boreman, F.P., Barentsen, R. *et al.* (1993). Relationships between attitude toward menopause, well-being, and medical attention among women aged 45–60 years. *Maturitas*, **17**, 77–88.
53. Hemmonki, E., Topo, P., Malin, M., Kangas, J. (1993). Physicians views on hormonal therapy around and after menopause. *Maturitas*, **16**, 163–173.
54. Welbush, J. (1993). The climacteric kaleidoscope: Questions and speculation. *Maturitas*, **16**, 157–162.

55. Nactigall, L.E. (1990). Enhancing patient compliance with hormone replacement therapy at menopause. *Obstet. Gynecol.*, **75**, 775–835.
56. Derby, C.A., Hume, A.L., McFarland, *et al.* (1993). Correlates of postmenopausal estrogen use and trends through the 1980's in two Southeastern New England Communities. *Am. J. Epidemiol.* **137**, 1125–1135.
57. MacLennan, A.H., MacLennan, A., Wilson, D. (1993). The prevalence of oestrogen replacement therapy in South Australia. *Maturitas*, **16**, 175–183.
58. Creasman, W.T. (1991). Estrogen replacement therapy: is previously treated cancer a contraindication? *Obstet. Gynecol.*, **77**, 309–312.
59. Theriault, R.L., Vassilopoulou-Sellin, R. (1991). A clinical dilemma: estrogen replacement therapy in postmenopausal women with a background of primary breast cancer. *Ann. Oncol.*, **2**, 709–717.
60. Hutchinson-Williams, K., Gutmann, L. (1991). Estrogen replacement therapy (ERT) in high-risk cancer patients. *Yale. J. Biol. Med.*, **64**, 607–626.
61. Marchant, D.J. (1993). Estrogen-replacement therapy after breast cancer. Risk versus benefits. *Cancer*, **71**, 2169–2176.
62. Powles, T.J., Hukish, T., Casey, S., O'Brien M. (1993). Hormone replacement therapy after breast cancer. *Lancet*, **342**, 60–61.
63. Stoll, B.A. (1989). Hormone replacement therapy in women treated for breast cancer. *Eur. J. Cancer Clin. Oncol.*, **25**, 1909–1913.
64. Wile, A.G., Opfell, R.W., Morgileth, D.A. (1993). Hormone replacement therapy in previously treated breast cancer patients. *Am. J. Surg.*, **165**, 372–375.
65. Disaia, P.J., Odicino, F., Grosen, E.A. *et al.* (1993). Hormone replacement therapy in breast cancer. *Lancet*, **342**, 1232, (letter).
66. Theriault, R.L., Vassilopoulou-Sellin, R. (1994). Estrogen replacement therapy in younger women with breast cancer. *J. Natl. Cancer Inst.*, (In press).
67. Vassilopoulou-Sellin, R., Theriault, R. (1994). A randomized prospective trial of estrogen replacement therapy in women with a history of breast cancer. *J. Natl. Cancer Inst.*, (In press).
68. Lufkin, E.G., Org, S.J. (1994). Relative value of transdermal and oral estrogen therapy invarious clinical situations. *Mayo Clin. Proc.*, **69**, 131–135.
69. Guidelines for counselling postmenopausal women about preventive hormone therapy. (1992). American College of Physicians. *Ann. Int. Med.*, **117**, 1038–1041.
70. Sporrong, T., Hellgren, M., Samsioe, G., Mattsson, L.-A. (1989). Metabolic effects of continuous estradiol-progestin therapy in postmenopausal women. *Obstet. Cynecol.*, **73**, 754–758.
71. MacLennan, A.H., MacLennan, A., Wenzel, S., Chambers, H.M., Eckert, K. (1993). Continuous low-dose oestrogen and progestogen hormone replacement therapy: a randomised trial. *Med. J. Aust.*, **159**, 102–106.
72. Casper, R.F., Chapdelaine, A. (1993). Estrogen and interrupted progestin: A new concept for menopausal hormone replacement therapy. *Am. J. Obstet. Gynecol.*, **168**, 1188–1196.
73. Christiansen, C., Riis, B.J. (1990). Five years with continuous combined oestrogen/progestogen therapy. Effects on calcium metabolism, lipoproteins, and bleeding pattern. *Brit. J. Obstet. Gynaecol.*, **97**, 1087–1092.
74. Stevenson, J.C., Cust, M.P., Gangar, K.F. *et al.* (1990). Effects of transdermal versus oral hormone replacement therapy on bone density in spine and proximal femur in postmenopausal women. *Lancet*, **335**, 265–269.
75. Whitehead, M.I., Fraser, D., Schenkel, L., Crook, D., Stevenson, J.C. (1990). Transdermal administration of oestrogen/progestagen hormone replacement therapy. *Lancet*, 335, 310–312.

Chapter 19

Clinical Programs for Breast Cancer Protection

MAUREEN M. HENDERSON and ANNE McTIERNAN

The primary care provider is responsible for promoting the general health of patients and has a pivotal function in assessing a woman's risk of breast cancer and telling her what steps she can take to lower her risk. Every woman needs to be given advice of this type from childhood to her terminal years, and in different countries, a variety of health professionals such as internists, pediatricians, family practitioners, gynecologists, mid-level practitioners and nurses, will contribute. However, long-term continuity of preventive care is essential and this should be the task of the primary health care provider.

Breast Cancer Risk Assessment in Practice

Breast cancer continues to be a major cause of mortality and morbidity among women, particularly in Western Europe and North America [1, 2]. Assessment is now being used in daily practice to identify groups of women at high risk for inclusion in clinical prevention trials, and to identify women who might benefit from intensive schedules of breast screening [3–5]. Translation of risk assessment from research into clinical practice could formalize what is already done instinctively by many primary care providers.

For maximum safety, breast cancer risk assessment must begin in late adolescence and continue at intervals throughout a woman's life. For most women, it will start on the first occasion she discusses a method of birth control with her physician. In ideal circumstances the promotion of good health as an adult will be part and parcel of a comprehensive well-child program given to all girls, obviating formal breast cancer risk assessment during childhood and adolescence.

Women at very high risk for breast cancer may benefit from the services that can be offered through a high risk clinic. Several such clinics have been opened in the United States in the past few years [6, 7]. These clinies have recruited women with

Basil A. Stoll (ed.), Reducing Breast Cancer Risk in Women, 177–183.
© 1995 *Kluwer Academic Publishers. Printed in the Netherlands.*

a family history of breast cancer, and have offered an array of medical services such as breast screening, breast health information and genetic and psychological counseling. Some clinics offer further services for women with positive screening results, such as ultrasonography, biopsies, and surgical and oncologic evaluation and treatment. Women at high risk for breast cancer not only need genetic counseling, but also psychosocial and risk-avoidance counseling. Studies have shown a relationship between a family history of breast cancer and a tendency to perceive breast cancer risk as even higher than the calculated probability [8, 9].

Programs for Breast Cancer Protection

Some of the recommended measures for prevention of breast cancer are those recommended for the promotion of general health and the prevention of other diseases, and would be part of routine pediatric, adolescent, reproductive adult and geriatric practice.

Childhood and Adolescence

Girls who undergo early first menses (ages 10–12 years), and who have early regular ovulation (within one year after onset of menarche), have been found to be at increased risk of developing postmenopausal breast cancer [10, 11]. Heavy body mass and low levels of exercise increase the likelihood of early first menses and the establishment of early regular ovulation [12, 13]. Pediatricians and family practitioners should therefore monitor girls' weight and exercise profiles, and actively intervene to maintain them within a healthy range.

High body mass during adolescence and young adult life is problematically associated with the risk of postmenopausal breast cancer. Since all of the evidence suggests that premenopausal breast cancer is associated with below average body mass from adolescence to the menopause [14], girls and young women recognized as having a high risk for early breast cancer (e.g. girls with a first degree relative with premenopausal breast cancer) should maintain their body mass at an average rather than a high or particularly low level.

Since the breast is a radio-sensitive organ, and since excessive radiation exposure has been shown to increase risk of breast cancer [15–18], especially when the exposure is before age 20 years [16, 19, 20], it is prudent to avoid unnecessary radiation exposure, especially in the ages surrounding menarche and adolescence, when the breast is undergoing rapid cellular division and growth.

Drinking alcohol in adolescence and young adulthood may be as strong a risk factor as drinking alcohol later in life [21]. The use of alcohol is associated with the use of tobacco so that prevention of the use of tobacco products as well as prevention of moderate or heavy use of alcohol should be part of general health prevention counseling, including prevention of breast cancer. If alcohol exerts its influence by increasing bioavailable estrogens [22], this effect could be particularly harmful during these years when the breast tissues are highly susceptible.

Early Adulthood, Reproductive Years

That an early first full-term pregnancy protects against the development of post-menopausal breast cancer has been known for several decades. Women who undergo their first full-term pregnancy after age 30 almost double their risk of developing breast cancer, compared with women who have their first full-term pregnancy before age 20 [10]. Advising women to begin their families early in life may not be compatible with contemporary normative social behavior. Even so, women may be receptive to advice to avoid delaying the start of their families beyond age 25 to 30, if at all possible.

Abortion before her first full-term pregnancy may also increase a woman's risk of early breast cancer [23, 24]. Young women with other risk factors for the disease (i.e. family history of breast cancer or history of benign breast disease), might be advised that early abortion may further increase [25] their risk. It is not known how early abortion aggravates breast cancer risk.

For women with a family history of breast cancer, the use of estrogen- or progesterone-based oral contraceptives should be discussed. Breast cancer incidence in young women has been found in several studies to be increased in long-term users of oral contraceptives as compared with non-users [26–28].

Several studies have shown that breast-feeding lowers the risk of premenopausal breast cancer, and the amount of protection appears to increase with increasing number of months of breast-feeding [29–31]. This protection afforded by breast-feeding seems to be independent of the effect on breast cancer risk of numbers of full-term pregnancies and age at first full-term pregnancy. Information on this protective effect could be given to women as an additional benefit of choosing to breast-feed rather than bottle-feed their infants.

Breast self-examination [BSE] and yearly clinical breast examination have been considered as methods of early breast cancer detection [32]. However, BSE has not been recommended for general use by the U.S. Preventive Services Task Force [33]. Its reservations are based on current lack of evidence of BSE efficacy in terms of mortality reduction.

Clinical breast examination is another screening modality that has been advocated. There is no evidence at this time that routine radiographic screening decreases deaths from breast cancer in women under age 50 [34]. The benefits of good clinical examination may be greater than most physicians have appreciated. The most recent scientific evaluation suggests that annual clinical breast examination provides a sound basis for early detection and successful treatment [34] in both premenopausal and postmenopausal women.

Peri- and Early Postmenopausal Years

Women who are at high risk for breast cancer might be advised to avoid prolonged use of hormone replacement therapy. Although studies have not given consistent estimates for risk of breast cancer associated with hormone replacement therapy use in women with benign breast disease or a family history of breast cancer [35], estimates have been as high as 1.5 to two-fold in the latter group of women [36]. The Women's Health Initiative will provide information about the relationship to breast cancer risk, as well as the benefits, of combined replacement therapy [37]. Meanwhile, judicious use, as well as serious consideration of long-term use, is necessary.

Use of regular screening mammograms has been found to decrease deaths from breast cancer by up to 30% among women aged 50 and over [38–40]. Yet, many of the older postmenopausal women who could benefit best from mammographic screening are not getting screened, or are being inadequately screened [41]. The U.S. National Cancer Institute recommends screening mammograms every one to two years in women aged 50 and over [42]. This is in line with recommendations adopted by major comprehensive U.S. health programs [43] and the Canadian National Service Programs [44].

Dietary recommendations for prevention of cancer differ from those for coronary heart disease. First, they emphasize total fat reduction without changing the proportions of saturated and polyunsaturated fats usually eaten. Second, they include a goal of eating at least five servings of fruit and vegetables and at least six servings of grain a day. Third, they propose lower absolute levels of total fat consumption. Currently, the standing recommendation for breast cancer prevention is for less than 30% of calories from fat [45] and most preventive programs suggest a fat intake between 25 and 30% of daily calories.

Older Years

Very high prevalence of obesity among postmenopausal women is reported in the United States and shows no signs of improvement. There is no doubt that obesity, and increasing degree of obesity, raises the breast cancer risk of postmenopausal women. What is still unclear is the importance of abdominal fat and of relatively rapid weight gain and weight loss, as well as any role for insulin. The steady maintenance of an appropriate body mass by judicious eating and exercise lifestyle cannot be too strongly emphasized. It is also prudent to monitor carbohydrate metabolism.

The low fat, high fruit and vegetable eating pattern should be encouraged throughout the older years in spite of the commonly observed increasing preference for foods made with fat and sugar. Dietary recommendations to prevent heart disease have been easier to handle in this regard because changing the ratio of polyunsaturated to saturated fat eaten has been successful in lowering CHD rates without any major reduction in the total grams of fat eaten.

Besides improving the likelihood of extended survival, the early detection and treatment of breast cancer through mammographic screening in the older years is likely to improve the quality of life in older women with breast cancer [46].

Conclusion

Much of the future of prevention of breast cancer incidence and deaths will lie with the primary care provider. Assessment of breast cancer risk will become part of the assessment of general health risks, and will stretch from childhood through old age. Giving advice about choices and actions for preventing breast cancer will also be an important task for the primary care provider.

It is relatively simple, and may be productive in public health terms, to incorporate breast cancer risk assessment and reduction into routine health monitoring and promotion, clinical surveillance and services. The establishment of more formal identification and risk reduction clinical protocols is required for women who are assessed as being at extremely high risk. The authors are developing plans for a high risk clinic to serve women who have volunteered to collaborate in epidemiological and cancer prevention research studies. Their approach relies heavily upon the existence of lifelong medical records or of easily linked periodic records. It will be most easily adapted for use within national, regional, or local systems providing comprehensive health services.

Acknowledgments

Alicia Cerna for preparation of the manuscript and Barbara Cochrane, Ph.D., for advice on the psychosocial literature.

References

1. Parkin, D., Muir, C., Whelan, S. *et al.* (1992). *Cancer Incidence in Five Continents*, Vol. VI. IARC Scientific Publications., No. 120, Lyon.
2. Harris, J., Lippman, M., Veronesi, U., Willett, W. (1992). Breast Cancer (Part 1). *N. Engl. J. Med.*, **327**, 320–328.
3. Taplin, S., Thompson, R., Schnitzer, C. *et al.* (1990). Revisions in the risk-based breast cancer screening program at Group Health Cooperative. *Cancer*, **56**, 812–818.
4. National Surgical Adjuvant Breast and Bowel Project (NSABP) (1992). *Protocol P–1: A Clinical Trial to Determine the Worth of Taxmoifen for Preventing Breast Cancer.*
5. Oza, A., Boyd, N.F., (1993). Mammographic parenchymal patterns: a marker of breast cancer risk. *Epidemiol. Rev.*, **15**, 196–208.
6. Halper, M., Roush, G., Diemer, K. (1989). Recruitment procedures for a high-risk breast cancer detection clinic. In *Adv. Cancer Control: Innovations and Research.* Alan R. Liss, Inc., New York, 183–189.

7. Biesecker, B., Boehnke, M., Calzone, K. *et al.* (1993). Genetic counseling for families with inherited susceptibility to breast and ovarian cancer. *J. Am. Med. Assoc.*, **269**, 1970–1974.

8. Lerman, C., Trock, B., Rimer, B. *et al.* (1991). Psychological side effects of breast cancer screening. *Health. Psychol.*, **10**, 259–267.

9. Dean, C., Roberts, M., French, K. *et al.* (1986). Psychiatric morbidity after screening for breast cancer. *J. Epidemiol. Comm. Health*, **40**, 71–75.

10. Kelsey, J.L., Gammon, M.D., John, E.M. (1993). Reproductive factors and breast cancer. *Epidemiol. Rev.*, **15**, 36–47.

11. Henderson, B., Bernstein, L. (1991). The international variation in breast cancer rates: an epidemiological assessment. *Breast Ca. Res. Treat.*, **18**, S11–S17.

12. Frisch, R., von Gotz-Welbergen, A., McArthur, J. *et al.* (1981). Delayed menarche and amenorrhea of college atheletes in relation to age of onset of training. *J. Am. Med. Assoc.*, **246**, 1559–1563.

13. Vihko, R., Apter, D. (1986). The epidemiology and endocrinology of the menarche in relation to breast cancer. *Cancer Surv.*, **5**, 561–571.

14. London, S., Colditz, G., Stampfer, M. *et al.* (1989). Prospective study of relative weight, height, and risk of breast cancer. *J. Am. Med. Assoc.*, **262**, 2853–2858.

15. Land, C.E., Boice, J.D., Jr., Shore, R.E. *et al.* (1980). Breast cancer risk from low-dose exposures to ionizing radiation: results of parallel analysis of three exposed populations of women. *J. Natl. Cancer Inst.*, **65**, 353–376.

16. Boice, J.D., Jr., Preston, D., Davis, F.G. *et al.* (1991). Frequent chest x-ray fluoroscopy and breast cancer incidence among tuberculosis patients in Massachusetts. *Radiat. Res.*, **125**, 214–222.

17. Shore, R.E., Hempelmann, L., Kowaluk, E. *et al.* (1977). Breast neoplasms in women treated with x-rays for acute postpartum mastitis. *J. Natl. Cancer Inst.*, **59**, 813–822.

18. Hoover, R. (1997). Cancer induced by cancer treatment. In Fortner, J., Rhoads, J. (eds.), *Accomplishments in Cancer Research. General Motors Cancer Research Foundation.* J.B. Lippincott Company, Philadelphia, 229–241.

19. Tokunaga, M., Land, C.E., Yamamoto, T. *et al.* (1987). Incidence of female breast cancer among atomic bomb survivors, Hiroshima and Nagasaki, 1950–1980. *Radiat. Res.*, **112**, 243–272.

20. Miller, A.M., Howe, G.R., Sherman, G.J. *et al.* (1989). Mortality from breast cancer after irradiation during fluoroscopic examinations in patients being treated for tuberculosis. *N. Engl. J. Med.*, **321**, 1285–1289.

21. Hiatt, R., Klatsky, A., Armstrong, M. (1988). Alcohol consumption and the risk of breast cancer in a prepaid health plan. *Cancer Res.*, **48**, 2284–2287.

22. Reichman, M., Judd, J., Longcope, C. *et al.* (1993). Effects of alcohol consumption on plasma and urinary hormone concentrations in premenopausal women. *J. Natl. Cancer Inst.*, 722–727.

23. Parazzini, F., LaVecchia, C., Negri, E. (1991). Spontaneous and induced abortions and risk of breast cancer. *Int. J. Cancer*, **48**, 816–820.

24. Remennick, L. (1990). Induced abortion as cancer risk factor: a review of epidemiological evidence. *J Epidemiol. Community Health*, **44**, 259–264.

25. Andrieu, N., Clavel, F., Gairard, B. *et al.* (1994). Familial risk of breast cancer and abortion. *Cancer Det. Prev.*, **18**, 51–55.

26. Wingo, P.A., Lee, N.C., Ory, H.W. *et al.* (1991). Age-specific differences in the relationship between oral contraceptive use and breast cancer. *Obstet. Gynecol.*, **78**, 161–170.

27. Malone, K.E., Daling, J.R., Weiss, N.S. (1993). Oral contraceptives in relation to breast cancer. *Epidemiol. Rev.*, **15**, 80–97.

28. White, E., Malone, K., Weiss, N. *et al.* (1994). Breast cancer among young U.S. women in relation to oral contraceptive use. *J. Natl. Cancer Inst.*, **86**, 505–514.

29. Byers, T., Graham, S., Rzepka, T. *et al.* (1985). Lactation and breast cancer: evidence for a negative association in premenopausal women. *Am. J. Epidemiol.*, **121**, 664–674.

30. McTiernan, A., Thomas, D.B. (1986). Evidence for a protective effect of lactation on risk of breast cancer in young women: results from a case-control study. *Am. J. Epidemiol.*, **124**, 353–358.

31. Newcomb, P., Storer, B., Longnecker, M. *et al.* (1994). Lactation and a reduced risk of premenopausal breast cancer. *N. Engl. J. Med.*, **330**, 81–87.

32. Anonymous. (1980). Guidelines for the cancer-related checkup: recommendations and rationale. *CA*, **30**, 194–240.

33. US Preventive Services Task Force. (1989). *Guide to Clinical Preventive Services*. Williams and Wilkins: Baltimore.

34. Fletcher, S.W., Black, W., Harris, R., Rimer, B., Shapiro, S. (1993). *Report of the International Workshop on Screening for Breast Cancer*. National Cancer Institute, Bethesda, Maryland.

35. Brinton, L., Schairer, C. (1993). Estrogen replacement therapy and breast cancer risk. *Epidemiol. Rev.*, **15**, 66–79.

36. Grady, D., Rubin, S., Petitti, D. *et al.* (1992). Hormone therapy to prevent disease and prolonged life in postmenopausal women. *Ann. Int. Med.*, **117**, 1016–1037.

37. Kirschstein, R. (1993). Largest U.S. clinical trial ever gets under way. *J. Am. Med. Assoc.*, **270**, 1521.

38. Council on Scientific Affairs. (1989). Mammographic screening in asymptomatic women aged 40 years and older. *J. Am. Med. Assoc.*, **261**, 2535–2542.

39. Shapiro, S., Venet, W., Strax, P. *et al.* (1982). Ten-to-fourteen year effect of screening on breast cancer mortality. *J. Natl. Cancer Inst.*, **69**, 349–355.

40. Tabar, L., Duffy, S., Burhenne, L. (1993). New Swedish breast cancer detection results for women aged 40–49. *Cancer*, **72**, 1437–1448.

41. Rakowski, W., Rimer, B., Bryant, S. (1993). Integrating behavior and intention regarding mammography by respondents in the 1990 National Health Interview Survey of Health Promotion and Disease Prevention. *Pub. Health Rep.*, **108**, 605–624.

42. Shapiro, S. (1994). The call for change in breast cancer screening guidelines. *Am. J. Pub. Health.*, **84**, (editorial) 10–11.

43. Taplin, S., Thompson, R.S., Carter, A.P., Schnitzer, F. (1989). Cost effectiveness in program delivery. *Cancer*, (Suppl.), 2682–2689.

44. Miller, A., Baines, C., To, T., Wall, C. *et al.* (1992). Canadian National Breast Screening Study: 1. breast cancer detection and death rates among women aged 40 to 49 years. *Can. Med. Assoc. J.*, **147**, 1459–1476.

45. Butrum, R., Clifford, C., Lunza, E. (1988). NCI dietary guidelines rationale. *Am. J. Clin. Nutr.*, **48**, (Suppl.).

46. Morrison, A. (1992) Cancer of the breast. In *Screening in Chronic Disease*. Oxford University Press, New York, New York.

Chapter 20

Nurses' Role in Educating Women on Risks

NINA ENTREKIN and LISA SUMMERLOT

Educating patients and the community at large about the importance of disease prevention and the value of early detection is an integral part of the nurses' role. Women of all ages and in all walks of life need accurate information about breast cancer risk if they are to make appropriate decisions and lifestyle choices. Nurses are in an ideal position to provide this education. Numerous studies have demonstrated the commitment that nurses have shown to educating women about breast cancer risk and the importance of early detection [1–13].

In order to meet the new challenges, nurses will need to educate themselves about the rapidly changing information on breast cancer risk. They will need to develop the tools which are required to accurately assess breast cancer risk. They will have to find the ways to bring this information to women, and to develop the skills needed to present the information in a meaningful way.

Educating Women Who Feel at Increased Risk

The perception of risk by people is not necessarily based on actual statistical risk. Fear may be greater than, or less than, an actual threat. What is presented in the news can affect what is perceived as a threat. It has been found that if people choose to engage in activities which put them at risk, they tend to minimize that risk. Risk perception is highest for risks which are seen as being outside of one's control and with the potential for being fatal [14].

Many women believe that their risk of breast cancer is extraordinarily high and some believe that their risk is 100%. They may make all kinds of important life choices based on their belief that they are destined to get breast cancer [15, 16]. Most often, these women have had a mother or sister die of breast cancer and have been told that their risk is influenced by the diagnosis in their first-degree relative.

185

Basil A. Stoll (ed.), Reducing Breast Cancer Risk in Women, 185–192.
© 1995 *Kluwer Academic Publishers. Printed in the Netherlands.*

Once they connect the perception of their personal risk to an emotional event as significant as the death of a family member, it is extremely difficult for them to put this risk into a realistic perspective. They are faced with a threat which is outside of their control and which has fatal potential. Highly publicized risk factors featured by the media only serve to reinforce to these women that they are destined to get breast cancer.

Nurses who encounter this population of women might be tempted to try to determine whether their fear is realistic or not. If 90% of breast cancer is not hereditary, there are many women whose diagnosis of breast cancer does not increase the risk to their relatives. Even in hereditary breast cancer, the risk is not 100% [17]. It is a logical assumption that providing these women with reassuring statistics will help to allay their fears.

What these women need first and foremost, however, is validation that their feelings are normal, understandable and shared by many women in the same situation. Explanations and statistical facts which contradict their feelings will not only fall on deaf ears, but may be viewed as an insensitive negation of what, to these women, is a powerful reality.

Women with a very high level of distress need psychological and educational interventions which require the involvement of a health care team. Referral to a risk counseling setting, where the emotional aspects of risk perception are addressed along with risk analysis and education, is indicated. High risk clinics or programs should develop support groups for women who struggle with similar fears. Nurses need to know what resources are available in their community to meet the special needs of these women. Indeed, nurses may be the ones who create such resources.

The fears of women who feel at greatly increased risk must be addressed. Studies have shown that a little fear may motivate women to engage in appropriate early detection behaviors. On the other hand, women who have a very high level of distress about their breast cancer risk will often not engage in these potentially life-saving procedures [16].

Educating the Average Woman on Risk

The average woman's breast cancer risk increases dramatically as she gets older and 82% of the breast cancers in the United States are diagnosed in women over age 50 [18]. Some researchers believe that all women over age 35 are at high risk of breast cancer [6]. The majority of these women, however, feel so safe that they are not seeking mammograms according to recommended guidelines [5]. Women with a false sense of security may be the very ones at risk of dying of breast cancer.

The size at which a breast cancer is found has significant implications for a woman's prognosis. In one study of breast cancers diagnosed at 1 cm or less, 95% of women were alive 12 years after diagnosis [19]. Studies have shown that if all women over 50 had screening mammograms as recommended, the mortality from breast cancer could decrease by 30% [5].

Often it is the media who define who is at risk of breast cancer. Studies which show even slight increases in risk make the news, and women use the findings of such studies to define the level of their personal risk. If the study finding does not apply to them, their false sense of security is reinforced. The fact that women over 50 are at an increased risk of breast cancer does not make headlines. This results in women getting the wrong idea about who is at increased risk.

Nurses in all primary care settings are in contact with women over age 50. If they take responsibility for educating all women about realistic breast cancer risk and early detection, they can be powerful agents of change. An understanding of cultural, ethnic, and age-related factors which affect how women receive educational messages is important [3, 4, 6, 9, 13]. Nurses must stay apprised of current research regarding healthy lifestyle choices such as low fat, high fiber diets, regular exercise, and stress reduction. They must learn to evaluate studies so that they can help women put highly publicized risk information into perspective.

Actions speak louder than words. As role models, if nurses do not follow the recommended schedule of mammography and clinical examinations, they cannot expect their patients to do so. One study found that only 26% of nurses practiced regular BSE [3]. Nurses who did not perform consistent monthly breast self examinations were found to be ineffective BSE teachers [2]. Given that 80–90% of breast cancers are discovered by women themselves [6], the above findings have significant implications.

Nurses who care for older women have a special responsibility to ensure that their patients receive appropriate screening. The findings of one study suggest that, as women get older, concern for increasing numbers of chronic complaints may divert their attention from the importance of screening examinations [4]. It should be the responsibility of every nurse who sees elderly women to make sure that screening recommendations are being followed in this population. Instruction in breast self-examination may need to be modified to take into account physical limitations and age-related prejudices that might influence compliance in performing BSE [20].

Nurses are also valuable assets to cancer-control organizations. Whether they participate in community lectures, health fairs, high school breast health classes or any number of other community-sponsored events, their expertise helps to authenticate the information that is provided about breast cancer risk and the importance of early detection.

Educating Women Who Are at Increased Risk

The first responsibility that nurses have to women who are at increased risk is to develop and use assessment tools which give an accurate picture of that woman' risk. Figure 1 contains elements of a sample nursing assessment. These elements can be used to elicit basic breast cancer risk-related information when interviewing women. A detailed personal and family history is perhaps the most helpful mechanism for establishing risk. Unfortunately, it is often incomplete, ignored or

PERSONAL HISTORY

Height:_____ Weight:_____ Age: _____

Number of Children:_____ Age at Birth of First Child:_____

Age at First Menses:_____ Still Menstruating:_____Yes _____No

Check if Applies: _____ Hysterectomy; When_____

_____ Ovaries Removed

Oral Contraceptive Use:_____Yes _____No Type:_____

Years of Oral Contraceptive Use:_____

Hormone Replacement Therapy:_____Yes _____No Type:_____

Duration of Therapy:_____

Patient's Perception of Her Breast Cancer Risk:

_____Below Average _____Average _____Above Average

MEDICAL HISTORY

Age at First Mammogram:_____ Date of Most Recent Mammogram:_____

Date of Last Clinical Breast Exam:_____

Practices Breast Self Examination:_____Yes _____No

History of Benign Breast Disease:_____Yes _____No

Date(s) and Findings of Any Breast Biopsies:_____

History of Breast Cancer:_____Yes _____No Age at Diagnosis:_____

History of Other Cancers:_____Yes _____No Type of Cancer:_____

Age at Diagnosis:_____

FAMILY HISTORY OF CANCER

_____No Family History of Breast Cancer

First Degree Relatives With Breast Cancer:

  Mother: _____ Age at Diagnosis:_____

  Sister(s) :_____ Age at Diagnosis:_____

  Daughter(s):_____ Age at Diagnosis:_____

Second Degree Relatives With Breast Cancer:

  Maternal Aunts:_____ Age at Diagnosis:_____

  Maternal Grandmothers:_____ Age at Diagnosis:_____

  Paternal Aunts:_____ Age at Diagnosis:_____

  Paternal Grandmothers:_____ Age at Diagnosis:_____

History of Other Family Members With Cancer:_____

Figure 1. Sample nursing assessment.

the information which is gathered is not acted on [21]. If nurses were instrumental in just this one area of providing reliable family history information, they could contribute significantly to cancer control [21, 22].

The assessment should include information about menstrual and reproductive history, hormone therapy, screening activities, and a thorough family history. The family history should detail current ages, ages at death, and ages at diagnosis of all cancers which occurred in at least two generations. Maternal and paternal histories are equally important [1]. Wherever a patient enters the health care system the nurse is often the team member who conducts the initial assessment. This is true of doctor's offices, acute care settings, nursing homes and home health. Even in the hospice setting a careful history may identify families at increased risk.

Nurses must educate themselves on the current status of risk-related information in order to understand the significance of assessment data. If a woman has had a biopsy which shows atypical hyperplasia, what does that mean in terms of her breast cancer risk? What does it mean if a family history demonstrates breast cancer in multiple generations at young ages with an incidence of bilateral breast cancer present? How is that family history different from one where there is cancer present, but only in elderly family members or only one family member affected? Once genetic testing becomes available, who will be the appropriate candidates for genetic testing, and what will this mean to that woman and her family? The nurse must also act as the liaison who reports pertinent information to the rest of the health care team, and the patient advocate who makes sure the information is acted upon.

Nurses must be aware of current clinical trials, and which of their patients might be eligible to participate. They will need to assess their communities for risk-counseling services and identify which patients might benefit from a personalized, thorough assessment of breast cancer risk. In this population of women who are at increased risk, the importance of following recommended screening guidelines must be stressed and systems put into place to assure compliance. This includes addressing the special needs of the elderly, the culturally diverse and medically-uneducated women.

Women who are at increased risk will have unique emotional needs. Unresolved grief and anger surrounding the death of a close family member may surface during the family history assessment. Women feel very vulnerable not only because the threat of cancer carries with it connotations of pain, disfigurement and death, but also because of the social stigma associated with the cancer diagnosis [23]. These women should be referred to cancer-risk counseling where feelings can be sorted out and validated, and where information and education can take place in a setting which helps women make sense out of confusing statistics [18]. The nurse may act as the advocate and liaison between the patient, counselors, and perhaps even family members. Risk information is sensitive information which may affect insurability, employability, social status, and family relationships. The confidentiality of such information must be protected by all members of the health care team.

Women at risk may ask nurses for advice about choices like hormone replacement, reproductive issues, or prophylactic surgery. Nurses are used to being sought out for their expert opinion, and it may be very tempting to advise women about what to do. In advising women at increased risk, however, there are no easy or absolute answers. The non-directive approach where all available information is provided and a woman is supported in whatever option she chooses for herself, is the only appropriate approach. No one should decide for her.

As genetic information and genetic terminology become more commonplace in many practice settings, nurses must become sensitive to how some of the terms they use may be interpreted by patients. A woman who has many relatives diagnosed with breast cancer will not consider that her family history is a 'positive' one. If someone has inherited a defective gene, does that make this person a 'defective' human being? If a gene mutation is present, is the person with the gene a 'mutant'? Does a 'pedigree' carry with it the connotation of something connected to dogs and horses? Nurses must learn to think of how such terms sound to their patients.

Educating Women Who Have an Established Hereditary Risk

The localization of the BRCA1 gene on chromosome 17 is imminent. Once this gene has been isolated and cloned, it is only a matter of time before a test is available which will determine with a reasonable degree of accuracy that a woman has inherited this gene. Women who carry this gene will have an 85% risk of breast cancer over their lifetime and a significantly elevated risk of ovarian cancer [17]. What women must realize before they are referred for testing is that the advances of science which give them this information have far outstripped the advances which provide them with reasonable options for protection.

These women who are at very high risk currently have the option of choosing close surveillance or prophylactic surgery [24]. Both of these options carry with them their own anxiety-producing implications. Close surveillance is not prevention, it is trying to find a cancer early enough so that the woman has a reasonably good prognosis. Breast cancers occur frequently in very young women in BRCA1 families. For these women, prophylactic bilateral mastectomy and oophorectomy is a grim option. It is common knowledge that neither of the procedures offer 100% protection in average women [24, 25] and there is no way to know how much protection is afforded to BRCA1 carriers.

Even though the gene has yet to be cloned, linkage analysis has allowed some research centers to postulate carrier status in members of certain families. The experience of these researchers has confirmed what we have learned about the counseling needs of some of the other adult-onset hereditary diseases such as Huntington's disease: the ethical, psychosocial and legal implications are enormous [26]. Even though extensive pre- and post-test counseling are a part of the testing process, there are many individuals who require continued long-term support. Survivor guilt may affect those who have not inherited the gene and they will require as much psychological support as those with the gene [17].

When the test for the BRCA1 gene becomes available, nurses may be the ones closest to the women who might consider being tested. In order to support these women in this decision making process, nurses must be aware of the issues involved and the resources that are available. If women do choose to be tested, nurses may be involved in assessing how well these women are coping with both positive and negative test results.

Conclusion

In order to prepare nurses for their expanding role as breast cancer risk educators, both formal academic and continuing nursing education programs should focus on primary prevention as well as on early detection of breast cancer [27]. A new program to train nurses as cancer risk counselors has been developed in the US by Dr. Patricia Kelly, Director of Medical Genetics and Cancer Risk Screening for Salick Health Care, Inc. This intensive and thorough program is designed to help nurses understand risk and to apply findings in a clinically relevant way.

Employers will need to provide nurses with access to the tools and knowledge needed as well as the time to participate in breast cancer risk education. While a recent study found a distressing lack of participation by nurses in cancer prevention and detection activities, 66% of the nurses surveyed believe these activities to be part of their professional role. It was suggested that hospitals and other agencies need to modify their employment policies to include clear expectations for cancer prevention and detection activities by nurses. With such changes in policy will come changes and expanding horizons in nursing practice [28].

References

1. Kelly, P.T. (1993). Breast cancer risk: the role of the nurse practitioner. *Nurse Practitioner Forum.*, **4**, 91–95.
2. Post-White, J., Carter, M., Anglim, M.A. (1993). Cancer prevention and early detection: nursing students' knowledge, attitudes, personal practices, and teaching. *ONF*, **20**, 743–749.
3. White, L.N., Spitz, M.R. (1993). Cancer risk and early detection assessment. *Seminars in Oncology Nursing*, **9**, 188–197.
4. Warren, B., Pohl, J.M. (1990). Cancer screening practices of nurse practitioners. *Cancer Nursing*, **13**, 143–151.
5. Crooks, C.E., Jones, S.D. (1989). Educating women about the importance of breast screenings: the nurses role. *Cancer Nursing*, **12**, 161–164.
6. Frank-Stromberg, M., Rohan, K. (1992). Nursing's involvement in the primary and secondary prevention of cancer. *Cancer Nursing*, **15**, 79–108.
7. Nevidjon, B. (1986). Cancer prevention and early detection: reported activities of nurses. *ONF*, **13**, 76–80.
8. Brody, J. (1986). Cancer education: how nurses can help. *ONF*, **13**, 18–20.
9. Frank-Stromberg, M. (1986). The role of the nurse in early detection of cancer: population sixty-six years of age and older. *ONF*, **13**, 66–74.
10. Heyman, E., Tyner, R., Phipps, C. *et al.* (1991). Is the hospital setting the place for teaching breast self-examination? *Cancer Nursing*, 14, 35–40.
11. White, L.N. (1986). Cancer prevention and detection: from twenty to sixty-five years of age. *ONF*, **13**, 59–64.

12. Sawyer, P.F. (1986). Breast self-examination: hospital-based nurses aren't assessing their clients. *ONF*, **13**, 44–48.
13. Nielsen, B.B. (1989). The nurse's role in mammography screening. *Cancer Nursing*, **12**, 271–275.
14. Slovic, P. (1987). Perception of risk. *Science*, **236**, 280–285.
15. Kelly, P.T. (1991). *Understanding Breast Cancer Risk*. Temple University Press, Philadelphia.
16. Kash, K.M., Holland, J.C., Halper, M.S., Miller, D.G. (1992). Psychological distress and surveillance behaviors of women with a family history of breast cancer. *J. Natl. Cancer Inst.*, **84**, 24–30.
17. Bieseker, M.S., Boehnke, M., Calzone, K. *et al.* (1993). Genetic counseling for families with inherited susceptibility to breast and ovarian cancer. *J. Am. Med. Assoc.*, **269**, 1970–1974.
18. Kelly, P.T. (1992). Informational needs of individuals and families with hereditary cancers. *Seminars in Oncology Nursing*, **8**, 288–292.
19. Tabar, L., Fagerberg, G., Day, N., Duffy, S., Kitchin, R. (1992). Breast cancer treatment and natural history: new insights from results of screening. *Lancet*, **339**, 412–416.
20. Coleman, E.A., Riley, M.B., Fields, F., Prior, B. (1991). Efficacy of breast self-examination teaching methods among older women. *ONF*, **18**, 561–566.
21. Lynch, H.T., Follett, K.L., Lynch, P.M. *et al.* (1979). Family history in an oncology clinic. *J. Am. Med. Assoc.*, **242**, 1268–1272.
22. Weber, W. (1993). Cancer control by family history. *Anticancer Research*, **13**, 1197–1202.
23. McGuire, D.B. (1979). Familial cancer and the role of the nurse. *Cancer Nursing*, **12**, 443–452.
24. Blum, J., Tomlinson, G. (1994). New insights on hereditary breast cancer. *Contemporary Oncology*, **1**, 23–31.
25. King, M.L., Rowell, S., Love, S.M. (1993). Inherited breast and ovarian cancer: What are the risks? What are the choices? *J. Am. Med. Assoc.*, **269**, 1975–1980.
26. Huggins, M., Block, M., Wiggins, S., *et al.* (1992). Predictive testing for Huntington disease in Canada: Adverse effects and unexpected results in those receiving a decreased risk. *Am. J. Med. Genet.*, **42**, 508–515.
27. Fernsler, J.I. (1989). Counseling women with respect to lifestyles, life events, and breast cancer risks. *AAOHN Journal*, **37**, 158–165.
28. Entrekin, N., McMillan, S. (1993). Nurses' knowledge, beliefs, and practices related to cancer prevention and detection. *Cancer Nursing*, **16**, 431–439.

PART FOUR

PERSPECTIVES AND VIEWPOINTS

Chapter 21

Women's Perspectives on Breast Cancer Protection

JEANMARIE MARSHALL

American women are alarmed about increasing breast cancer rates over the last 50 years. They want to feel they have some control over their health and to know what they can do to reduce the likelihood that they will get breast cancer or any other type of cancer. When patients consult with their doctors about prevention or how to reduce their risk, they are most often told about early detection – breast self-examination and mammography. When women considered at high risk want information about protection, they hear about early detection, the future availability of genetic testing, low-fat diet, prophylactic mastectomies, the Tamoxifen trials, among other things. Is any of this actually protection against breast cancer?

Both women with breast cancer and those who don't have it are asking the medical community tough questions about the disease and want to know why breast cancer is on the increase. Many feel that medical research has focused too much on detection and treatment, and little attention has been paid to the causes of the disease. Some women with cancer have become activists and are publicly challenging the research priorities of the cancer establishment (the National Cancer Institute, American Cancer Society, and cancer research centers) in the US. In light of recent news reports of falsified data in the National Surgical Adjuvant Breast and Bowel Project (NSABP) led by Dr. Bernard Fisher at the University of Pittsburgh, as well as the withholding of crucial information by the NCI in the tamoxifen prevention trials about the risk of uterine cancer, women are not only confused and angry, but also losing faith in cancer research.

This chapter addresses four major topics which came up most often in interviews with women about breast cancer protection: genetic factors, concerns about possible environmental links, mammography and early detection, and the economics of reducing risk. Other concerns such as diet, prophylactic mastectomies, and breast-feeding were also raised in these discussions.

Basil A. Stoll (ed.), Reducing Breast Cancer Risk in Women, 195–204.
© 1995 *Kluwer Academic Publishers. Printed in the Netherlands.*

This chapter reflects the opinions and feelings of women ranging in age from 34 to 70 with the majority being over 40 (70%). Most of the women did not have breast cancer (87%) although a few did, and some had a family history of breast cancer. The women interviewed live mainly on the east coast of the United States in urban, suburban, and rural areas, and represent various socio-economic backgrounds.

Hopefully, this chapter will shed some light on women's concerns and anxieties about breast cancer prevention and what the medical and scientific community can do to address those concerns.

Are Women Ready for Genetic Testing?

The long-awaited discovery of the breast cancer gene may be considered a break-through in medical research, but what are the implications for women who are considered high risk? How will they feel about the prospect of a positive test result if there is little they can do to prevent the disease? What effect, if any, will genetic testing have for women who do not have a family history, given that hereditary breast cancer accounts for only 5–10% of all cases.

Some of the women interviewed had strong opinions about the genetic marker test and question whether it is a really a breakthrough. After all, hereditary breast cancer is 'a very small part of the overall problem', according to one woman.

Tina L. may be a candidate for genetic testing. Her mother was diagnosed with breast cancer when Tina was ten and died of it thirteen years later. Tina is a 35-year old mother of two small boys and has carefully thought about her risk of breast cancer and what her options are.

"I would not want to have the test. If I tested negative, it would be a false sense of security. So I won't get hereditary breast cancer. Big deal! It's only like 5% of all breast cancers. What about the other 95%? A negative test wouldn't mean that I'm not at risk."

"Let's say I took the test and it was positive. I would first wonder about the accuracy of the test. If it was accurate, then what? What would the knowledge of a positive test result really do for me? It would put a big black cloud of gloom and doom over my head that would not be there if I didn't have the test results. What could I do with that information to help me? Even if the test was wrong, as long as I believed it was correct, maintaining hope would be difficult. You can't live without hope."

"With a positive test result, what action could I take? I wouldn't change my lifestyle. I already have a low-fat diet, I breast-fed my babies, I exercise, I do relaxation work. I take very good care of myself. I wouldn't do anything different except wake up in a cold sweat at night."

"Would I get mammograms more often with a positive test result? No. I'm 35-years old and I've had one mammogram. I know the effectiveness of mammography screening in women my age is not so good. There are a lot of false negatives. I heard one study showed that mammography misses like 40 or 50% of breast cancers in women under 50."

"I believe that prevention starts earlier than early detection. Early detection is not prevention!" states Tina whose feelings were echoed by others.

Ellen C. is a 55-year old woman with breast cancer diagnosed five years ago. Her sister, mother, and aunts have also been stricken with the disease. She too is critical of the test.

"I think genetic testing only has value if women can actually to do something to prevent this disease. What good is it to have the knowledge if you can't prevent it? If it had been available to me before my diagnosis, I would not have chosen to do the test. I would not use it to *plan my life*, only to *save my life*. Unless I could do something to protect myself, the test would be of no use to me. Personally, I would not want the knowledge of a positive test result."

"I hear about women getting prophylactic mastectomies as a prevention. I was seriously considering this surgery before my diagnosis. I think the researchers need to be doing studies to find out if prophylactic mastectomies do any good. Women will need to have clear information about their options if they do test positive."

Lydia W. is 42 and has thought about the genetic test since her mother was diagnosed recently with breast cancer.

"With genetic testing, if it only applies to 5% of all breast cancer cases, then I don't consider it very important."

"I would do the test if there was breast cancer in my family for say, two or three generations. But with only my mother getting it recently as an older woman, I don't have strong feelings about it being hereditary. It was probably environmental, but who knows?"

While many don't consider the test a good option for women, others see the soon-to-be available genetic test as a new means of having more information to help make decisions.

Debbie N., age 37, is concerned because her sister was diagnosed 16 years ago at the age of 29. "There's a part of me that would do it, although it would not be a priority for me. A negative test would give me peace of mind, but maybe I wouldn't want to expend that effort because I might not even have a family history. I feel I'm reducing my risk by going to the doctor regularly, doing self-exams and mammograms."

Lesley N. is 36 and was diagnosed with breast cancer at the age of 31. Her mother died of the disease when Lesley was only five. She feels the test could be useful if she were to have children: "If I had a daughter, I would consider getting the test done for her."

Pat W., 52, has no family history but would consider getting tested: "If I tested positive for the gene, I would take more precautions, be more proactive, follow studies more carefully. If I were to have a granddaughter, I feel the test could be valuable information for her."

While the discovery of the breast cancer gene could expand our general under-standing of the disease, the sense is that women will not welcome the genetic marker test until there is truly something they can do about preventing breast cancer.

Women's Concerns about the Breast Cancer and the Environment

Breast cancer clusters exist throughout the US but are more common in the highly industrialized northeast and north central states. Stories about high breast cancer rates linked to chemical plants on Long Island, toxic waste dumps on Cape Cod, widespread spraying of DDT and other pesticides, and hazardous waste sites across the US have been reported in the national and international press. Evidence of a possible link between high breast cancer rates and organochlorines in the environment has inspired legislation in a number of states to restrict the sale, manufacture, and use of chlorine.

Clearly, environmental factors are emerging as an important part in the equation of women's risks and environmental factors may be preventable.

Environment as used in this chapter includes not only air, water, and soil, but also our diets, living and working conditions, products we put on our bodies, and medical procedures. That means that the air we breath, the food we eat, the water we drink, the radiation to which we are exposed, where we live, the work we do – these may be responsible for at least 75% of all breast cancers, as well as all cancers.

Women want to know what is causing the breast cancer epidemic, what role environmental toxins play, and what can be done to prevent this killer disease. They are asking these questions and not getting good answers from their physicians, so many women are educating themselves and looking into pollutants in their communities.

Laura B. feels there has been too much emphasis on genetics in the research and not enough focus on environmental factors. "I believe the genetic links are being overplayed. It's only like 5%. Families live in certain areas and have similar diets and favorite foods. If these foods are chemically polluted, it could mimic a genetic history. Families move away, and take their diet preferences with them. It looks genetic and it's not. The only people who are reproducing must be the ones with the faulty gene? Are we to believe this? How could it be true? The percentages don't work. Breast cancer is going up. Other women without the faulty gene are still having babies."

She has concerns about exposure to pollutants in our food, soil, and water. "I have a problem. There are no federal regulations monitoring the amount of pollutants and additives like chlorine and fluoride. I think about the food I eat and food fats, and what could have been sprayed on them. Certain pesticides stay in soils when we plant and then they continue to add more poisons in the soil. After 20 years of spraying, we have to wonder what is in the soil."

"I believe that supplementing your diet with anti-oxidants can help detoxify these chemicals. But why should we have to detoxify our environment?"

Suzanne M. wonders about chemicals in the environment: "I'm not sure what role they play with breast cancer but I have always been leery of chemicals in the environment. Food additives scare me. What about the bovine growth hormone in our milk or the spraying of apples? Has there been any studies?"

Some raised concerns about the use of anti-perspirants with aluminum chlorhydrate and its effect on the body.

"I was reading about how researchers were looking into hormonal contraceptives that women could apply in a cream form onto their armpits because the skin of our underarms has the highest absorption rate of anywhere on our body. That got me thinking. What happens when we put aluminum chlorhydrate/zirconium trichlorohydrex and other harsh chemicals in the form of anti-perspirant and deodorant on our bodies daily?" asked Lydia W.

"We are sternly warned not to use these products if our skin is broken, irritated, or if a rash develops. Shaving keeps underarms perpetually scraped and irritated, perhaps providing even readier access of the chemicals to our lymph nodes and system. Could there be a link? I don't know but I think it should be looked at."

Another woman raised concerns about the ingredients in anti-perspirants: "I've heard that aluminum chlorhydrate can affect the brain. Also, aluminum has been linked to Alzheimers which women get at a higher rate than men. We need to be investigating these things."

Because of their concern about the affect these chemicals might have on their bodies, these women no longer use anti-perspirants. Now they use deodorant which does not contain aluminum chlorhydrate.

Many women raised concerns about exposure to pollutants in their communities. Mary Lou H., age 63, lives in Falmouth on Cape Cod in Massachusetts where high rates of cancer have been reported. "I worry about where I live. Falmouth was one of five towns in which they found high rates of breast cancer near Otis Air Force Base where they've been dumping toxic fuels into the sand. Flumes of toxic waste move so many feet a year underground, polluting our wells and our water. The water supply here is highly chlorinated. I can smell it in the water. Then there's the Pilgrim Nuclear Power Plant not far from here in Plymouth. It's been leaking radiation. It was just shut down again last year. Boston Edison always says, "oh it's just something minor," but you just don't know what's going on. Why should we believe them?"

Recently, women with cancer have become active around the issue of cancer and the environment. Because breast cancer research has focused almost entirely on treatment and detection, there has been little focus on the environmental causes. Cancer activists are challenging the priorities of the National Cancer Institute and the American Cancer Society, and demanding that the government, medical and scientific communities look more closely at possible environmental links.

In February of 1993, women's cancer groups, women's organizations, and environmentalists from Canada, Mexico, and across the US came together for a meeting in Austin, Texas to launch a campaign called Women, Health and The Environment: Action for Cancer Prevention. The activists are calling for a phase-out of the widespread use of chlorine, among other things. Research has shown possible evidence of a link between the increase in breast cancer rates and the rapid proliferation of organochlorines into the environment. Organochlorines are chlorine-based derivatives and many of them, such as DDT, PCBs, and dioxin, are known carcinogens.

The activists are not alone in their call for a chlorine phase-out. In October 1993, the American Public Health Association, the nation's premier public health organization, voted that "chlorine-containing organic compounds are found to pose public health risks" and approved a resolution that these chemicals should be treated as a class and subject to a broad phase-out. In early 1994, the Clinton Administration unveiled a clean water plan eliminating most uses of chlorine.

Ellen C., a cancer activist from Boston, attended the meeting in Austin organized by Greenpeace and the Women's Environment and Development Organization (WEDO). "Women from all over North America representing various ethnic and racial groups, social classes, and ages came together to talk about women, cancer, and the environment, and plan a strategy for political action. We want the government regulatory agencies to stand up to the polluters and start taking action on the damage that is being done to our communities. This campaign is about our health, our children's health, and most importantly, our future."

Mammography: Is Early Detection Early Enough?

Although mammography and breast self-exams are neither prevention nor a cure for breast cancer, some women feel that mammography is the only protection there is and finding a cancerous lump early will increase their odds for survival.

Many women observe the American Cancer Society guidelines recommending a mammogram every one to two years for women between 40–49 and every year for women over 50. Debbie N., a 37-year old woman, feels that getting a mammogram gives her some peace of mind. "I've been getting a mammogram every year and a half since I was 29. My doctor recommended it because of my sister's diagnosis. I consider myself high risk because of, not only family history, but also I don't have children and I grew up on Long Island where there are high rates of breast cancer."

However, some women are becoming increasingly confused and disillusioned with screening mammography. Women under 50 are concerned about the conflicting information they're receiving from the American Cancer Society and the National Cancer Institute about the effectiveness of the test for their age group. Although the controversy about mammography for younger women raged in the medical community for many years, it is only recently that women learned there is evidence that screening mammograms do not reduce mortality rates in younger women. Researchers speculate that this is because certain breast cancers tend to be especially aggressive in premenopausal women, and early detection through mammography may not do any good.

Many women spoke about mammography not being protection. Terri T., a 65-year old woman discusses the drawbacks to screening mammography: "Mammograms are for early detection, for getting it early, but not for prevention. Who knows? Even if you have the test, you could still get breast cancer. There are no guarantees and no easy answers for this one."

Laura B. expressed concern about its effectiveness: "By the time they find a knot in the breast, cancer is already in your body. It's too little, too late. The test may help to extend your life, but it probably won't save your life."

Ellen C. was in her 40s when her breast cancer was missed by mammography. "I was a high risk person because of family history. The mammogram showed no problem and then shortly thereafter, cancer was discovered. The films were mis-read by the radiologist. My sister had a mammogram which showed nothing and then, six months later discovered a 5 cm. lump."

"When I became politically active around breast cancer, I talked with many women in their 40s who had similar experiences with mammography missing their cancer. We just can't trust this test. It offers no security at all."

In spite of a distrust of mammography for younger women, research shows the test can be a good screening tool for women over 50; however, older women are not getting the message because the ads promoting mammography often depict younger women, some in their 20s and 30s, and ignore older women who are at the greatest risk. According to a recent poll, only half of the women over 50 in the US have had one or more mammograms.

"No, I don't go every year for a mammogram, but my doctor finally insisted," said one 63-year old woman. "I was 58 for the first one. But I still do self-exams regularly."

The mammography ads not only target young women, but often make misleading claims. Ellen C. calls them unethical. "One ad I read by the American Cancer Society stated, "Early detection results in cure nearly 100% of the time." How can they make a statement like this? Why are the regulatory agencies and medical associations allowing these misleading ads?"

Women are bombarded with messages about how 'safe' mammography is, yet no minimum dose of radiation has been proven safe with respect to breast cancer. Some women express concern about the exposure to the radiation. "You're taking this sensitive area – the breast, and radiating it. How can this be safe?" asked Laura B.

Another woman questioned her physician about the safety. "I asked my doctor about the radiation exposure. I find that doctors have a tendency to always have an answer, even if they don't know. She responded, "There's very little radiation exposure from a mammogram. It's no more radiation than you would get from walking around every day." What does that mean? I wonder what is a safe dose? Do they really know?" Others echoed this sentiment.

Until the medical community develops a more accurate and safer test, women will continue to rely on mammography for early detection. However, many feel that early detection is too late and mammography has been oversold.

The Economics of Reducing Risk

In the United States, there are more than 36 million people without health insurance and another 50 million underinsured. A disproportionate number of the uninsured are women and many of them are single heads of households. When a woman without health insurance is diagnosed with breast cancer, the lack of insurance becomes an important risk factor. According to a recent study at Brigham and Women's Hospital in Boston, breast cancer patients with no coverage or Medicaid (US government-funded health insurance for the poor and disabled) tend to learn of their disease at later stages and have poorer survival rates than women who have private insurance.

Accessibility to quality health care regardless of one's ability to pay is at the forefront of the health care reform debate in the US. What role does economies play in how women think about breast cancer protection? What are the financial costs associated with prevention?

Concerns were raised about accessibility to affordable health care and to healthy foods that have not been sprayed with pesticides.

For women who don't have health insurance, a visit to the doctor may be put off because of inability to pay for it. Katherine is a 43 year old lawyer and is uninsured because she could not afford her health insurance premiums. "My finances are tight. If I could afford to get a mammogram every year, I would. My gynecologist reminds me and I keep promising her I'll do it."

Dr. Harold Michlewitz, a gynecologist in Brockton, Massachusetts sees many poor and working-class women in his practice. "Poor women are less apt to get regular mammograms because they're less likely to go in for their checkups."

Other women raised concerns about diet and the affordability of healthy foods. Suzanne M. feels a good diet could reduce her risk of cancer but finds the costs of eating well too expensive. "I can't afford to buy all organic because my groceries costs more than $200/week for my family of five. I don't buy much junk food, mostly meat, vegetables, and dairy. I look carefully at the price of things. The spraying of pesticides on the food concern me, but I just cannot afford to buy organic."

Tina L. states, "I think a good low-fat diet with organic foods may help reduce risk. I know that organic food is difficult to get. People who are poor have difficulty getting healthy food and fresh vegetables."

It is important for the medical community to acknowledge poverty and lack of health insurance as a risk factor for breast cancer.

Conclusion

Women are in need of better information from their physicians regarding breast cancer protection. Many are confused about conflicting reports from the medical community regarding research on treatment and detection and skeptical about what to believe. In spite of 25 years of optimistic public relations pronouncements from the cancer establishment – 'We are winning the war on cancer', deaths from breast cancer have not decreased and treatments offered to patients are the same today as they were 50 years ago – surgery, radiation, and chemotherapy (or slash, burn, and poison, as they are called by breast cancer activists).

Women want answers. They deserve to know what is causing the disease and how to protect themselves from it. As Rachel Carson wrote in her 1962 book *Silent Spring*, "For those in whom cancer is already a hidden or visible presence, efforts to find cures must of course continue, but for those not yet touched by the disease and certainly for the generations as yet unborn, prevention is the imperative need."

Acknowledgements

Many thanks to all the women who gave their time for interviews and to the women of the Women's Community Cancer Project of Cambridge, Massachusetts for their help and support.

References

American Cancer Society (1994). *Cancer Facts & Figures.*

Arditti, R., Schreiber, T. (1993). Killing us quietly: cancer, the environment, and women. In Stocker, M. (ed.), *Confronting Cancer, Constructing Change: New Perspectives on Women and Cancer*, Third Side Press, Chicago, 231–235.

Baines, C.J. (1992). Women and breast cancer: is it really possible for the public to be well informed? *Can. Med. Assoc. J.*, **146**, 2147.

Carson, R. (1962). *Silent Spring.* Fawcett Publications, Greenwich, Connecticut.

Clorfene-Casten, L. (1993). *The Environmental Link to Breast Cancer.* Ms., May/June, 52–56.

Cowley, G. (1993). Family matters: the hunt for a breast cancer gene. *Newsweek*, 12/6/93, 46–52.

Epstein, S. (1992). Cancer establishment ignores evidence on avoidable causes of breast cancer. *Environment & Health*, November/December, 15–16.

Hardisty, J., Leopold, E. (1993). Cancer and poverty: double jeopardy for women. In Stocker, M., (ed.), *Confronting Cancer, Constructing Change: New Perspectives on Women and Cancer.* Third Side Press, Chicago, 213–215.

Ince, S. (1994). Cancer's missing link. *Vogue*, January, 140–141.

Kolata, G. (1993). Studies say mammograms fail to help many women. *New York Times*, 2/26/93, 1.

Marshall, J. (1993). Who needs a mammogram? *Lear's*, October, 56–58.

McQuiston, J.T. (1994). Cancer study renews old concerns. *New York Times*, 4/13/94, B6.

Randall, T. (1993). Varied mammogram readings worry researchers. *JAMA J. An. Med. Assoc.*, **269**, 2616.

Saltus, R. (1993). Breast cancer, DDT tie is cited. *Boston Globe*, 4/21/93.

Schemo, D.J. (1994). Long Island breast cancer is possibly linked to chemical sites. *New York Times*, 4/13/94, 1.

Steingraber S. (1993) How the breast cancer activists of Long Island are changing the focus of science. *Sojourner*, November.

Steingraber, S. (1991). Lifestyles don't kill. carcinogens in air, food, and water do: imagining political responses to cancer. In Stocker, M., (ed.), *Cancer as a Women's Issue: Scratching the Surface.* Third Side Press, Chicago, 91–102.

Thornton, J. (1993). *Chlorine, Human Health, and The Environment: The Breast Cancer Warning.* A Greenpeace report.

Tyson, R. (1994). Chlorine targeted for cutback. *USA Today*, 2/2/94, 1.

R.L. Genetic counselling: a preview of what's in store. *Science*, 1/29/93, 259–624.

Winslow, R. (1992). Breast cancer takes a bigger toll among poor. *Wall Street Journal*, 6/19/92, B1

Chapter 22

A Patient's View of Breast Cancer Trials

HAZEL THORNTON

In September 1991 I was invited to participate in the UK Randomised Trial for the Management of Screen-detected Ductal Carcinoma In Situ (DCIS) of the Breast. The invitation was given when I went to receive my diagnosis, two weeks after excision biopsy following the finding of an abnormality after routine mammographic screening of 50–64 year olds.

Two and a half years later, I am still trying to clarify my ideas and justify my refusal to participate in that trial. I have acquired greater knowledge and understanding of the many facets that need to be examined to understand current attempts to address the appalling scourge of breast cancer by means of the randomised controlled trial. I am perhaps well-placed to try and make observations from the patient's viewpoint on the ability of trials to contribute to reducing the risk of breast cancer in women.

The profession's view of 'patient involvement in breast cancer trials' is almost invariably a consideration of involving the patient, or providing a choice, in what the profession wants to offer the patient. This is not at all the same as patients defining what they perceive to be their preferred outcomes, and then being able to express these by being involved in the design of trials to ensure that the aims reflect their desired outcome. The profession would do well to consider this concept, for "if – and only if – a patient's aim about treatment is identical with the aim implied by the study, can consent to participation be regarded a reasonable choice" [1].

Frequently the profession imagines that the patient will be satisfied by being offered a choice *within what they have devised*. I have come to believe that it is a radical step for them to contemplate that the public should have a say in defining the direction and balance of research: the balance between basic research and research into treatments, or the balance between finding a cure and avoiding risks, or of identifying the questions that need to be addressed in specific trials. I refer to trials where there is choice and flexibility to define variable preferred outcomes which take into account 'quality of life' versus 'survival gains' [2, 3]

205

Basil A. Stoll (ed.), Reducing Breast Cancer Risk in Women, 205–208.
© 1995 *Kluwer Academic Publishers. Printed in the Netherlands.*

and accommodate the very different requirements of women according to their attitudes, age, circumstances, responsibilities and preferences.

The clinician/researcher, must, of necessity, view breast cancer data *objectively* in order to make rational judgements for enhancing the length and quality of life for all patients with breast cancer who come before him, whilst attempting to empathize with the individual needs of the individual patient. The cancer patient's reactions are inevitably intensely *subjective* at the moment she is given her diagnosis and asked to participate in a trial [4]. How then can a partnership, with true patient involvement, be brought about? This inequality of patient/profession must be overcome if we are to establish a partnership between the profession and the patient, with a shared responsibility.

To make a useful contribution, patients will need to face unpleasant realities; learn to appreciate uncertainty; be educated to understand the dilemmas and problems of clinical research and the dilemmas of obtaining consent [4]; understand the need for trials to evaluate new treatments and assess the value of established ones (demand quality); be aware of the diversity of opinion within the profession and be prepared to work hard to acquire an understanding of all aspects of research activity, preferably when they are well [5, 6] so that they may effectively participate in the shared responsibility and debate [7].

The profession too must work hard to make this mutual education productive and come to terms with a new approach where patients may exercise a shared responsibility in research, even though this may be constructively critical of the direction and quality of research currently being undertaken. It must learn not to be dismissive and patronising of patients' views of research. It must examine the proposition that patients may question the wisdom of the current direction of research with its emphasis on ever-proliferating trials of treatment [7].

The requirement of informed consent confers both benefit (with the acceptance of responsibility) and harm to the patient, the clinician, and to the doctor–patient relationship, particularly when it comes as a shock to a patient who has just received a life-threatening diagnosis. Where the seeking of consent to participate in a trial comes as a complete shock, it is because of the gross mismatch of experience with expectation, bringing with it the first inkling that some of the responsibility for furthering our understanding of this disease is being put upon the patient's shoulders.

The whole history of medicine until the technological revolution of this century was based on the idea that suffering humanity went to the medical profession not only for the relief of pain and for care, but also to obtain the comfort that is derived from sharing one's worst fears with one who is experienced, confident and knows what to do to help. Technology has brought with it technicians and a touching belief that we can fix it, or, if it wasn't fixed properly, then it must be someone's fault and we should litigate!

Too often these 'rights' are not matched by the litigating patient with an appraisal of that patient's responsibilities both in terms of a desire for health (as opposed to fixing the illness) and in terms of involvement in determining the direction of medical technology. For this, society as whole rather than the profession should bear the responsibility. Fallibility is disallowed when judging technology, yet the appraisal of health technologies on the human body takes little account of the fact that confidence and hope in one's physician are vital ingredients in the recipe for care. Today's aim is to cure by our faith in technology.

What are we actually achieving by striving to thwart death a little longer, to improve 'survival percentages' by evermore insulting and toxic attacks which do not 'cure'? What are we achieving by constantly enrolling patients in trials comparing an absolutely endless possibility of permutations of surgery, chemotherapy, radiotherapy and endocrine manipulations? Is it not time that the patient stood back and surveyed this technological war on the cancer which lays waste the battleground of the body?

Questions continually arise in my mind concerning the value and effect of these trials for breast cancer sufferers and potential breast cancer sufferers. The suspicion in my mind is that we have become unbalanced in our attempts to deal with this disease. We continually attempt to deal with it in a mechanistic fashion, overlooking the interaction of the mind with the body, the harm we may be indirectly inflicting by our absorption and preoccupation with earlier and earlier screening measures based on an incorrect biological assumption, and our lack of knowledge about causes.

Might fear of cancer have caused reason to fly out the window? Might we not be in danger of anxiety and fear causing a reaction of panic to a systemic disease where the cause is unknown and where the treatments on offer are often worse than the disease, such that an oncologist can proudly announce that the patient who had died of chemotherapy-induced lung disease, died 'cancer-free' [2]? Do not such efforts demonstrate a lack of balance in our efforts to control cancer? Is it not time for the patient to examine the current breast cancer industry and become involved in defining its direction?

Risk-limiting exercises against this background are fraught with the likely possibility that misguided attempts increasingly cause non-sufferers to suffer. That those who will ultimately suffer are made to suffer for far longer than they need, with a minimal survival gain and a worsened quality of life. As Skrabanek expresses it: "The destination is the same, but many women are forced to board the phantom train, destined to crash, a few stations earlier" [8]. The 'time-span' of breast cancer is constantly being enlarged forward and backward: forward by refinements of aggressive treatments which benefit some and not all, and which cannot be targeted accurately; and backwards through treating non-invasive non-precursors of invasive breast cancer, back through habits, lifestyles, diets, reproductive patterns, all the way back to our genetic inheritance.

Let patients therefore critically view breast cancer trials, take responsibility by examining the questions these trials are addressing, and always ask the question, 'is this trial addressing a question we really want the answer to?' The proposition is that "if – and only if – a patient's aim about treatment is identical with the aim implied by the study, can consent to participation be regarded as a reasonable choice" [1].

If this criterion of quality was applied by all women invited to participate in breast cancer trials, by those educated to understand the issues, we would have trials that reflected the preferred outcomes of patients.

References

1. Widder, J. (1994). Randomising means, not aims in clinical trials. *Lancet*, **343**, 359.
2. Astrow, A.B. (1994). Rethinking cancer. *Lancet*, **343**, 494–495.
3. Fallowfield, L.J. Hall, A., Maguire, G.P., Baum, M. (1990). Psychological outcomes of different treatment policies in women with early breast cancer outside a clinical trial. *Brit. Med. J.*, **301**, 575–580.
4. Thornton, H.M. (1992). Breast cancer trials – a patient's viewpoint. *Lancet*, **339**, 44–45.
5. Baum, M. (1993). New approach for recruitment into randomised controlled trials. *Lancet*, **341**, 812–813.
6. Thornton H. (1993). A 'ladyplan' for trial recruitment – everyone's business! *Lancet*, **341**, 796–797.
7. Thornton, H. (1994). *The Patients' Role in Research*. Conference, Brugge, April 1994.
8. Skrabanek, P. (1989). Mass mammography. The time for reappraisal. *Intl. J. Technology Assessment in Healthcare*, **5**, 423–430.

Chapter 23

Should We Aim at Prevention in Youth?

A. LINDSAY FRAZIER and GRAHAM A. COLDITZ

There is increasing evidence that the exposures which determine breast cancer risk occur early in life, particularly in the interval between the onset of menstruation and first childbirth. The effect of migration on cancer incidence rates supports this notion. The rates of colon cancer and breast cancer are both substantially lower among the Japanese than among Americans. Upon immigration to the United States, rates for both increase to the level of residents. However, the shift occurs almost immediately for colon cancer, suggesting that exposure at any age establishes risk whereas for breast cancer, the increased incidence is largely delayed until the second generation, suggesting that exposures during childhood and early adulthood are required to increase the likelihood of breast cancer [1].

This evidence for the window of vulnerability between first menuses and first birth is grounded in the biology of breast tissue development. During the time between menarche and first birth, the cells of the breast are undergoing rapid proliferation and differentiation. Each round of cell division offers potential for the occurrence and propagation of a mutation in the DNA, setting the stage for future malignancy. However, once the cells have undergone terminal maturation as a result of first full term pregnancy, DNA-damaging exposures become more irrelevant. Experiments in animals suggest that the time between menarche and first pregnancy is the most vulnerable period for carcinogenic exposure [2].

The following discussion reviews evidence that certain toxic exposures which occur early in life confer an increased risk of breast cancer in adult life. It also considers whether it is feasible to decrease breast cancer risk by shortening the interval between onset of menstruation and first childbirth, particularly by delaying the onset of menstruation.

Basil A. Stoll (ed.), Reducing Breast Cancer Risk in Women, 209–216.
© *1995 Kluwer Academic Publishers. Printed in the Netherlands.*

Table 1. Exposures during childhood and young adulthood that increase risk of breast cancer

---

Chest irradiation
Onset of alcohol consumption before age 30
Uptake of smoking before age 30
Use of oral contraceptives for > 4 years before first pregnancy
Decreased physical activity leading to earlier age at menarche
'Overnutrition' leading to earlier age at menarche
Delayed childbearing, fewer number of children, and increased number
    of years between each child
Lifetime duration of lactation < 3 months

Risk Exposure during Adolescence and Early Adult Life

Age at the time of exposure has been shown to be pivotal in determining the subsequent risk of breast cancer in studies of irradiation, alcohol consumption, cigarette smoking, and oral contraceptive use. The younger the age at exposure, the greater is the risk. In fact, in several instances, *only* early exposure generates risk (Table 1).

Irradiation at an Early Age

Girls who undergo irradiation of the chest at a young age have an increased risk of breast cancer. This observation has been replicated in a number of settings. Women who survived the atomic bomb in Hiroshima or Nagasaki have an increased risk of breast cancer, dependent both on age and dose [3]. Elevation in risk is seen with doses as low as 0.5 Gy. of radiation. The relative risk (i.e. the rate of breast cancer in women who have been exposed divided by the rate in those women never exposed) is the highest for girls who were under the age of 4 at the time of the bombings. Risk decreases with age of exposure until age 40, when the number of cases observed is no greater than that expected among unexposed women.

Routine X-ray examinations were common in the treatment of tuberculosis. An analysis of 31,710 women treated in Nova Scotia sanitariums between 1930 and 1952 who had undergone pneumotherapy showed an overall excess of mortality from breast cancer (relative risk of 1.36) [4]. The age of the patient at the first exposure to radiation determined the amount of risk conferred. Girls irradiated between the ages of 10 and 14 had a relative risk of 4.46 of developing breast cancer. Radiation between the ages of 15 and 24 resulted in a relative risk of 1.77. For women over age 35 at the time of exposure, the relative risk dropped to 1.1, barely distinguishable from the general population. No excess deaths due to breast cancer were observed in the first five years after the exposure. The peak in incidence did not occur until 25 to 34 years after the initial radiation [4].

The treatment of Hodgkin's Disease includes irradiation of disease within the chest. In a retrospective review of all patients treated for Hodgkin's Disease at Stanford University between 1961 and 1990, 25 cases of breast cancer were discovered among 885 women treated during the time period [5]. Overall, the relative risk for developing breast cancer was 4.1. Again, however, the risk was entirely dependent on the age at exposure. Girls under age 15 at the time of treatment had a relative risk of 1.36. For those treated between the ages of 15 and 24, the relative risk dropped to 1.9. Treatment between age 24 and 29 still conferred an elevation in risk (7.3), but no excess risk of developing breast cancer was observed among the 300 women treated over the age of 30. The incidence of breast cancer after treatment for Hodgkin's disease began to rise 5 years after treatment, but peaked between 15 and 20 years.

These examples of the risk of breast cancer after radiation emphasize the importance of the age at which the exposure occurs. Although important for understanding the susceptibility of developing breast tissue, the amount of radiation in each case far exceeds the amount received by a normal individual during a lifetime.

Alcohol Consumption at an Early Age

Multiple studies have linked the consumption of alcohol to breast cancer [6]. The risk shows a dose-response relationship. The Nurses' Health Study has examined the effect of alcohol consumption among women. For women who drank 15 grams of alcohol per day (>1 drink) and had no other risk factors, the relative risk of breast cancer was 2.5 when compared to women who never drank [7]. The degree of risk conferred by this moderate alcohol consumption is actually greater than from a family history of breast cancer (relative risk of 1.8) [8].

Several studies have explored the effect of early drinking habits (as compared to current drinking habits) on the risk of breast cancer. All have found a significant impact of consumption at a younger age. In a case-control study which asked participants to estimate consumption at three different age periods (<30 years, 30–49 years and >50 years.) The entire elevation in risk associated with drinking was confined to the earliest time period [9]. Another study observed that women who started to drink before age 25 had a relative risk of breast cancer of 1.8 (adjusted for reproductive history, family history and age) compared to women whose first exposure to alcohol occurred after age 25 [10].

In a study of 303 women who developed breast cancer, the women were asked to estimate the time in their lives when they drank the most [11]. Women who reported drinking the most before age 30 had nearly twice the relative risk (2.6) of breast cancer when compared to women who reported drinking more in later periods of their lives (1.4). In a third case-control study, consumption between the ages of 18 and 35 conferred a greater relative risk (relative risk of 2.2), than drinking after age 35 (relative risk of 1.8) [12].

Smoking at Early Age

Current smoking as an adult has not been related to incidence of breast cancer in numerous studies. Most studies show either no association or, at most, a small increase in relative risk. However, several studies which have examined age at the commencement of smoking have demonstrated an elevation in risk for early initiators. In three studies, the elevation in risk was modest (relative risk of 1.3) [13–15], but in a fourth, the association between early smoking and risk of breast cancer was more pronounced. Among women who were heavy smokers (>25 cigarettes per day), those who started to smoke before the age of 16 had a 70–80% greater chance of breast cancer [16].

Use of Oral Contraceptives at an Early Age

The association between use of oral contraceptives (OCs) and breast cancer risk provides another example of an apparent age-dependent risk. Overall, women who have used birth control pills have no higher risk of breast cancer than women who have never taken OCs [17]. However, several studies have suggested that prolonged use prior to first pregnancy (i.e. before age 25) does elevate risk [18, 19].

A meta-analysis summary of the thirteen case-control studies which have been published on this subject calculated the relative risk equal to 1.72 for women who had been exposed to oral contraceptives for at least four years before their first full-term pregnancy [20]. These data combined with the importance of reproductive factors in the genesis of breast cancer suggest that the breast is particularly sensitive to hormonal events between first menses and first pregnancy.

Can We Modify Age at Onset of Menstruation?

Delayed age at first menses and early age at first child-birth have both been shown to confer protection from breast cancer in numerous epidemiologic studies. Though some have hypothesized that these events 'set' hormone levels that influence later risk, the data is not convincing [21–23]. Rather, the emerging hypothesis is that the shorter the interval between first menses and first birth, the less DNA damage is accumulated and the smaller the subsequent risk of malignancy. Some who are concerned about the rising incidence of breast cancer suggest hormonal regulation as a means of modifying risk factors. One group of researchers propose to mimic early menopause by preventing ovulation through monthly injections of a gonadotropin-releasing hormone agonist [24].

We would suggest that the reduction in risk possible from more socially-based prevention strategies offers greater hope for reduction in incidence than such high-tech, high-cost proposals. In addition, the long-term effects of prolonged hormonal manipulation on the incidence of diseases such as osteoporosis, cardiovascular disease and endometrial cancer, is not known and is worrisome.

In the Western world, the age at first menses has decreased from age 17 to age 12.8 over the past two centuries [25]. Each year of decrease raises the risk of breast cancer by 4% [26]. This drop in age at first menses is attributed to better nutrition (i.e. higher caloric intake) and the eradication of the major childhood diseases. More precisely, the decreased age at first menses is due to a shift in energy balance – a change in both calories consumed and calories expended. In the developed world, total caloric intake has increased, but caloric expenditure has also decreased. Children spend less energy through physical activity. The shift from a predominately rural to urban lifestyle, the advent of television and the relative unsafety of the playground have all contributed to a more sedentary lifestyle for children.

There are no studies relating nutrition during childhood to the risk of breast cancer and the recall of past diet is in any case plagued by error and bias [27]. However, adult height reflects the adequacy of childhood nutrition and is often used as a proxy. Many studies have linked adult stature to risk of breast cancer, (for review see [28]).

Adult stature is determined in part by genetic disposition but also by nutrition during childhood. Certainly, stunting of growth due to inadequate nutrition during childhood is known to occur and explains most of the variability when comparing the average height in the less developed world with that in the developed world. Even in the developed world, there is considerable variability in height, in part determined by the social conditions that influence nutrition during childhood. For instance, in a national sample in Britain of 13,000 children who were measured at age 7, a span of 13 cm was found when comparing those children in the uppermost socioeconomic level to those in the lowest [29].

There is sufficient variability even in the developed world to examine the relation between childhood nutrition, height and risk of breast cancer. Taller women have been shown repeatedly to be at greater risk for breast cancer. The observation has been made in both case-control and prospective studies in both the United States and Europe and the effect is, in general, stronger among postmenopausal women [28]. The NHANES I study, which is one of the largest cohorts to examine this issue, obtained baseline measurements on 7413 women between 1971 and 1975. The original cohort was recontacted between 1982–1984. The relative risk of having developed breast cancer in the interim was 2.1 for women in the top quartile of height compared to those in the lowest [30].

Could social changes be modified to decrease the risk of breast cancer? First, it is necessary to recognize that the 'better' childhood nutrition of the 20th century is in truth overnutrition. A survey of over 20,000 Americans, shows that from 1976 to 1991, total energy intake among Americans increased by 100–300 kcal per person, concurrent with an increase in obesity. We continue to eat more and more. Second, we could advocate more energy expenditure via more vigorous physical activity. Increasing physical activity among youth would have a positive impact on many diseases beyond breast cancer, beginning with those linked to obesity such as diabetes and cardiovascular disease.

Can the average age at first menses (or menarche) be shifted to a later age through more vigorous physical activity? A prospective study of the determinants of age at menarche was conducted in Germany among 261 girls selected through a random sample of households [31]. Girls were asked about their level of physical activity at baseline and follow-up. Those in the highest quartile of activity had a delayed menarche (relative risk of 'early' menarche 0.3). Frisch has observed that delayed menarche is common among athletes [32]. Frisch has also reported that the 2776 women who were not college athletes had a significantly higher lifetime risk of breast cancer (relative risk of 1.8), than the 2622 women who participated in sports during college life [33].

Delayed menarche is associated with both lower lean body mass and lower percentage of total body weight due to fat. It is estimated that a girl must have at least 17% of total body weight due to fat before menarche can occur. Frisch suggests that the protective effect of leanness and delayed menarche against breast cancer may operate through a number of different mechanisms [34]. First, percent body fat influences estrogen synthesis and leaner women make a less potent form of estrogen – a catechol estrogen. Second, all women increase the percent of weight due to fat during the interval from menarche to completion of growth, but the rate of increase in fat is lower for women in whom menarche occurs later. The implication is that lean women stay lean. Lastly, women with later menarche also have a longer delay before the return of menstruation when breast feeding.

Implications for Breasts Cancer Prevention

There are basically two different strategies for breast cancer prevention. The first has been the predominant strategy for the last several decades: identify high risk individuals and target screening and intervention to them. The success of this strategy depends on at least two premises: (1) that high risk individuals can be identified early enough to make a difference in the natural history of the disease. (2) that the percentage of the disease attributable to high risk individuals is large enough, that changing the course of their disease will change the overall incidence of the disease in the whole population.

We argue that this 'high-risk' strategy will not result in major reductions in incidence of breast cancer for two reasons. First, the identification of women at high risk of breast cancer is largely determined by a positive family history and only 15% of breast cancer occurs in such women [8].

Therefore 85% of women who will develop breast cancer will not benefit from interventions targeted at high-risk individuals. Second, if the critical time for exposures that determine risk is between the age at menarche and the time of first pregnancy, it will not yet be apparent which girls are at high risk due to family history because the girl's mothers, for the most part, will not be old enough to have developed breast cancer yet.

We propose that the alternative prevention strategy, targeting the entire population for change, will be more likely to affect the incidence of the disease. Small shifts across the entire population can result in a greater change for the population as a whole, than just targeting a small subpopulation of those at highest risk.

Conclusion

This review of the data suggests that the interval from first menses to first birth is critical to the development of breast cancer. If the studies are reinforced by further research, appropriate intervention strategies become apparent. Increasing physical activity among young women would have a large public health benefit, potentially affecting the incidence of osteoporosis, cardiovascular disease and diabetes, as well as breast cancer.

References

1. Buell, P. (1973). Changing incidence of breast cancer in Japanese–American women. *J. Natl. Cancer Inst.*, **51**, 1479–1483.
2. Russo, J., Gusterson, B.A., Rogers, A.E. *et al.* (1990). Biology of disease: comparative study of human and rat mammary tumorigenesis. *Laboratory Investigation*, **62**, 244–278.
3. Tokunaga, M., Land, C., Yamamoto, T. *et al.* (1987). Incidence of female breast cancer among atomic bomb survivors, Hiroshima and Nagasaki, 1950–1980. *Radiation Res.*, **112**, 243–272.
4. Miller, A.B., Howe, G.R., Sherman, G.J. *et al.* (1989). Mortality from breast cancer after irradiation during fluorscopic examinations in patients being treated for tuberculosis. *N. Engl. J. Med.*, **321**, 1285–1289.
5. Hancock, S.L., Tucker, M.A., Hoppe, R.T. (1993). Breast cancer after treatment of Hodgkin's disease. *J. Natl. Cancer Inst.* **85**, 25–31.
6. Rosenberg, L., Metzger, L., Palmer, J. (1993). Alcohol consumption and risk of breast cancer: a review of the epidemiologic evidence. *Epidemiol. Rev.*, **15**, 133–44.
7. Willett, W.C., Stampfer, M.J., Colditz, G.A. *et al.* (1987). Moderate alcohol consumption and the risk of breast cancer. *N. Engl. J. Med.*, **316**, 1174–1180.
8. Colditz, G., Willett, W., Hunter, D. (1993). Family history, age and risk of breast cancer: prospective data from the Nurses' Health Study. *J. Am. Med. Assoc.*, **270**, 338–343.
9. Harvey, E.B., Schairer, C., Brinton, L.A., Hoover, R.N., Fraumeni, J.F., Jr. (1987). Alcohol consumption and breast cancer. *J. Natl. Cancer Inst.*, **78**, 657–661.
10. Van't Veer, P., Kok, F.J., Hermus, R.J.J. Sturmans, F. (1989). Alcohol dose, frequency and age at first exposure in relation to the risk of breast cancer. *Int. J. Epidemiol.*, **18**, 511–517.
11. Hiatt, R.A., Klatsky, A.L., Armstrong, M.A. (1988). Alcohol consumption and the risk of breast cancer in a prepaid health plan. *Cancer Res.*, **48**, 2284–2287.
12. Young, T.B. (1989). A case-control study of breast cancer and alcohol consumption patterns. *Cancer*, **64**, 522–558.
13. O'Connell, D.L., Hulka, B.S., Chambless, L.E., Wilkinson, W.E., Deubner, D.C. (1987). Cigarette smoking, alcohol consumption, and breast cancer risk. *J. Natl. Cancer Inst.*, **78**, 229–234.
14. Brinton, L., Schairer, C., Stanford, J. *et al.* (1986). Cigarette smoking and breast cancer. *Am. J. Epidemiol.*, **123**, 614–622.
15. Adami, H.-O., Lund, E., Bergstrom, R. *et al.* (1988). Cigarette smoking, alcohol consumption and risk of breast cancer in young women. *Br. J. Cancer*, **58**, 823–837.

16. Palmer, J.R., Rosenberg, L., Clarke, E.A. *et al.* (1991). Breast cancer and cigarette smoking: a hypothesis. *Am. J. Epidemiol.*, **134**, 1–13.
17. Prentice, R.L., Thomas, D.B. (1987). On the epidemiology of oral contraceptives and disease. *Adv. Cancer Res.*, **49**, 285–401w.
18. Pike, M.C., Henderson, B.E., Casagrande, J.T., Rosario, I., Gray, G.E. (1981). Oral contraceptive use and early abortion as risk factors for breast cancer in young women. *Br. J. Cancer*, **43**, 72–76.
19. McPherson, K., Vessey, M.P., Neil, A. *et al.* (1987). Early oral contraceptive use and breast cancer: Results of another case-control study. *Br. J. Cancer*, **56**, 653–660.
20. Romieu, I., Berlin, J.A., Colditz, G.A. (1990). Oral contraceptives and cancer; review and meta-analysis. *Cancer*, **66**, 2253–2263.
21. Bernstein, L., Pike, M., Ross, R., Henderson, B. (1991). Age at menarche and estrogen concentrations of adult women. *Cancer Causes Control*, **2**, 221–225.
22. MacMahon, B., Trichopoulos, D., Brown, J. *et al.* (1982). Age at menarche, urinary estorgens and breast cancer risk. *Int. J. Cancer*, **30**, 427–431.
23. Apter, D., Reinila, M., Vihko, R. (1989). Some endogenous characteristics of early menarche, and risk factors for breast cancer, are preserved into adulthood. *Int. J. Cancer*, **44**, 783–787.
24. Spicer, D., Shoupe, D., Pike, M. (1991). GnRH agonists as contraceptive agents: predicted significantly reduced risk of breast cancer. *Contraception*, **44**, 289–305.
25. Van Wieringen, J. (1986). Secular growth changes. In Faulkner, F., Tanner, J. (eds.), *Human Growth: A Comprehensive Treatise*, Plenum Press, New York and London, 307–331.
26. Kvale, G., Heuch, I. (1988). Menstrual factors and breast cancer risk. *Cancer*, **62**, 1625–1631.
27. Friedenreich, C.M., Slimani, N., Riboli, E. (1992). Measurement of past diet: review of previous and proposed methods. *Epidemiol. Rev.*, **14**, 177–196.
28. Hunter, D., Willett, W. (1993). Diet, body size and breast cancer. *Epidemiol. Rev.*, **15**, 110–132.
29. Goldstein, R. (1971). Factors influencing the height of seven year old children; results of the National Child Development Study. *Human Biology*, **43**, 92–111.
30. Albanes, D., Jones, D.Y., Schatzkin, A., Micozzi, M.S., Taylor, P.R. (1988). Adult stature and risk of cancer. *Cancer Research*, **48**, 1658–1662.
31. Merzenich, H., Boeing, H., Wahrendorf, J. (1993). Dietary fat and sports activity as determinants for age at menarche. *Am. J. Epidemiol.*, **138**, 217–224.
32. Frisch, R., Von Gotz-Welbergen, A., McArthur, J. *et al.* (1981). Delayed menarche and amenorrhea of college athletes in relation to age of onset of training. *J. Am. Med. Assoc.*, **246**, 1559–63.
33. Frisch, R., Wyshak, G., Albright, N. *et al.* (1985). Lower prevalence of breast cancer and cancers of the reproductive sustem among former college athletes compared to non-athletes. *Br. J. Cancer*, **52**, 885–891.
34. Frisch, R. (1987). Body fat, menarche, fitness and fertility. *Human Reproduction*, **2**, 521–533.
35. Rose, G. (1992). *The Strategy of Preventive Medicine*. Oxford University Press, New York.

Chapter 24

Role and Limitations of Mammography in Screening

ANTHONY B. MILLER

It is important to recognize that screening for breast cancer at the current stage of knowledge serves only to reduce the risk of breast cancer mortality, not the risk of developing breast cancer. This places screening for breast cancer on a different plane when compared to screening for cancer of the cervix. Cervical cytology, though capable of detecting invasive cancer early, largely aims to detect the precursors of cancer of the cervix in order to reduce the incidence of invasive cancer [1]. However, earlier detection of breast cancer by mammography does not result in a reduction in the incidence of breast cancer.

This chapter considers the value of mammography in reducing mortality from breast cancer when used alone or in combination with clinical breast examination (CBE) in women under and over the age of 50. It also consider whether alternatives to mammography are likely to be of value in reducing breast cancer mortality.

Mammography in the Reduction of Breast Cancer Mortality

Mammography is widely regarded as the most effective method for the detection of breast cancer. However, even for those cancers for which clinical trials have demonstrated efficacy of screening, some of those who do not die of the cancer would not have died in the absence of screening. It is the proportion that would die of their disease in the absence of screening who really benefit from screening.

The initial report of the Health Insurance Plan (HIP) trial [3] showed an effectiveness of the combination of mammography plus CBE annually in women age 50–64 on entry in to the trial, but provided no evidence that breast cancer screening was effective in women age 40–49. Subsequently, long-term follow-up of the HIP study suggested similar efficacy in younger and older women [4, 5], but the num-

217

Basil A. Stoll (ed.), Reducing Breast Cancer Risk in Women, 217–221.
© 1995 *Kluwer Academic Publishers. Printed in the Netherlands.*

bers of breast cancers detected by mammography screening in women age 40–49 upon entry were low [6]. Analysis of breast cancer mortality in the BCDDP [7, 8], comparing the observed numbers of deaths with those expected from national data on cancer incidence and survival, showed little evidence of a benefit from screening in the 40–49 age group, but lower breast cancer mortality than expected in women over the age of 50. Studies in Europe have largely confirmed the HIP findings of benefit for women age 50 or more, but were largely negative for women age 40–49 [1].

More recently, some evidence on the efficacy of breast cancer screening in women under the age of 50 suggests a very delayed benefit compared to women aged 50 or more. The Swedish overview analysis combined the data from the Two-county, Malmö, Stockholm and Gothenberg trials by age at entry [9]. The overview suggested a 10–13% reduction in breast cancer mortality beginning about 10 years after initiation of screening in women under the age of 50. It was however, not statistically significant, and it is not clear how much of the benefit occurred through screening women once they reached the age of 50. In women age 50–69 on entry, the overview analysis showed a significant 30% reduction in breast cancer mortality. For women age 70–74, there was no evidence of benefit, but only two screens had been given and the numbers of women studied were few. All the Swedish trials used mammography alone.

The UK trial 10 year report [10] provided findings by age. Like the Malmö trial, women were recruited from the age of 45, so that findings for women age 45–49 on entry were available. The relative risk for this age group was 0.74 (95% CI 0.54–1.01). This finding was of borderline significance, but there is more uncertainty about it than the randomized trials as it was based on a geographic comparison. For women over the age of 50, there appeared to be little evidence of benefit for those age 50–54 on entry, but about a 22–23% reduction in breast cancer mortality for those age 55–64 on entry.

It is therefore clear that there is little evidence of the effectiveness of mammography in reducing breast cancer mortality in women under the age of 50, at least in the first 10 years after initiation of screening. There is however, consistent evidence for benefit in women over the age of 50 (or in the UK study, over the age of 55). This is a similar conclusion to that reached three years ago [1].

Canadian National Breast Screening Study (NBSS)

One of the suggestions made to explain a lack of effect of the European studies in women under the age of 50 is that they evaluated mammography every 2 years and that screening every year is necessary for effectiveness in women age 40–49 [11]. This is one of the reasons why the Canadian National Breast Screening Study (NBSS) findings have been greeted with surprise, as double-view mammography was used, given every year, combined with good CBEs and the teaching of breast self-examination [12, 13].

Screening of women age 40–49 with yearly mammography and CBE, detected considerably more node negative and small breast cancers than did usual care, but had no impact on mortality from breast cancer in the first 7 years. Again, screening women age 50–59 with yearly mammography in addition to CBE, detected considerably more node negative and small breast cancers than screening with CBE alone, but had no impact on mortality from breast cancer in the first 7 years from entry. This finding can only be explained by mammography selectively detecting good-prognosis cancers.

It is somewhat startling to realise that in spite of the improvements in mammography from the 1960s to the 1980s (when the most recent trials were run) there has been no increase in the estimated effect of breast cancer screening. A recent combined analysis suggests a modest 24% reduction in breast cancer mortality overall for women age 50–74 [14]. It is by no means certain that even earlier diagnosis than achieved in these trials or in the NBSS will result in benefit. All that may be achieved may be the earlier detection of even more good prognosis cancers, the poor prognosis cancers still being fatal even though lead time has been gained. The NBSS has demonstrated that the only indicator of outcome that can be used to indicate possible benefit before breast cancer mortality data are available, is a reduction in the cumulative prevalence of advanced (node positive) breast cancers.

Alternatives to Mammography in the Reduction of Breast Cancer Mortality

Among the alternatives to mammography that have been considered for breast cancer screening are thermography, ultrasound, CBE and breast self examination (BSE). Thermography was shown to be too insensitive and non-specific to be used for breast screening in the 1970s [7]. Ultrasound is now recognised as of value in the diagnosis of breast abnormalities but not for screening. The preceding section hinted that some of the benefits ascribable to mammography in the combination with CBE and or BSE may be due to the simpler modalities. If this were shown to be so, this could be of considerable importance in many developing countries which cannot afford mammography-based screening programs for breast cancer [15].

As far as BSE is concerned, the UK study utilized classes to teach BSE in two cities and evaluated mortality from breast cancer [16]. There was no significant reduction in mortality from breast cancer over a 10 year period, though compliance with invitations to attend BSE classes was poor [16]. There have also been two case-control studies reported [17, 18] which did not associate BSE with reduced risk of developing advanced breast cancer, although in one [17] the authors noted a possible effect of BSE in reducing the prevalence of advanced breast cancer in the small number of women who appeared to be BSE compliers. Recently a cohort study of BSE compliers has been reported from Finland [19]. This study shows a 29% reduction in breast cancer mortality in the study population compared to that expected from the general population of Finland.

For CBE, the evidence that breast cancer mortality reduction will follow from good physical examinations is very indirect, and largely based on the lack of differential between the allocated groups in the 50–59 age group comparison in the NBSS. Some indirect support also comes from one of the case-control studies of BSE [17], where there appears to be a lower risk of developing advanced breast cancer for those who had one or more CBE in the five years preceding the diagnosis of breast cancer, compared to those who had none.

Conclusion

Most current breast screening programs have been planned on the expectation of a 30% or greater breast cancer mortality reduction in the age group screened. The recent data suggest, that such benefit may be obtainable by high quality programs from mammography alone in women over the age of 50. However, the contribution of mammography to breast cancer mortality reduction, beyond that of careful physical examination of the breasts, may be less than has been assumed.

References

1. Miller, A.B., Chamberlain, J. Day, N.E. *et al.* (1990). Report on a workshop of the UICC project on evaluation of screening for cancer. *Int. J. Cancer*, **46**, 761–769.
2. Miller, A.B. (1985). Principles of screening and of the evaluation of screening programs. In Miller, A.B. (ed.), *Screening for Cancer*. Academic Press, Orlando, 3–24.
3. Shapiro, S., Strax, P., Venet, L. (1971). Periodic breast cancer screening in reducing mortality from breast cancer. *J. Am. Med. Assoc.*, **215**, 1777–1785.
4. Chu, K.C., Smart, C.R., Tarone, R.E. (1988) Analysis of breast cancer mortality and stage distribution by age for the Health Insurance Plan clinical trial. *J. Natl. Cancer Inst.*, **80**, 1125–1132.
5. Shapiro, S., Venet, W., Strax, P., Venet, L. (1988). Periodic screening for breast cancer. In *The Health Insurance Plan Project and Its Sequelae, 1963–1986*. The Johns Hopkins University Press Baltimore.
6. Miller, A.B. (1991). Is routine mammography screening appropriate for women 40–49 years of age? *Am. J. Prev. Med.*, **7**, 55–62.
7. Beahrs, O.H., Shapiro, S., Smar, C. (1979). Report of the working group to review the National Cancer Institute, American Cancer Society Breast Cancer Detection Demonstration Projects. *J. Natl. Cancer Inst.*, **62**, 640–709.
8. Morrison, A.S., Brisson, J., Khalid, N. (1988). Breast cancer incidence and mortality in the breast cancer detection demonstration project. *J. Natl. Cancer Inst.*, **80**, 1540–1547.
9. Nyström, L., Rutqvist, L.E., Wall, S. *et al.* (1993). Breast cancer screening with mammography: overview of Swedish randomized trials. *Lancet*, **341**, 973–978.
10. UK Trial of Early Detection of Breast Cancer Group. (1993). Breast cancer mortality after 10 years in the UK trial of early detection of breast cancer. *The Breast*, **2**, 13–20.
11. Kopans, D.B. (1992). Response (letter). *J. Natl. Cancer Inst.*, **84**, 1367–1368.
12. Miller, A.B., Baines, C.J., To, T., Wall, C. (1992). The Canadian National Breast Screening Study: breast cancer detection and mortality in women age 40–49 on entry. *Can. Med. Assoc. J.*, **147**, 1459–1476.

13. Miller, A.B., Baines, C.J., To, T. *et al.* (1992). The Canadian National Breast Screening Study: breast cancer detection and mortality in women age 50–59 on entry. *Can. Med. Assoc. J.*, **147**, 1477–1488.

14. Wald, N.J., Chamberlain, J., Hackshaw, A. (1993). Report of the European Society for Mastology Breast Cancer Screening Evaluation Committee. *The Breast*, **2**, 209–216.

15. Miller, A.B. (1989). Mammography: a critical evaluation of its role in breast cancer screening, especially in developing countries. *J. Publ. Health Policy*, **10**, 486–498.

16. UK Trial of early detection of breast cancer group (1988). First results on mortality reduction in the UK trial of early detection of breast cancer. *Lancet*, **ii**, 411–416.

17. Newcomb, P.A., Weiss, N.S., Storer, B.E. *et al.* (1991). Breast self-examination in relation to the occurrence of advanced breast cancer. *J. Natl. Cancer Inst.*, **83**, 260–265.

18. Muscat, J.E., Huncharek, M.S. (1991). Breast self-examination and extent of disease: a population-based study. *Cancer Detect. Prevent.* **15**, 155–159.

19. Gastrin, G., Miller, A.B., To *et al.* (1994). Incidence and mortality from breast cancer in the Mama program for breast screening in Finland, 1973–1986. *Cancer*, **73**, 2168–2174.

Chapter 25

The Mind and Breast Cancer Risk

BETH LEEDHAM and BETH E. MEYEROWITZ

The notion that psychosocial factors may influence cancer development has enjoyed popularity for centuries but evidence to support most of these claims has been lacking. Recently, however, psychosocial oncologists have begun careful research designed to explore the role of psychological factors in cancer risk. This research has explored hypotheses ranging from the traditional view that cancer may be caused by experiences of depression or life stress to more sophisticated hypotheses on the role that psychological factors might play in immune function.

Research suggests that people's response to challenge may affect whether and how they develop cancer. In one of the earliest studies, a group of patients with various types of cancer was assessed for their psychologic adjustment [1]. Interviews showed four coping attitudes; positive adaptation, giving-up, dependence and lack of acceptance. High scores on the giving-up factor were found to be associated with worse concurrent distress, worse concurrent illness and shorter survival time.

This work is consistent with experimental research on helplessness in animals. In a classic study, rats injected with tumor were randomly assigned to escapable shock, inescapable shock, or no-shock conditions. Although animals in the shock conditions were exposed to identical stressful stimuli, those who were unable to respond actively by escaping developed significantly more tumors than those in the other groups [2].

The 'fighting spirit' is the conceptual opposite of helplessness and hopelessness. Greer [3] interviewed 69 early stage I breast cancer patients, three months after undergoing a simple mastectomy. Patients' responses grouped into several categories: denial or minimizing; fighting spirit, which consisted of active coping and optimism; stoic acceptance, which consisted of fatalism; helplessness/hopelessness; and anxious preoccupation, which was marked by fear of recurrence. Baseline responses were found to be related to prognosis at five-, ten-, and fifteen-year follow-ups, in that significantly more of the patients who initially responded with the fighting spirit pattern were surviving [4].

Basil A. Stoll (ed.), Reducing Breast Cancer Risk in Women, 223–229.

Research has also linked depressed mood with worse prognosis in cancer patients. Thus, Levy and colleagues [5] reported on 36 recurrent breast cancer patients who completed psychological assessments during hospitalization and were then followed-up until death. Controlling for disease-free interval before recurrence, number of metastatic sites, and disability status, it was found that both worse mood and hostility predicted shorter survival times. Positive mood, in fact, was a better predictor of survival time than the physicians' estimates of prognosis or the number of metastatic sites.

In another study on patients with earlier disease, Levy and colleagues [6] obtained baseline physiological and psychological assessments from 90 operable breast cancer patients, whom they then followed for five years or more. Although initial psychological distress did not predict the likelihood of recurrence, higher levels of distress predicted *earlier* recurrence, independent of any influence by tumor stage, immune function, tumor size and estrogen receptor status.

Expression of Distress

Other research suggests that the patient's ability to express distress may modify the impact of cancer. In 50 patients with various cancers, Blumberg [7] noted that personality profiles could distinguish a group of patients with 'fast-moving' cancers from a group in remission. He characterized individuals with worse prognoses as 'serious, over-cooperative, over-nice, over-anxious, painfully sensitive, passive, apologetic personalities' who repressed their distress and anxiety. Those in remission appeared to be 'successful in either avoiding or reducing excessive emotional stress' by expressing negative feelings. Consequently, patients in remission appeared more poorly adjusted.

Derogatis and colleagues [8] supported Blumberg's characterization of the 'successful' cancer patient. Thirty-five metastatic breast cancer patients completed baseline psychological assessments and were then followed-up until death. Few clinical differences emerged between those who died within one year of baseline, and those who lived one year or longer. However, it was noted that those who survived longer expressed significantly *more* distress, depression, anxiety, and hostility at baseline examination than did the short-term survivors. Long-term survivors also had significantly more negative attitudes toward their physicians, and their physicians had evaluated them as significantly less well-adjusted than patients who died quickly.

Not all available data concur but mounting evidence suggests that active expression of emotions is related to cancer incidence and prognosis. In one of the most striking studies, Grossarth-Maticek and colleagues [9] interviewed 1353 Yugoslavs in 1965–66 and tracked the subjects until 1976. Cancer incidence in those scoring highest on the 'rationality/antiemotionality' scale (which measured suppression of aggression) was 40 times that for those scoring lowest on this measure.

There has been controversy in the literature over these findings, and some researchers have failed to find a relationship between emotional suppression/expression and cancer outcome [4, 10]. However, numerous other studies, using a variety of designs and measures of emotional suppression, various samples (i.e. cancer-free individuals and cancer patients), and in some cases adjusting for clinical factors [11], have found consistent relationships between cancer incidence and prognosis and the suppression of strong emotion [12].

Reflecting that this type of behavior appears to be the opposite of the Type A coronary-prone behavior pattern, Temoshok and Heller [13] developed the Type C (cancer-prone) concept. Unlike Type A individuals, who openly express competitiveness, impatience and hostility, and who are at increased risk for cardiovascular disease, individuals with the Type C response pattern are characterized as prone to cancer and as suppressing negative emotions and responding to challenges in an unassertive, passive, and compliant fashion.

To provide empirical support for this concept, Kneier & Temoshok [14] compared 20 melanoma patients to 20 cardiovascular disease patients and 20 disease-free control subjects, on measures of emotional suppression. The melanoma group appeared most likely to suppress emotion, as shown by both paper-and-pencil assessments and the discrepancy between self-reported and physiological measures of arousal. The cardiovascular group appeared least likely to suppress emotions. These differences did not appear to be caused by variations in disease-related anxiety, since degree of suppression did not vary with individual prognosis.

Several questions about the Type C construct remain open. Research has not firmly demonstrated the reliability and validity of Type C as a stable pattern. It is also possible that Type C might predict outcome for only certain individuals. Some well-constructed studies have failed to link Type C responses to disease progression in patients with advanced cancer, suggesting that the effects of Type C may be dwarfed by the pathologic process in very ill patients [10, 15].

It is also unclear exactly how Type C might influence cancer outcome. Although some authors have suggested a link between emotional suppression and endocrine or immune function [16], a study by Temoshok *et al.* [17] points to behavior as a likely mediator, possibly by delay in seeking diagnosis.

Life Stress

The research linking passive behavior to worse cancer prognosis begs the question of stress. What is the relationship of life stress to cancer incidence and progression, and can the pattern of results on the role of passivity be explained by stress?

Animal research has demonstrated a link between stress and increased growth of virally-induced tumors and has also shown increased tumor growth in stressed animals exposed to known environmental carcinogens. However, other research has failed to find a causal relationship between stress and cancer growth in animals, while in some cases, it has demonstrated that stress can inhibit tumor growth [18].

Findings in humans have been similarly inconclusive although some research has linked stress to both increased incidence of cancer as well as worse prognosis in cancer patients [19]. Ramirez *et al.* [20] matched fifty recurrent breast cancer patients to 50 patients in remission, based on treatment, tumor stage and sociodemographic factors. Patients recalled the number and types of stress experienced since diagnosis. Women in the recurrence group recalled significantly more stressful life events than those in remission, such that the relative risk of relapse was 5.67 for patients who had experienced a severe stress, such as bereavement. Although provocative, such findings are limited by a correlational, retrospective design.

Epidemiologic data and several well-designed prospective studies have failed to demonstrate a link between stressful events and cancer risk or prognosis in humans. Given the ambiguous results in both animal and human studies, Fox [18, 21] has concluded that any link between stress and cancer is likely to be small and dependent on responses to stress, rather than on stress itself. It is possible, for example, that cancer patients who express their reactions to a stressor and who respond to it actively, have a better prognosis than those who suppress their emotional reactions and respond with depression, helplessness, hopelessness, and passivity. Such an interaction between stress and coping could explain the mixed findings on relationship between stress and human cancer.

In summary, the research on coping, emotions, and personality at first appears disparate, but the pattern of data suggests that passive response may predict increased cancer risk and worse prognosis. It is unclear whether it is the passive response which increases cancer risk, or if such responses are markers of a more stable, underlying personality trait which affects cancer outcome.

Health Behavior

Good health behavior can improve the chances for cancer survival. One estimate suggests that in the United States, early detection could increase five-year survival rates for the most common cancers by 20% [22]. However, a woman's intention to adopt a healthier lifestyle, perform self-examination or comply with doctors' orders does not necessarily translate into action. Change in health care behavior depends on the individual's appraisal of personal susceptibility to the condition, beliefs about the severity of the condition, obstacles limiting the individual's ability to perform a certain type of action, and other factors [23–25]. There are several ways in which health care professionals can help to change health care behavior both in cancer patients and healthy women at risk for cancer.

First, health care professionals can encourage self-protective behavior such as breast self-examination, and health education may be all that is needed to spur a person to action. However, there may be many reasons other than ignorance why a given individual fails to practice good health-care behavior. She may underestimate her own susceptibility to breast cancer, for example, or feel helpless to effect lasting changes in her lifestyle. She may feel incompetent to perform an accurate breast self-examination or else feel that prevention or early detection are ineffective. In some cases, the prospect of developing cancer may seem so threatening that an individual may reduce the threat by denying her own risk altogether.

Health professionals can try to change these potentially harmful attitudes and beliefs. Recent research on a national sample in the United States demonstrates that among women who had not had a breast examination in the past two years, over two-thirds had visited a physician during that time [26]. Some of these physician visits represent missed opportunities for cancer screening.

Second, there is a need for social support for cancer patients and their relatives. Health professionals should help patients get the support they need by learning about and recommending support groups. They should be aware of emotional problems patients may experience and should suggest specific coping strategies based on the successful experiences of previous patients [27].

Third, health care professionals should encourage an active response pattern in patients. Because the exact nature of the passivity-cancer link remains unclear, interventions aimed at changing passive response patterns are premature, but people should feel free to ask questions and voice their concerns. When patients are encouraged to ask questions during routine visits to the physician, they report greater satisfaction with the visit and greater feelings of control [28].

Health professionals need to allow people to express their negative feelings. Interested patients should be given as much control over the treatment process as is feasible while patients who prefer to have the physician maintain complete control should be allowed to make that decision.

Fourth, medical professionals can help patients by making appropriate referrals to mental health professionals when needed. It is especially important to reassure the reluctant patient, who may fail to seek help in the belief that mental health services are only for the mentally ill. Relaxation therapy and hypnosis are often effective in reducing stress and lessening symptoms [29] and individual or group therapy can improve medical adherence in noncompliant patients [29]. Cognitive therapy for depression and anxiety is effective and may be superior to other treatment including pharmacotherapy [30–33], while cognitive-behavioral interventions have been designed specifically to aid cancer patients in problem solving [34].

Some patients benefit from cancer support groups, which can help patients combat feelings of isolation and provide different types of information and support than those available from health care providers or family members [35]. Family therapy can also improve social support and can provide help to patients' spouses and children, who are often-forgotten 'second-order patients' [36].

Conclusion

We make the following recommendations to clinicians involved in breast cancer prevention:

Include psychologists and other behavioral scientists in interdisciplinary teams. There is an increasing literature on mind-body interrelationships that can influence efforts to prevent breast cancer. By inviting psychosocial oncology researchers to serve on teams, health care professionals can stay current on this research. It also may be beneficial to include behavioral scientists as collaborators or consultants when developing intervention and research programs for breast cancer prevention.

Become aware of mental health practitioners in your community who are experienced in psychosocial oncology. It may be tempting to assume that common sense can guide counseling and that special training is unnecessary to provide optimal psychological care. It is, however, likely that specific training is required for counseling breast cancer patients and healthy women at risk for breast cancer.

Be proactive in raising psychological issues and providing referrals. People frequently avoid 'burdening' their health care team with their fears and concerns. Individuals who are passive in their approach to health care (as people prone to cancer may be), are likely to be especially vulnerable to this problem.

References

1. Davies, R.K., Quinlan, D.M., McKegney, F.P., Kimball, C.P. (1973). Organic factors and psychological adjustment in advanced cancer patients. *Psychosom. Med.*, **35**, 464–471.
2. Visintainer, M.A., Seligman, M.E.P., Volpicelli, J. (1983). Helplessness, chronic stress, and tumor development. *Psychosom. Med.*, **45**, 75–79.
3. Greer, S., Morris, T., Pettingale, K.W. (1979). Psychological response to breast cancer: effect on outcome. *Lancet*, **ii**, 785–787.
4. Greer, S. (1991). Psychological response to cancer and survival. *Psychol. Med.*, **21**, 43–49.
5. Levy, S.M., Lee, J., Bagley, C., Lippman, M. (1988). Survival hazards analysis in first recurrent breast cancer patients: seven-year follow-up. *Psychosom. Med.*, **50**, 520–528.
6. Levy, S.M., Herberman, R.B., Lippman, M. *et al.* (1991). Immunological and psychosocial predictors of disease recurrence in patients with early-stage breast cancer. *Behav. Med.*, **17**, 67–75.
7. Blumberg, E.M., West, P.M., Wells, F.W. (1954). A possible relationship between psychological factors and human cancer. *Psychosom. Med.*, **16**, 277–286.
8. Derogatis, L.R., Abeloff, M.D., Melisaratos, N. (1979). Psychological coping mechanisms and survival time in metastatic breast cancer. *J. Am. Med. Assoc.*, **242**, 1504–1508.
9. Grossarth-Maticek, R., Bastiaans, J., Kanazir, D.T. (1985). Psychosocial factors as strong predictors of mortality from cancer, ischaemic heart disease and stroke: the Yugoslav prospective study. *J. Psychosom. Res.*, **29**, 167–176.
10. Jamison, R.N., Burish, T.G., Wallston, K.A. (1987). Psychogenic factors in predicting survival of breast cancer patients. *J. Clin. Oncol.*, **5**, 768–772.
11. Hislop, T.G., Waxler, N.E., Coldman, A.J. *et al.* (1987). The prognostic significance of psychosocial factors in women with breast cancer. *J. Chron. Dis.*, **40**, 729–735.
12. Gross, J. (1989). Emotional expression in cancer onset and progression. *Soc. Sci. Med.*, **28**, 1239–1248.
13. Temoshok, L., Heller, B.W. (1981). *Stress and 'Type C' Versus epidemiological risk factors in melanoma*. Proceedings of the 89th Annual Convention of the American Psychological Association.
14. Kneier, A.W., Temoshok, L. (1984). Repressive coping reactions in patients with malignant melanoma as compared to cardiovascular disease patients. *J. Psychosom. Res.*, **28**, 145–155.

15. Cassileth, B.R., Lusk, E.J., Miller, D.S., Brown, L.L., Miller, C. (1985). Psychosocial correlates of survival in advanced malignant disease? *N. Engl. J. Med.*, **312**, 1551–1555.
16. Pettingale, K.W., Greer, S., Tee, D.E.H. (1977). Serum IgA and emotional expression in breast cancer patients. *J. Psychosom. Res.*, **21**, 395–399.
17. Temoshok, L., Heller, B.W., Sagebiel, R.W. *et al.* (1985). The relationship of psychosocial factors to prognostic indicators in cutaneous malignant melanoma. *J. Psychosom. Res.*, **29**, 139–153.
18. Fox, B.H. (1983). Current theory of psychogenic effects on cancer incidence and prognosis. *J. Psychosoc. Onc.*, **1**, 17–31.
19. Levenson, J.L., Bemis, C. (1991). The role of psychological factors in cancer onset and progression. *Psychosomatics*, **32**, 124–132.
20. Ramirez, A.J., Craig, T.K.J., Fentiman, I.S. *et al.* (1989). Stress and relapse of breast cancer. *BMJ*, **298**, 291–293.
21. Fox, B.H., Temoshok, L., Dreher, H. (1987). Mind-body and behavior in cancer incidence. *Advances*, **5**, 41–60.
22. American Cancer Society. (1994). *Cancer Facts and Figures*. American Cancer Society, Atlanta, Georgia.
23. Becker, M.H. (1924). The health belief model and personal health behavior. *Health Educ. Mono.*, **2**, 324–473.
24. Rippetoe, P.A., Rogers, R.W. (1987). Effects of components of protection-motivation theory on adaptive and maladaptive coping with a health threat. *J. Pers. Soc. Psychol.*, **52**, 596–604.
25. Weinstein, N.D. (1980). Unrealistic optimism about future life events. *J. Pers. Soc. Psychol.*, **39**, 806–820.
26. Makuc, D.M., Fried, V.M., Kleinman, J.C. (1989). National trends in the use of preventive health care by women. *Am. J. Public Health*, **79**, 21–26.
27. Meyerowitz, B.E. (1983). Postmastectomy coping strategies and quality of life. *Health Psychol.*, **2**, 117–132.
28. Thompson, S.C., Nanni, C., Schwankovsky, L. (1990). Patient-oriented interventions to improve communication in a medical office visit. *Health Psychol.*, **9**, 390–404.
29. Lipsey, M.W., Wilson, D.B. (1993). The efficacy of psychological, educational, and behavioral treatment: confirmation from meta-analysis. *Am. Psychol.*, **48**, 1181–1209.
30. Beck, A.T. (1993). Cognitive therapy: past, present, and future. *J. Consult. Clin. Psychol.*, **61**, 194–198.
31. Elkin, I., Shea, M.T., Watkins, J.T. *et al.* (1989). National Institute of Mental Health treatment of depression collaborative research program. *Arch. Gen. Psychiat.*, **46**, 971–982.
32. Dobson, K.S. (1989). A meta-analysis of the efficacy of cognitive therapy for depression. *J. Consult. Clin. Psychol.*, **57**, 414–419.
33. Klosko, J.S., Barlow, D.H., Tassinari, R., Cerny, J.A. (1990). A comparison of alprazolam and behavior therapy in treatment of panic disorder. *J. Consult. Clin. Psychol.*, **58**, 77–84.
34. Weisman, A.D., Sobel, H.J. (1979). Coping with cancer through self-instruction: a hypothesis. *J. Hum. Stress.*, **5**, 3–8.
35. Taylor, S.E., Falke, R.L., Shoptaw, S.J., Lichtman, R.R. (1986). Social support, support groups, and the cancer patient. *J. Consult. Clin. Psychol.*, **54**, 608–615.
36. Rait, D., Lederberg, M. (1989). The family of the cancer patient. In Holland, J.C., Rowland J.H. (eds.), *Handbook of Psycho-oncology: Psychological Care of the Patient with Cancer*, Oxford University Press, New York, 585–597.

Chapter 26

Avoidable Environmental Links to Breast Cancer

DEVRA LEE DAVIS and H. LEON BRADLOW

Established risk factors do not account for current patterns of breast cancer and of other hormonally-related tumors. There is also an increasing frequency of reproductive dysfunction, including reduced estimated sperm counts in males, and reproductive failure, endometriosis and fibroid tumors in females. For breast cancer, a common link binds most of the known risk factors, and that is a cumulative elevated lifetime exposure to estrogen [1, 2]. The proportion of estrogen receptor positive breast cancers is also increasing [3].

This chapter assesses experimental and epidemiologic evidence that a portion of breast cancers presenting today may be due to avoidable environmental factors which alter the body's estrogen production or its biologic activity. These environmental factors are referred to as xeno-estrogens. Discussion in this chapter is restricted to environmental chemical, biologic and physical exposures to such agents but dietary and pharmaceutical agents can also function as xeno-estrogens.

The increasing incidence of breast cancer has stimulated interest in possible environmental factors [4]. Over 30 years ago, Rachel Carson raised public awareness about the ability of environmental chemicals to disrupt hormones in wildlife. She noted that DDT thinned the eggshells of many birds, and substantially reduced their ability to reproduce [5]. "In brief, the argument for the indirect role of pesticides in cancer is based on their proven ability to damage the liver and to reduce the supply of B vitamins, thus leading to an increase in the 'endogenous' estrogens, or those produced by the body itself. Added to these are the wide variety of synthetic estrogens to which we are increasingly exposed those in cosmetics, drugs, foods and occupational exposures. The combined effect is a matter that warrants the most serious concern."

Debate has persisted about whether DDT poses any serious threat to human health, despite a number of studies indicating an elevated tumor rate in exper-

Basil A. Stoll (ed.), Reducing Breast Cancer Risk in Women, 231–235.
© *1995 Kluwer Academic Publishers. Printed in the Netherlands.*

imentally-exposed animals. One recent study found that DDT-exposed workers had increased rates of pancreatic cancer [6]. Despite these findings, DDT was not restricted in Australia until 1987, and is still heavily used in many developing countries.

Effects of Xeno-Estrogens

Recently, a series of papers have hypothesized that avoidable environmental exposures may explain some of the puzzling patterns in breast cancer. Xeno-estrogens can elevate the endogenous production and biological activity of estrogens, and thereby increase the risk of breast cancer [7]. They may also reduce the risk of the disease by favorably altering estradiol metabolism. Some pesticides, fuels and engine exhausts, plastics, and natural products can alter the body's natural levels of estrogen. Cell culture and animal studies demonstrate the ability of a number of organochlorine compounds to affect hormonal metabolism, especially estradiol production. Ortho-para-DDT actually is more potent than the body's own estrogen in inhibiting the binding of estradiol to tissue cells. With respect to PCBs, a number of isomers are anti-estrogenic, while others are potent estrogens.

Xeno-estrogens can affect not only total estrogen levels overall but also metabolic pathways. Two competing enzyme systems control metabolism of estradiol by two mutually exclusive pathways: pathway I inserts a hydroxyl (OH-) radical at the 2-carbon position and yields the catechol estrogen 2-hydroxyestrone (2-OHE_1), a weakly anti-estrogenic metabolite; pathway II adds an OH- at the 16 position and yields 16α-hydroxyestrone ($16\alpha\text{-OHE}_1$). The second pathway creates a fully potent metabolite which increases tumor growth, DNA damage and cell proliferation [8].

A number of experimental studies and clinical studies indicate that 16α-hydroxylation (the second pathway) may be a biological marker of risk for breast cancer and may directly contribute to the initiation and progression of the disease. Earlier work has noted that $16\alpha\text{-OHE}_1$ levels were significantly elevated in patients with risk factors for breast cancer, compared to those without known risk factors [9, 10]. Neither age, menopausal status, nor stage of progression of disease modifies these differential levels of $16\alpha\text{-OHE}_1$; thus, levels of $16\alpha\text{-OHE}_1$, appear to constitute an intrinsic biomarker for breast cancer [11].

A number of experimental mammary carcinogens have been shown to enhance the production of $16\alpha\text{-OHE}_1$ or suppress 2-OHE_1, including DMBA, Benz-α-pyrene (BP), ras and myc oncogenes, mouse mammary tumor virus (MMTV) and the human papilloma virus (HPV). In contrast, compounds that stimulate 2-OHE_1, or suppress $16\alpha\text{-OHE}_1$, appear to reduce genetic damage and cell proliferation. Thus, I-3-C has specific antigrowth effects in estrogen receptor positive human breast cancer cells, and increases Pathway I, while reducing Pathway II [7]. Additional epidemiologic support for the protective role of I-3-C comes from studies that find that the risk of breast cancer is lowest in women from countries where the consumption of I-3-C rich cabbage is highest [12].

Naturally varying levels of these endogenous estrogen metabolites may explain some reported ethnic and geographic variations in breast cancer. Thus, one study found that Asian women, who have much lower rates of breast cancer, generally have higher levels of 2-OHE$_1$ and low levels of 16α-OHE$_1$ [13]. Diets high in soy products, cruciferae and other vegetables could be relevant, and other dietary and environmental exposures also may explain these findings.

There is mounting evidence that a number of different classes of chemical compounds may affect estradiol metabolism. Public attention recently has focused on DDT and its metabolites but this is likely to be only one of many important avoidable environmental causes of breast cancer that affect cumulative estrogen production and metabolism. A number of other chemical agents have potent effects on hormone levels. In addition, to the recently studied DDT and other organochlorine compounds, plasticizers, such as bisphenol-A (BPA) [14] and nonylphenol [15] have been shown to be strongly estrogenic both in human breast cells and in whole animals studies.

Other compounds with demonstrated estrogenic activity include the animal growth stimulant zearalone, and the synthetic estrogen Diethyl Stilbestrol [16]. The latter is known to be more estrogenic than estradiol. As to fuels, engine exhausts and other widespread air pollutants, many of their key ingredients, such as benzene and polycyclic aromatic hydrocarbons, have been shown to have potent estrogenic activity, and also to increase mammary tumors in animals [17].

Several recent prospective reports [18–20] have found significantly higher levels of some pesticides in women with breast cancer relative to control subjects, while one retrospective analysis did not find such an association [21]. Wolff and colleagues [18] found that women in the top 10% of exposure to some organochlorine pesticides had four times more breast cancer, when compared with those in the lowest 10%. Other studies have been negative, but have usually involved small numbers of persons studied, with insufficient attention to information that may be relevant, such as duration of breastfeeding and age at first pregnancy. Dewailly [19] recently found that women whose breast cancers were estrogen receptor positive had a fourfold excess risk of breast cancer if they also had incurred higher levels of exposure to DDT.

A recent study on this issue [21] was conducted in the USA on 150 cases of breast cancer and 150 controls using blood samples stored for nearly 30 years. No significant difference in organochlorine residues was found in the three ethnic groups between cases and controls (African Americans, whites, and Asian Americans.) However, when whites and African-American women are analyzed as two separate groups, those with higher levels of exposure to organochlorine compounds had risks of breast cancer that were 2 to 3 times greater than those without such past exposures. Patterns in Asian women differed completely, consistent with other observations.

Could organochlorine pesticides explain part of the recent patterns of breast cancer? We must accept that a number of other chemicals also affect estrogen levels experimentally, including plasticizers, volatile materials in fuels, pharmaceuticals, and plant estrogens, some of which are given to cattle. In addition, up to ten million American women received the synthetic estrogen Diethyl Stilbestrol (DES) during pregnancy, and millions more have been exposed to much lower levels of this compound when it was used as a growth stimulant in cattle and chickens.

Effect of Electromagnetic Fields (EMF)

Preliminary evidence suggests that EMF may directly or indirectly affect breast cell growth by some as yet unestablished mechanism. Some experimental studies have found that light at night or EMF interferes with the secretion of the hormone, melatonin, in the brain [22]. Others [23] have found that melatonin directly inhibits the proliferation of human breast cancer cells. Thus, factors that reduce melatonin could be expected to increase breast cell proliferation.

Conclusion

A growing body of experimental and epidemiologic evidence indicates that some breast cancer cases are due to avoidable environmental exposures that increase estrogen production, and thereby lead to the development of breast cancer.

References

1. Harris, J.R., Lippman, M.E., Veronesi, U., Willett, W. (1992). Breast cancer (first of three parts). *N. Engl. J. Med.*, **327**, 319–328.
2. Pike, M.C., Spicer, D.V., Dahmoush, L., Press M.F. (1993). Estrogens, progestogins, normal breast cells, and breast cancer risk. *Epidemiol. Rev.*, **15**, 17–35.
3. Glass, A., Hoover, R. (1990). Rising incidence of breast cancer: relationship to stage and receptor status. *J. Natl. Cancer Inst.*, **82**, 693–696.
4. Krieger, N. (1989). Exposure, susceptibility, and breast cancer risk: a hypothesis regarding exogenous carcinogens, breast tissue development, and social gradients, including black/white differences in breast cancer incidence. *Breast Cancer Res. Treat.*, **13**, 205–223.
5. Garson, R. (1961). *Silent Spring*, Riverside Press, Cambridge, Mass.
6. Garabrant, D.H., Held, J., Longholz, B. *et al.* (1992). DDT and related compounds and risk of pancreatic cancer. *J. Natl. Cancer Inst.*, **84**, 764–771.
7. Davis, D., Bradlow, H.L., Wolff, M. *et al.* (1993) Medical hypothesis: xenoestrogens as preventable causes of breast cancer. *Environ. Health Perspect.*, **101**, 372–377.
8. Telang, N.T., Suto, A., Wong, G.Y., Bradlow, H.L., Osborne, M.P. (1992). Induction by estrogen metabolite 16α-hydroxyestrone of genotoxic damage and aberrant proliferation in mouse mammary epithelial cells. *J. Natl Cancer Inst.*, **84**, 634–638.
9. Schneider, J., Kinne, D., Fracchia, A. *et al.* (1982). Abnormal oxidative metabolism of estradiol in women with breast cancer. *Proc. Natl. Acad. Sci. USA*, **79**, 3047–3051.
10. Osborne, M.P., Karmali, R.A., Bradlow, H.L. *et al.* (1988). Omega-3 fatty acids: modulation of estrogen metabolism and potential for breast cancer prevention. *Cancer Invest.*, **6**, 629–6318.
11. Schneider, J., Huh, M.M., Bradlow, H.L. Fishman, J. (1984). Antiestrogen action of 2-hydroxyestrone of genotoxic damage and aberrant proliferation in mouse mammary epithelial cells. *J. Biol. Chem.*, **259**, 4840–4845.

12. Kohlmeier, L., Dortschy, R. Brassica consumption and colon cancer. *Intl. J. Epidemiol.*, (In press).
13. Goldin, B.R., Gorbach, S.L. (1988). Effect of diet on the plasma levels, metabolism and excretion of estrogens. *Am J. Nutrition*, **48**, 787–790.
14. Krishnan, A.V., Bisphenol, A. (1993). An estrogenic substance is released from polycarbonate flasks during autoclaving. *Endocrinology*, **132**, 2279–2286.
15. Soto, A.M., Justica, H., Wray, J.W., Sonnenschein, C. (1991). P-nonylphenol, an estrogenic xenobiotic released from 'modified' polystyrene. *Environ. Health Perspect*, **92**, 167–173.
16. Rall, D.P., McLachlan, J.A. (1980). Potential for exposure to estrogens in the environment. In McLachlan, J.A. (ed.), *Estrogens in the Environment*, Elsevier–North Holland, New York, 199–203.
17. Morris, J.J., Seifter, E. (1992) The role of aromatic hydrocarbons in the genesis of breast cancer. *Med. Hypotheses*, **38**, 177–184.
18. Wolff, M.S., Toniolo, P.G., Lee, E.W., Rivera, M., Dubin, N. (1993). Blood levels of organocholorine residues and risk of breast cancer. *J. Natl. Cancer Inst.*, **85**, 648–652.
19. Dewailly, E., Dodin, S., Verreault, R. *et al.* (1994). High organochlorine body burden in women with estrogen receptor–positive breast cancer. *J. Natl. Cancer Inst.*, **86**, 232–234.
20. Falck, F., Jr., Ricci, A., Jr., Wolff, M.S., Godbold, J., Deckers, P. (1992). Pesticides and poly-cholorinated biphenyl residues in human breast lipids and their relation to breast cancer. *Arch. Environ. Health*, **47**, 143–146.
21. Krieger, N.K., Wolff, M.S., Hiatt, R.A. *et al.* (1994). Breast cancer and serum organochlorines: A prospective study among white, black and Asian Women. *J. Natl Cancer Inst.*, **86**, 589–99.
22. Stevens, A.J.E. (1987). Electric power use and breast cancer, a hypothesis. *Am. J. Epidemiol.*, **125**, 556–561.
23. Wilson, S.T., Blask, D.E., Lemus-Wilson, A.M. (1992). Melatonin augments the sensitivity of MCF-7 human breast cancer cells to tamoxifen *in vitro*. *J. Clin. Endocrinol. Metab.*, **75**, 669–670.

Chapter 27

Asking the Right Questions

BASIL A. STOLL

Increasing numbers of women are asking what they can do to reduce their risk of developing breast cancer. Such questions become intense when a woman has a long history of breast problems or when a close relative has developed the disease. Similar questions come from women concerned about an average risk of developing the disease. Their desire for information and the measures they are prepared to undertake, are often greater than those of women at a far higher risk.

The dilemma for a woman is that the clinician is now able to quote an odds ratio on her risk of developing breast cancer but can offer much less certainty on the effectiveness of the protective measures available. While recent research has enabled us to recognize a woman's increased risk, our means of preventing breast cancer have not kept pace. This discrepancy will become increasingly obvious in the very near future when genetic testing for breast cancer becomes available. It can reveal women with a 80–90% chance of developing breast cancer at some future time.

Information Should Control Anxiety Not Increase It

This dilemma is the theme which pervades all the chapters in this book. For many women, information and education about their individual risk of breast cancer will help to combat anxiety if it is given in a *personal perspective*. This means that the clinician must help to identify for each woman individually the potential benefits and risks of each protective option offered, whether it involves a change in life style or a medical or surgical procedure. This must involve considerable time spent in asking and answering questions.

Some women are natural information-seekers and they will search out every scrap of information about their problem. Such information-seeking is a way of seeing their problem in perspective, and they aim to relieve anxiety by evaluating

237

Basil A. Stoll (ed.), Reducing Breast Cancer Risk in Women, 237–242.

the scientific certainties (on uncertainties) behind the advice they have been given. Women seeking advice on breast cancer risk are frequently given a mass of technical information, or else a handful of written information, which leaves them numb and uncomprehending. This is information overload – it is both misleading and meaningless. The aim must be to provide each woman with the information necessary to permit an informed decision in her particular circumstances. The identification of increased breast cancer risk in a woman should bring her a guide to protective measures and an informed choice, not merely bad news.

Who is to provide counselling?

Any time now, the availability of genetic testing for breast cancer is likely to be announced. It will be associated with considerable newspaper and magazine publicity and will lead to considerable questioning by women worried about their breast cancer risk. The answers which they receive need to be accurate because in the USA, as in other Western countries, women are widely misinformed about the many factors which influence a woman's risk and what can be done for a woman at high risk. Their knowledge is often distorted by emotive or sensational items in the press or other media.

Practically every chapter in this book makes it clear that for the woman who is at a high risk of breast cancer, education and support require sensitive *personal counseling* by trained professionals. Even the smallest community in the country should be able to offer this facility. The greatest degree of risk is related to a history of premenopausal breast cancer in mother or sister. The relatives of such patients should be given the highest degree of priority. Those with biopsy evidence of cancer precursor lesions in a breast deserve almost equal priority. But every woman should be given access.

The aim of the skilled counselors should be to;
(1) Correct misapprehensions and misinformation.
(2) Provide an assessment of the degree of a woman's risk. Genetic testing might be discussed if a woman wanted a greater degree of certainty.
(3) Discuss the possibility of protective measures such as early ovariectomy or mastectomy for a woman with very high risk. These procedures offer 50–99% chance of long-term protection from breast cancer.
(4) Offer support and understanding for emotional problems. Offer family or individual counseling as desired by the woman.
(5) Know all the resources available for suitable diagnosis and management in the community and ensure access to such resources irrespective of a woman's ability to pay.
(6) Advise on lifestyle changes to those women who wish to take an active part in their own protection. Our current state of knowledge suggests that hereditary risk of breast cancer will dwarf lesser risk factors and therefore make changes in lifestyle less relevant.

(7) For women without obvious hereditary risk, discuss control of lifestyle including fat intake, general diet, avoidance of obesity, choice of oral contraceptive or hormone replacement therapy and participation in trials of pharmacologic agents. Such women may be best educated in groups in order to avoid overloading the counselors.

The woman who decides to take action should be given all the necessary information to help her make an informed choice. There is no correct decision for low, moderate or high degrees of risk. It depends on what value a woman attaches to the hoped-for reduction of risk, in relation to the anxieties involved in the monitoring plan or protective procedure. One woman may prefer a more drastic program with a high likelihood of reducing risk while another may choose a less complex program with only a fair chance of success.

The safety of each protective measure is of paramount importance and each woman weighs the risks from her personal viewpoint, according to her age and state of health. Assessment of risk is different when the same measure is being considered for clinical trial in healthy women in the population, when a far stricter criterion of safety is demanded because public safety is concerned. Each woman decides on her best option based on her knowledge of the clinical data for the measure and her own value judgement. The clinician merely explains the risks and benefits of each option in relation to her physical factors, and tries to help each women find a program which fits in best with her personal needs and anxieties.

Patient autonomy is now seen as a moral imperative, yet a mere twenty years ago, the phrase was almost unknown. Apart from social pressures, several major changes in medical practice have led doctors to reevaluate the longstanding assumption that all patients want to be treated in a paternalistic manner. Informed consent grew mainly as a result of medical advances. The patient had to be given all necessary information if she was to choose between a number of treatment options.

How Many People Would Change Their Life Styles?

A moderate degree of risk reduction is possible from changes in a woman's life style, diet or childbearing program. Advice of this type will not be complied with unless a woman is carefully educated on the nature of breast cancer and also wishes to play an active role herself in the reduction of cancer risk. Compliance is on the whole, less likely if her understanding of the disease is limited, her education or economic background poor, or if the influence of family and friends is negative. If women regard themselves as being at risk but can see no positive or useful action to take, they often take refuge in denial. A very high level of fear may paralyse the will and inhibit a woman's ability to react logically.

At the present time, few primary care doctors or other health professionals devote much time to the education of patients in behavior which may reduce their risk of disease in general, and breast cancer in particular. Some physicians justify this by minimizing the importance of some of the risk factors discussed in this book or by doubting the effectiveness of change in lifestyle as a protective measure. They claim that they devote little time to cancer prevention advice mainly because they believe that they cannot help patients change in this respect, and they often quote smoking as an example. They claim that most patients either do not want, or else would not follow, their advice in respect to breast cancer prevention.

This may be true for some. In modern society, people derive most of their knowledge about health hazards from the popular media. Highly publicized risk factors are more likely to be seen as a threat to health than daily routine risks. A European survey in 1987 showed that 54% of the population ascribed a major role in cancer deaths to radioactivity, 44% to pollution, 34% to a person's occupation, 30% to alcohol, 27% to sunshine, 24% to heredity and 17% to psychological stress. In fact, even the most dangerous of these risk factors is responsible for less than 5 per cent of cancer deaths.

People are constantly encouraged to take responsibility for their own health but it is human nature to believe that the major factors which threaten one's health lie mainly outside one's control. People whose lifestyle puts them at risk to disease (smokers for example) tend to minimize the effects of their behaviour. We tend to accept news items which reinforce our own prejudices on preconceived notions. Some people prefer to believe that radioactivity, pollution on occupation outweigh all other factors in increasing cancer risk because it absolves them of responsibility for regulating their lifestyle or diet.

The first step in advising lifestyle change in a woman at increased breast cancer risk is to determine how threatened she believes herself to be if action is not taken. If she considers the risk small, the benefit of changing her lifestyle may appear to her less important than the disadvantages. With regard to suggested lifestyle constraints such as having babies at a young age, it is unlikely that a generation of women which has fought hard for its freedom to control reproductive activity, will find this acceptable. Thus, while many would regard pharmacologic manipulation of hormonal levels as being unnatural (even if its efficacy is proved), it may be the most practical approach in our present state of knowledge.

Are We Targeting the Right Women in Clinical Trials?

How accurate is the identification of a woman's breast cancer risk? At present, few physicians have the necessary expertise to evaluate the risk from familial and clinical factors. Even experts differ in defining the criteria for women at high risk, as shown by the different categories selected in different countries for evaluating Tamoxifen as a protective measure.

The highest degree of risk is shown clinically by a history of premenopausal breast cancer in mothers or sisters or evidence of precursor or precancerous change in a breast biopsy. Evidence of a lesser degree of risk includes advancing age and several characteristics in a woman's reproductive history or lifestyle. It is uncertain however, how these should be combined into a risk index for a woman. Genetic testing, when it is available will reveal the highest degrees of susceptibility but for that very reason, some women may prefer to avoid it.

The clinical trials of new protective methods not only have to prove their overall efficacy, but also to establish the type of risk for which they are individually best suited. It must be taken into consideration that none of the established risk factors for breast cancer accounts for a large percentage of the total incidence of the disease. All risk factors combined are thought to explain less than 30% of cases diagnosed in the population. It is also possible that women at high risk on account of genetic susceptibility may be a specific subset of cases, whose response to a particular preventive measure may not be typical of the main mass of breast cancer patients.

Are Current Clinical Trials Justifiable?

Further research is needed to pinpoint the preventable causes of breast cancer, but meanwhile, we must continue the clinical trials which are evaluating proposed measures of protection. Gene therapy to prevent breast cancer is likely to remain a dream for some time to come, although genetic linkage analysis will soon permit the screening of members of families at high risk. Because the media tend to highlight advances in medicine long before they are developed and tested, many women wrongly believe that they can postpone a decision on choosing from presently available preventive measures.

Current clinical trials involve administration of the antiestrogen Tamoxifen, suppression of ovarian activity by hormones or by surgery, administration of Vitamin A analogues (retinoids) and restriction of fat in the diet. Large scale trials of Tamoxifen have been started in the USA, Canada, Europe and Australia/New Zealand. One of the consequences of the setting up of these trials has been considerable publicity in the Western media leading to public interest in breast cancer prevention.

A series of molecular changes in breast tissue cells is responsible for the development of breast cancer. However, there is little doubt that estrogen is intimately involved in stimulating proliferation of normal breast cells and in promoting growth activity in initiated (but dormant) breast cancer cells. It has been shown that precursor lesions of breast cancer such as atypical hyperplasia and *in situ* cancer tend to disappear spontaneously at the time of the menopause, presumably as a result of the lower circulating estrogen levels. Such precancerous lesions are therefore not committed inexorably to continue developing into invasive cancers. A hormonal formula for oral contraceptives or hormonal replacement therapy which will block the development of breast cancer, is currently the subject of considerable research.

Currently available are clinical trials of estrogen inhibition either by ablation of ovarian activity on the administration of the antiestrogen Tamoxifen. Also under clinical trial is a Vitamin A analogue (retinoid) which inhibits cell proliferation and can cause premalignant lesions to disappear. In animals a combination of

Tamoxifen and retinoids has an additive effect on breast cancer, and we need to extend such trials to the prevention of human breast cancer. Combinations of agents which work by different mechanisms offer the potential of increasing effectiveness against cancer development, using a dose below the toxicity level for each agent when used individually. It is also hoped that the identification of biochemical or genetic markers which characterize the precursor stage of breast cancer, will soon permit more accurate study of the effect of chemopreventive agents during the developmental stage of breast cancer.

The development of scientific assessment by trials has created a conflict of interest for the clinician. He must care for the patient but must also take part in the evaluation of new treatments. Most clinicians believe that participation in clinical trials is the best way for patients to receive state-of-the-art care. However, the guiding principle must be that patients are informed when they are participating in research, must be told the risks and the benefits expected and must be free at any time to withdraw from the trials. This is the basis of informed consent, and the patient grants written permission whose moral purpose is not to protect the doctors from being sued but to involve the patient in the decision-making. The physician merely offers the opportunity for patients to enter a clinical trial. A woman should be given all available evidence to balance expected benefit against possible disadvantages and she must be able to *understand* the information.

Conclusion

Women in Western countries are confused about conflicting reports from the medical community on the efficacy of early detection and preventive approaches to breast cancer. Every woman is potentially at risk to breast cancer and it is a highly emotive problem. Until acceptable approaches to prevention can be offered, women will be exploited by bogus experts. This book concentrates less on the details of past research and more on what needs to be done in the immediate future.

Clearly, it is important to increase research into avoidable factors in the environment which may be increasing breast cancer risk. However, the underlying risk has probably been there since civilisation began and our best hope currently is research on blocking the progression of the disease from the precursor stage. While waiting for these advances, there is an urgent need to train selected professionals, especially nurses, in cancer risk counseling and make them available in every community hospital.

Index

Developments in Oncology

1. F.J. Cleton and J.W.I.M. Simons (eds.): *Genetic Origins of Tumour Cells*. 1980
   ISBN 90-247-2272-1
2. J. Aisner and P. Chang (eds.): *Cancer Treatment and Research*. 1980
   ISBN 90-247-2358-2
3. B.W. Ongerboer de Visser, D.A. Bosch and W.M.H. van Woerkom-Eykenboom (eds.):
   Neuro-oncology. Clinical and Experimental Aspects. 1980   ISBN 90-247-2421-X
4. K. Hellman, P. Hilgard and S. Eccles (eds.): *Metastasis*. Clinical and Experimental
   Aspects. 1980   ISBN 90-247-2424-4
5. H.F. Seigler (ed.): *Clinical Management of Melanoma*. 1982   ISBN 90-247-2584-4
6. P. Correa and W. Haenszel (eds.): *Epidemiology of Cancer of the Digestive Tract*. 1982
   ISBN 90-247-2601-8
7. L.A. Liotta and I.R. Hart (eds.): *Tumor Invasion and Metastasis*. 1982
   ISBN 90-247-2611-5
8. J. Bánóczy: *Oral Leukoplakia*. 1982   ISBN 90-247-2655-7
9. C.C. Tijssen, M.R. Halprin and L.J. Endtz: *Familial Brain Tumours*. A Commented
   Register. With an Introduction by F.J. Cleton. 1982   ISBN 90-247-2691-3
10. F.M. Muggia, C.W. Young and S.K. Carter (eds.): *Anthracycline Antibiotics in Cancer*.
    1982   ISBN 90-247-2711-1
11. B.W. Hancock (ed.): *Assessment of Tumor Response*. 1982   ISBN 90-247-2712-X
12. D.E. Peterson and S.T. Sonis (eds.): *Oral Complications of Cancer Chemotherapy*.
    1983   ISBN 90-247-2786-3
13. R. Mastrangelo, D.G. Poplack and R. Riccardi (eds.): *Central Nervous System
    Leukemia*. Prevention and Treatment. 1983   ISBN 0-89838-570-9
14. A. Polliack (ed.): *Human Leukemias*. Cytochemical and Ultrastructural Techniques in
    Diagnosis and Research. 1984 .   ISBN 0-89838-585-7
15. W. Davis, C. Maltoni and S. Tanneberger (eds.): *The Control of Tumor Growth and Its
    Biological Bases*. 1983   ISBN 0-89838-603-9
16. A.P.M. Heintz, C.Th. Griffiths and J.B. Trimbos (eds.): *Surgery in Gynecological
    Oncology*. 1984   ISBN 0-89838-604-7
17. M.P. Hacker, E.B. Douple and I. Krakoff (eds.): *Platinum Coordination Complexes in
    Cancer Chemotherapy*. 1984   ISBN 0-89838-619-5
18. M.J. van Zwieten: *The Rat as Animal Model in Breast Cancer Research*. A His-
    topathological Study of Radiation- and Hormone-induced Rat Mammary Tumors. 1984
    ISBN 0-89838-624-1
19. B. Löwenberg and A. Hagenbeek (eds.): *Minimal Residual Disease in Acute Leukemia*.
    1984   ISBN 0-89838-630-6
20. I. van der Waal and G.B. Snow (eds.): *Oral Oncology*. 1984   ISBN 0-89838-631-4
21. B.W. Hancock and A. Milford Ward (eds.): *Immunological Aspects of Cancer*. 1985
    ISBN 0-89838-664-0
22. K.V. Honn and B.F. Sloane (eds.): *Hemostatic Mechanisms and Metastasis*. 1984
    ISBN 0-89838-667-5
23. K.R. Harrap, W. Davis and A.H. Calvert (eds.): *Cancer Chemotherapy and Selective
    Drug Development*. 1984   ISBN 0-89838-673-X
24. C.J.H. van de Velde and P.H. Sugarbaker (eds.): *Liver Metastasis*. Basic Aspects,
    Detection and Management. 1984   ISBN 0-89838-684-5
25. D.J. Ruiter, K. Welvaart and S. Ferrone (eds.): *Cutaneous Melanoma and Precursor
    Lesions*. 1984   ISBN 0-89838-689-6

Developments in Oncology

26. S.B. Howell (ed.): *Intra-arterial and Intracavitary Cancer Chemotherapy.* 1984
   ISBN 0-89838-691-8
27. D.L. Kisner and J.F. Smyth (eds.): *Interferon Alpha-2.* Pre-clinical and Clinical
   Evaluation. 1985   ISBN 0-89838-701-9
28. P. Furmanski, J.C. Hager and M.A. Rich (eds.): *RNA Tumor Viruses, Oncogenes,
   Human Cancer and AIDS.* On the Frontiers of Understanding. 1985
   ISBN 0-89838-703-5
29. J.E. Talmadge, I.J. Fidler and R.K. Oldham: *Screening for Biological Response
   Modifiers.* Methods and Rationale. 1985   ISBN 0-89838-712-4
30. J.C. Bottino, R.W. Opfell and F.M. Muggia (eds.): *Liver Cancer.* 1985
   ISBN 0-89838-713-2
31. P.K. Pattengale, R.J. Lukes and C.R. Taylor (eds.): *Lymphoproliferative Diseases.*
   Pathogenesis, Diagnosis, Therapy. 1985   ISBN 0-89838-725-6
32. F. Cavalli, G. Bonadonna and M. Rozencweig (eds.): *Malignant Lymphomas and
   Hodgkin's Disease.* Experimental and Therapeutic Advances. 1985
   ISBN 0-89838-727-2
33. L. Baker, F. Valeriote and V. Ratanatharathorn (eds.): *Biology and Therapy of Acute
   Leukemia.* 1985   ISBN 0-89838-728-0
34. J. Russo (ed.): *Immunocytochemistry in Tumor Diagnosis.* 1985   ISBN 0-89838-737-X
35. R.L. Ceriani (ed.): *Monoclonal Antibodies and Breast Cancer.* 1985
   ISBN 0-89838-739-6
36. D.E. Peterson, E.G. Elias and S.T. Sonis (eds.): *Head and Neck Management of the
   Cancer Patient.* 1986   ISBN 0-89838-747-7
37. D.M. Green: *Diagnosis and Management of Malignant Solid Tumors in Infants and
   Children.* 1985   ISBN 0-89838-750-7
38. K.A. Foon and A.C. Morgan, Jr. (eds.): *Monoclonal Antibody Therapy of Human
   Cancer.* 1985   ISBN 0-89838-754-X
39. J.G. McVie, W. Bakker, Sj.Sc. Wagenaar and D. Carney (eds.): *Clinical and Experimental Pathology of Lung Cancer.* 1986   ISBN 0-89838-764-7
40. K.V. Honn, W.E. Powers and B.F. Sloane (eds.): *Mechanisms of Cancer Metastasis.*
   Potential Therapeutic Implications. 1986   ISBN 0-89838-765-5
41. K. Lapis, L.A. Liotta and A.S. Rabson (eds.): *Biochemistry and Molecular Genetics of
   Cancer Metastasis.* 1986   ISBN 0-89838-785-X
42. A.J. Mastromarino (ed.): *Biology and Treatment of Colorectal Metastasis.* 1986
   ISBN 0-89838-786-8
43. M.A. Rich, J.C. Hager and J. Taylor-Papadimitriou (eds.): *Breast Cancer.* Origins,
   Detection and Treatment. 1986   ISBN 0-89838-792-2
44. D.G. Poplack, L. Massimo and P. Cornaglia-Ferraris (eds.): *The Role of Pharmacology
   in Pediatric Oncology.* 1987   ISBN 0-89838-795-7
45. A. Hagenbeek and B. Löwenberg (eds.): *Minimal Residual Disease in Acute Leukemia.*
   1986 .   ISBN 0-89838-799-X
46. F.M. Muggia and M. Rozencweig (eds.): *Clinical Evaluation of Antitumor Therapy.*
   1987   ISBN 0-89838-803-1
47. F.A. Valeriote and L.H. Baker (eds.): *Biochemical Modulation of Anticancer Agents.*
   Experiemental and Clinical Approaches. 1986   ISBN 0-89838-827-9
48. B.A. Stoll (ed.): *Pointers to Cancer Prognosis.* 1987
   ISBN 0-89838-841-4; Pb. 0-89838-876-7

Developments in Oncology

Developments in Oncology

Previous volumes are still available

KLUWER ACADEMIC PUBLISHERS – DORDRECHT / BOSTON / LONDON